Mental Health Care Resource Book

Meenu Anand
Editor

Mental Health Care Resource Book

Concepts and Praxis for Social Workers and Mental Health Professionals

Springer

Editor
Meenu Anand
Department of Social Work
University of Delhi
New Delhi, Delhi, India

ISBN 978-981-97-1202-1 ISBN 978-981-97-1203-8 (eBook)
https://doi.org/10.1007/978-981-97-1203-8

This Springer imprint is published by the registered company Springer Nature Singapore Pte Ltd.
The registered company address is: 152 Beach Road, #21-01/04 Gateway East, Singapore 189721, Singapore

Paper in this product is recyclable.

This book is dedicated to my Late Parents who made me what I am today. I believe they are continuing to watch over me and encouraging me from up above through the stars.
I also dedicate this book to my husband and my son for their resolute love and support.

Preface

Mental health has emerged as an important intersecting discourse in relation to the contemporary socio-cultural ethos in society. As one of the popular buzzwords in the post-pandemic context, the discourse has gained significant impetus as the key to happiness and well-being. Promotion and protection of mental health and its bearing on fostering resilience to stress and adversity is being considered as vital for all sections of the population transcending the socio-cultural boundaries of gender, caste, class, race, and ethnicity. As a buoyant concept, mental health determines the differential balance, power, and control individuals have over their lives and governs their social functioning across personal, family, work, and community domains. The biological, psycho-social, and cultural determinants of mental health across various stages of lifespan determine an individual's protection as well as vulnerabilities to specific mental health risks and disorders. A holistic approach to mental health implies an understanding of the role of multiple actors, eclectic factors, and their interactions across all structures of society.

The theme of mental health has always intrigued and riveted me. During my professional work with grassroots organizations and my academic teaching, together spanning over twenty-six years, I have always felt inquisitive and enticed toward the subject. The more I have learnt, the greater has been the yen to gain a holistic understanding on the subject, particularly from a psycho-social and social work standpoint. I also have felt the acute scarcity of resources on the subject, especially from the indigenous context. This resource book on mental health care has taken over 7 years in the making. While the initial ideas about its extensive framework encircled my mind for 5 years, the actual writing and compilation took more than 2 years to take a definitive silhouette.

Through this resource book, I have tried to bring a balanced understanding of different facets and abridge the complex intertwining of illness and culture amidst the rising cases of mental disorders in the post-pandemic world. I have tried to ground the book on strong theoretical underpinnings, while situating an array of associated social and environmental determinants of mental health and well-being. I have also attempted to explore the ways in which the socio-cultural conditions structure the existence of people with diverse identities in addition to amalgamating practice-based skills and experiential narratives from the grassroots.

This book is also my humble attempt to bring positivity, optimism, and hope around the discourse of mental health. Adopting a strengths-based approach, the book offers a wellness, rather than psychopathological perspective and contains treatment models as well as practice-based skills that are evidence based. With my personal conviction and strong professional belief in the psycho-social aspects of mental health and inherent resilience among all individuals, this book highlights the broader social context in mental health care while questioning the hegemony of a psychiatric diagnosis and the pervasive dominance of medicalized lexis.

This resource book is a one-of-a-kind blend of theoretical perspectives, practice skills, as well as emancipatory praxis. The book is distinctive as it features practice-based skills and approaches utilized by mental health specialists while also embracing grassroots voices. All amalgamated together, I have made every endeavor to make it an unparalleled synthesis of scholarly understanding of mental health, practical expertise, and grassroots testimonies. I particularly anticipate that the experiential reflections will give the readers, the much-needed hope that recovery from vulnerabilities and mental disorders is very much possible without the boisterous psychiatric intransigence.

As one of its own kind, the resource book establishes the foundation for diverse Psy-professionals with varied expertise and skill set to provide an array of mental health services. I do believe that the book can contribute toward envisioning an innovative and invigorated role for social work in mental health care, as well as (re)claim its significant position and contribution. I also hope that the substantial competence of Psy experts specializing in psycho-social interventions would be acknowledged. I truly anticipate that this resource book will be advantageous to a wide spectrum of scholars and practitioners working in the fields of social work, psychology, sociology, gender studies, and social psychiatry.

New Delhi, India
20th March 2024

Dr. Meenu Anand

Acknowledgements

There is an array of individuals who have contributed in astounding and vibrant ways to the creation and development of this book. I'd like to begin by thanking Ms. Satvinder Kaur at Springer Nature for always encouraging my early ideas and offering insightful inputs. Her efforts to unify numerous domains in an eclectic manner have resulted in the publication of this book. I would also like to express my sincere thanks to Prof. Archana Dassi for laying my rock-solid professional foundation and always guiding me through various academic dilemmas and turmoils.

I assiduously thank Prof. Malashri Lal for being my constant inspiration and continually motivating me to dream high and write/publish outstanding work. My candid conversations with her always (re)ignited the embers inside me, especially during the times when I was feeling exasperated. The credit for the title of this book as well as one of the chapters that addresses women's mental health goes to her.

With much humility and gratefulness, I sincerely thank all the contributors for their persistent faith in me and for bearing with my insistent requests. I particularly thank Profs. R. S. Murthy, Vibhuti Patel, Mr. Amrit Bakhshy, Profs. Smita N. Deshpande, Saumya Uma, and Mohd. Tarique who despite their extremely challenging professional engagements, contributed to this resource book. I wish to express my earnest thanks to each and every contributor for their trust, kindness, and commitment toward enabling me to bring out this book.

I am indebted to my friend Prof. Nilima Srivastava for being an ongoing fount of emotional support and for always allowing me to express my sentiments whenever I have needed to over the past two decades of our friendship and affectionate camaraderie.

There are no words that can adequately convey my love, feelings, and gratitude to my family. Living with a dedicated scholar who frequently requires solitude and bountiful me-time to devote to writing and research is indeed challenging. Jitender, my husband, deserves credit for being alongside me and for bearing with my scholastic pressures. I've been able to focus on my writing because of his understanding and loving companionship. His much-needed accolades and constructive criticism have helped me maintain my work-life balance. Tanish, my son, deserves my gratitude for his unrelenting trust in me and my abilities as a professional. He is not just a close confidante but also my in-house partner for eloquent discussions on psychology and mental health. He also happily acceded to my request for providing his valued opinion on all the chapters/sections that I wrote for this book. Jitender and Tanish are truly my super-heroes, the core of my entire universe and I will always be grateful to them for embodying unconditional love, affection, and boundless inspiration.

Last but not the least, my special thanks to my students for sharing their personal chronicles, ideas, and incessant effervescence that ignites the very contours of my intellect. I am obliged to them for their love, warmth, and trust in me. With much humility, I sincerely hope that this resource book on Mental Health Care will facilitate them and many others in their academic and personal pursuits.

20th March 2024 Dr. Meenu Anand

Contents

Part I Overarching Conceptual Foundations

1 **Introduction** 3
Meenu Anand

2 **Understanding Mental Disorders, Mental Health and Well-Being** 25
R. Srinivasa Murthy

3 **Social and Cultural Determinants of Mental Health** 55
Vibhuti Patel

4 **Women's Mental Health: The Unchartered Terrain** 71
Meenu Anand

5 **Biopsychosocial Approach to Mental Health** 87
Ananya Mahapatra and Prerna Sharma

6 **Community Mental Health: Evolution, Current Status, and Future Perspectives** 101
K. R. Anish and P. Ginu George

7 **Contextualizing Law and Policy Framework on Mental Health** 115
Saumya Uma

Part II Practice Skills in Mental Health

8 **Skill Sets and Novel Approaches for Rehabilitation of Persons with Mental Disorders** 131
Smita N. Deshpande, Mary E. Hawk, and Vishwajit L. Nimgaonkar

9 **Therapeutic Alliance in Psychotherapy: Clinical Significance and Skills Training** 143
M. Manjula and Reshma Antony

10 Motivational Interviewing: Walking Towards Change 159
Prerna Srivastava and Kannappa V. Shetty

11 Practicing Social Skills Training in Mental Health 175
Pravin B. Yannawar

12 Group Therapy: Basic Concepts and Skills 189
Sangeetha Reddy Duvvur

13 Integrating 'Spirituality' in Social Work—Challenges and Opportunities 205
R. Srinivasa Murthy

Part III Experiential Insights from Praxis

14 The Banyan Journey: A Continuum in Community Mental Health Care 229
M. Namrata Rao, A. Lakshmi Ravikanth, Lakshmi Sankaran, Palaakshee Bansal, and Rima Chowdhury

15 The Indian Family Caregivers of Persons with Mental Illness—PwMI: Large Canvas, Beyond Family 251
Amrit Bakhshy

16 Three Decades of a Journey Towards Mental Health for All: The Story of IPH 271
Anuradha Sovani

17 Destitution, Mental Illness and Law: Issues, Challenges and Possibilities 287
Mohd. Tarique

18 Embrace All.... No Labels Attached: Reflections by OYA Foundation 299
Raheen Jummani

19 Conclusion 309
Meenu Anand

Editor and Contributors

About the Editor

Meenu Anand, Ph.D., teaches at the Department of Social Work, University of Delhi and has extensive professional experience and exposure to gender and mental health. Dr. Anand has been actively involved in working on issues related to gender, mental health, and education for more than twenty-six years. She has led several national and international projects on multifaceted developmental issues during her specialized work experience with various grassroots NGOs. Dr. Meenu Anand also specializes as a trainer and conducts various capacity-building and gender sensitization workshops for school and University teachers, bureaucrats, journalists, police personnel, NGO functionaries, and diverse stakeholders. She has been instrumental in the development of curriculum at the postgraduate level on gender for Women's Studies and Development Centre, University of Delhi, and has a vast publication in the form of books as well as research papers in national and international journals that seek to highlight issues related to gender, mental health, and social work within interdisciplinary frameworks. She is passionate about working and researching on gender and mental health. Among one of her prominent publications is the book 'Gender and Mental Health: Combining Theory and Practice' published by Springer Nature, Singapore in 2020.

Contributors

K. R. Anish is a registered mental health professional and academician with 23 years' experience He has served as Head of the Department of Social Work at Rajagiri College, Chairman of the Board of Studies of Mahatma Gandhi University, Kannur University, Rajagiri College of Social Sciences and Member of BOS of Sree Sankaracharya University and a number of autonomous colleges in Kerala. His areas of interest and research are intercultural competence, social work education, mental health interventions and migration. He has authored/edited four books and published articles in Scopus indexed journals. He also serves as an Editorial Board Member of Children and Youth Services Review (CYSR), Indian Journal of Health Social Work and reviewer of intentional journals; Social Work Education, Indian Journal of Social Work, The International Journal of Community and Social Development etc.

Reshma Antony is a trained clinical psychologist and currently pursuing her Ph.D. in NIMHANS. She has a keen interest in the therapeutic process from a clinician's perspective. She has worked with patients suffering from various psychological conditions and also completed her postgraduate thesis work on the psychologist's experience of empathy.

Amrit Bakhshy is father of a daughter living with a diagnosis of paranoid schizophrenia for over three decades. He has used his life experiences to bring to the attention of the larger society through his remarkable writings. Further, he has synthesized his and other caregivers' experiences into books and to contribute in changing the legislation and social welfare measures in India. He is a living example of how a challenge of life can be converted into an opportunity. He has been President Schizophrenia Awareness Association Pune (2010–2019), Chairperson Hospital Managing Committee, NIMHANS, Bangalore (2015–2018), Member Institutional Body NIMHANS Bangalore (2014–2018), Chairperson/member Ethics Committee, ILS Pune (2014–2020), Member, Committee of Experts to frame Rules and Regulations for Mental Healthcare Act 2017 (2018), Member Expert Group on Psychotic Disorders, International Consortium for Health Outcome Measurement, Invited by WHO's Department of Mental Health and Substance Abuse for Expert Advice to review the mental health related draft material, Member, International Advisory Board for PIECEs: Improving outcomes for people with psychosis in Pakistan and India. Books "Mental Illness and Caregiving" (English, Marathi, Hindi), The Mental Health Care Act 2017—Guide for Stakeholders.

Palaakshee Bansal works as Junior Research Assistant, Centre for Trauma Studies and Innovation, Banyan Academy of Leadership in Mental Health (BALM). Palaakshee holds a Master of Arts degree in Applied Psychology from Tata Institute of Social Sciences (TISS), class of 2022. As an emerging professional, she is dedicated to enhancing the lives of children and teenagers. With a background as a researcher at the Banyan Academy of Leadership in Mental health (BALM) and project fellow at N.C.E.R.T, she aspires to empower the youth through her psychology expertise.

Rima Chowdhury works as Junior Research Assistant, Centre for Trauma Studies and Innovation, Banyan Academy of Leadership in Mental Health (BALM). With a Master's in Applied Psychology, she has a focused interest in work with groups who are marginalised. She is passionate about the Existential School of Psychology, and aims to implement it while working with children and adolescents. Currently, she is working on field in rural Uttarakhand, to improve Government education.

Smita N. Deshpande is currently serving as Professor in the Department of Psychiatry at St John's National Academy of Health Sciences, Bengaluru, India. She served as the Head, Department of Psychiatry, ABVIMS-Dr. RML Hospital, New Delhi from July 2004 to September 2018. She is conducting Fogarty International Centre; NIH USA funded Training Programmes in Research in intervention, implementation and Psychiatric Genetics since 2004. Beginning with systems research in 1988, she conducted research in schizophrenia genetics since 1992. She led over 36 research projects in autism, schizophrenia genetics, clinical trials, psychosocial aspects, disability and rehabilitation in schizophrenia and Implementation research for Indian and international agencies such as the NIH, WHO, ICMR, DST and DBT. She participated in developing the Indian Scale for Assessment of Autism (ISAA) recognized by the Government of India for certifying disability for autism. She developed the Indian Autism Screening Questionnaire (2021). She was a member of developing ICMR human research guidelines for vulnerable groups in 2017. She led the groups in drafting guidelines for mental and neurological disabilities, and multiple disabilities for the Government of India for the Indian Rights of Persons with Disabilities Act. She is on the board of several international journals. She is Vice-Chair, World Psychiatric Association Section on genetics. She is an international trainer and Consultant for the World Health Organization for Tobacco Control.

Sangeetha Reddy Duvvur is a trained counselling psychologist who has been in private practice since 2007. She has worked as an affiliate professor teaching counselling skills and group therapy. She has extensive experience in conducting and training group therapy and has also served as an expert advisor and supervisor for group therapy service providers. Sangeetha Reddy received her Master's degree in Counselling from Montfort College and is also certified in gestalt therapy and existential-humanistic approach. She is invested in a practice emphasizing an integrative approach using gestalt, existential, humanistic, somatic, and trauma-informed orientations to work with the whole person and to ensure that therapy is personalized, collaborative, and unique to one as a client.

P. Ginu George is a Research Scholar and a Registered Mental Health Professional, Rajagiri College of Social Sciences.

Mary E. Hawk DrPH, LSW, is Associate Professor and Chair of Behavioral and Community Health Sciences at the University of Pittsburgh School of Public Health, USA. Her research foci include implementation and assessment of structural interventions to improve health outcomes for oppressed populations, including those with substance use and substance use disorders; program evaluation to enhance service delivery in health and public health settings; and the development of community-engaged approaches to optimize public health. Her work centers on approaches that advance health equity for historically excluded populations. She is Principal Investigator of a study funded by the National Institute of Mental Health (NIMH, USA) assessing the impact of a financial management intervention on antiretroviral treatment HIV adherence among unstably housed people living with HIV. She is Multiple Principal Investigator (MPI) of a study funded by the National Institute of Drug Abuse (NIDA, USA) investigating experiences of stigma in healthcare settings by people living with HIV who use drugs. She is co-founder of The Open Door, Inc., a harm reduction housing program created to improve health outcomes for chronically homeless people living with HIV who have untreated serious mental illness and harmful substance use, wherein she published the first study to explore viral suppression as a measure of housing program effectiveness. Finally, she is MPI on two training grants: a D43 Training Grant through Fogarty International/NIMH seeking to increase research capacity among Indian mental health professionals and an NIMH T32 Training grant titled *A Training Program to Address HIV Related Health Disparities in MSM*.

Ananya Mahapatra is currently working as a Specialist (Psychiatry) at Dr. Baba Saheb Ambedkar Hospital and Medical College, New Delhi. Her primary areas of interest are depression, anxiety, and social psychiatry. She has conducted and published research on stigma related to mental disorders, caregiver needs, and psychosocial issues related to psychiatric disorders in numerous national and international publications.

M. Manjula is a Professor of Clinical Psychology at the Department of Clinical Psychology, National Institute of Mental Health and Neuro Sciences (NIMHANS), Bangalore, Karnataka State. She completed her M.Phil. and Ph.D. in Clinical Psychology from NIMHANS and is been affiliated to NIMHANS as a faculty from 2007. She is a trained cognitive behaviour therapist and works in the Behavioural Medicine unit of the Department of Clinical Psychology. Her clinical and research work includes providing therapeutic services to the patients referred from within and outside the Institute; supervision of the therapeutic work of the trainees, training and teaching of the post graduate students, carrying out funded and non-funded research; supervising the post graduate and doctoral research of the students. Her areas of research interest include Cognitive behaviour therapies and third wave therapies across the anxiety, mood, stress and personality disorders; Process and outcome research in therapy; mental health interventions in youth. She has published around 75 papers in national and international journals; written 8 book chapters and 7 books and manuals. She has guided about 20 M.Phil. dissertations and 12 Ph.D. thesis. She has received funding for research projects from ICSSR, ICMR and DST. She has conducted more than 100 workshops for public (students, parents, women) and professionals (mental health professionals, BSF, Airforce, teachers, IT professionals, police, Fire fighters etc.).

R. Srinivasa Murthy has been a full-time academician/researcher from the time of completion of postgraduate training in 1975. He was a faculty member at PGIMER, Chandigarh (1975–1981) and the National institute of Mental Health and Neurosciences (NIMHANS) Bangalore (1982–2003). Prof. Murthy was Professor of Psychiatry at NIMHANS, from 1987 to 2003. He was Head of the Department of Psychiatry, from January 1988 to February 1997 with over 50 postgraduates and 40 academic staff. He has been a much-respected teacher and mentor to many of the current leaders in psychiatry in India. He was a staff of World health Organisation (WHO) during 2000–2001 (Chief Editor, World Health Report, 2001-Mental Health) and 2004–2006 (in the WHO-EMRO Office). Since retirement, he has provided honorary services to non-governmental organizations like the Association for the Mentally challenged (AMC) Bangalore (2008–2014), Sri Shankara Cancer Hospital and Research Centre (SSCHRC), Bangalore (2015–2016). He is currently working to develop and disseminate 'self-care skills' for emotional health with a special focus on persons living with a diagnosis of cancer and caregivers of persons living with developmental disabilities.

Vishwajit L. Nimgaonkar M.D., Ph.D. is a Professor of Psychiatry and Human Genetics at the University of Pittsburgh, where he directs the Program in Genetics and Psychoses. He also serves as the Associate Chief of Staff/Vice President of the Behavioral Health Service Line at the Veterans Administration Pittsburgh Health System. His research is focused on the causation and treatment of severe psychiatric illnesses, including genetic and environmental factors. His group also models the functional effects of identified risk factors using iPSC-based technologies. With funds from the NIH, Dr. Nimgaonkar oversees research projects and research training in the United States and India. Dr. Nimgaonkar' training includes Medicine (MBBS) from the University of Madras; Ph.D. (D.Phil.) from the University of Oxford, UK; psychiatric residency training at the Maudsley Hospital, London, UK, and post-doctoral training at the University of London, UK. He is a Member of the Royal College of Psychiatrists, a Fellow of the American College of Neuropsychopharmacology and a Diplomate of the American Board of Psychiatry and Neurology. Dr. Nimgaonkar has received a Rhodes scholarship, the Sir Dennis Hill Prize from the Institute of Psychiatry, London, the NIMH Independent Scientist Award, the Harry Levin Award for Clinical Excellence from Western Psychiatric Institute and Clinic and an Outstanding Mentorship Award from the Department of Psychiatry, University of Pittsburgh School of Medicine. He has published over 260 peer reviewed publications.

Vibhuti Patel is Retired Professor of TISS and SNDT Women's University, Mumbai and currently, Vice President of Indian Association for Women's Studies and Hon. Distinguished Faculty at Impact and Policy Research Institute, Delhi. She previously served as Director, Post Graduate Studies and Research at SNDT Women's University and Chairperson, Advanced Centre for Women's Studies, School of Development Studies, Tata Institute of Social Sciences. She is co-editor of *Gendered Inequalities in Paid and Unpaid Work of Women*, Springer, 2022. She has authored *Women's Challenges of the New Millennium (2002).* She has co-authored of *Indian Women: Change and Challenge (1985)* and *Reaching for Half the Sky (1985). She is* editor of two volumes, *Discourse on Women and Empowerment (2006)* and *Girls and Girlhoods at the Threshold of Youth and Gender (2009.* She is Editor of a peer-reviewed quarterly *Quest in Education* published Indian Council of Basic Education and c0-editor of an Interdisciplinary Women's Studies Annual Journal, *Urdhva Mula* published by Sophia Centre for Women's Studies and Development. She is associated with VACHA- A Resource Centre for Women and Girls, a community based organisation.

Raheen Jummani is a Clinical Psychologist, Art based therapist and Social Worker. She has been working from past 18 years, she has reached out to people from various backgrounds—Sex Workers and their Children, Children living in Slums and on Streets, People affected with HIV/AIDS, Cancer Patients, People having diverse Mental Health Disorders, Care Givers, Rape and Child Sexual Abuse Survivors, Children with Learning Difficulties and Domestic Violence Survivors. She has transformed her passion into reality and formulated 'Open Your Arms Foundation' which provides psychological services in Schools, NGO's, Shelter Homes and Rescue Homes. Raheen's doctrine is enhancement of humanity.

M. Namrata Rao is the Co-Lead, Centre for Trauma Studies and Innovation, Banyan Academy of Leadership in Mental Health (BALM). Namrata is a neuroscience graduate passionate about research in psychological trauma and developmental psychology. She began her career as a teacher working with vulnerable communities. Currently, she is involved in research, training and advocacy at BALM.

A. Lakshmi Ravikanth is the Co-Dean, Banyan Academy of Leadership in Mental Health (BALM). Engaged with the Banyan and (BALM) since their inception. At BALM, contributed to education training research and co-authored articles and papers. Is a practising counselor with keen interest in relationship counselling, supportive psychotherapy . Core interests are existential psychotherapy and other eclectic approaches, and ethics in practice

Lakshmi Sankaran is the Chair and Co-Lead, Centre for Trauma Studies and Innovation, Banyan Academy of Leadership in Mental Health (BALM). A counsellor and a mental health practitioner for 20 years, she joined BALM in 2013 as the chairperson of applied psychology and her academic interests include family counseling, ABT and substance use interventions.

Kannappa V. Shetty has a Master's in Social Work from Bangalore University and M.Phil. and Ph.D. from National Institute of Mental Health and Neuro Sciences (NIMHANS) where he was associated for almost one decade. He has completed Post-Doctoral Fellowship in University of Florida, USA. Currently, Dr. Shetty is working as Assistant Professor at the School of social work, Indira Gandhi National Open University (IGNOU), New Delhi. He has also worked as Assistant Professor in Dharwad Institute of Mental Health and Neuro Sciences (DIMHANS), Dharwad, Karnataka. His areas of interest include expressed emotion in Schizophrenia and BPAD, Poverty and Mental Health, Addiction disorders (Alcohol, Cannabis, Nicotine), Suicide Prevention, School Mental Health and Preventive and Promotive Mental health. As a Mental health professional, he has been extensively involved in Clinical, Training, Research in Mental Health field. He has published 40 articles in National and International journals and presented over 30 papers in conferences. He often writes articles for Kannada newspapers, gives talk in radio and TV and conducts trainings on different issues of mental health. He has been involved in street plays, short film, poetry, NSS etc.

Prerna Sharma is an Assistant Professor (Clinical Psychology), at the Center for Excellence in Mental Health, IHBAS, New Delhi. Her research interests include adolescent mental health and well-being, early parenting environment, personality disturbances, emotional and developmental trauma. Her therapeutic approaches are third wave therapies such as DBT, ACT, Schema therapy, Grief and Trauma work.

Anuradha Sovani Psychologist and Psychotherapist, is the Former Professor and Head, Department of Psychology, and Former Dean, Faculty of Humanities, SNDT Women's University; M.A., M.Phil., and Ph.D. from University of Mumbai; Chancellor's Gold Medallist. Trustee and Consultant, Institute for Psychological Health, Thane, Maharashtra, and National Core Committee member and Ethics Committee Chairperson for Association of Adolescent and Child Care India. She has as authored eleven books in the areas of Child Mental Health, Quality of Life, Couple relationships and Couple counselling, and Personality Disorders. Kindle publications include a book on Personality Accentuations, and "*Diary of a Novice Counselor*", and a series of illustrated children's stories heralding attitude change, "*Vik Stories*". She has published over 70 research papers in national and international journals, and book chapters in National and International publications.

Prerna Srivastava has completed her Masters in Technology (M.Tech) in Biotechnology and Masters in Arts (M.A) in Psychology. She has cleared NET in Life Sciences as well as in Psychology. She was associated with NIMHANS for 4 years. She has completed M.Phil. degree in Clinical Psychology from Institute of Psychiatry, Centre of Excellence (IOP-COE), Kolkata, West Bengal. She is currently in to private practice and her areas of interest are Empathy, Obsessive Compulsive Disorder, and Personality Disorders. She has co-authored 3 articles and 1 book chapter. She has a research experience of 4 years. She likes reading and creative writing.

Mohd. Tarique works extensively on the issues of homelessness and Destitution. He founded Koshish in 2006 at TISS after graduating in Social Work. Recognised as prestigious Ashoka Fellow for his innovative social initiative, Forbes India included him in '30 Under 30' list of Indians making significant impact. Presently he is serving on the Supreme Court appointed monitoring committee for shelters for urban homeless and task force on social protection for State Planning Commission, Chattishgarh.

Saumya Uma is a Professor of Law and the Director, Centre for Women's Rights at Jindal Global Law School, O. P. Jindal Global University, India. She has over 28 years' combined experience as an academic, legal practitioner, researcher, writer, trainer, campaigner and consultant. She teaches and researches at the intersections of gender, human rights and the law

Pravin B. Yannawar M.Phil. (NIMHANS, Bengaluru), Ph.D. (Delhi University), works as Assistant Professor, Department of Psychiatric Social Work, Institute of Human Behaviour and Allied Sciences, Delhi. With professional experience spanning over more than twenty five years, he is also the *Technical Consultant*, State Mental Health Authority (SMHA), New Delhi; *Nodal Officer*, Disability, IHBAS Delhi and *Manager*, Saksham, Model HWH/LSH at IHBAS Delhi. He has extensive professional experience and has worked with reputed organisations including Tata Institute of Social Sciences (TISS), Mumbai; Maharashtra Institute of Mental Health (MIMH), BJ Medical College, Pune and All India Institute of Medical Sciences (AIIMS), New Delhi. Dr. Yannavar has attended several National and International Conferences and published scientific research papers with various reputed journals.

Abbreviations

ABT	Arts Based Therapy
ACMI	Action for Mental Illness
AIDS	Acquired Immuno Deficiency Syndrome
AMC	Association for Mentally Challenged
AMEND	Association for Mentally Disabled
ANM	Auxiliary Nurse and Midwife
APA	American Psychological Association
ASHA	Accredited Social Health Activist
AUDIT	Alcohol Use Disorders Identification Test
AVV	Atma Viswas Vidyalaya
AYUSH	Ayurveda, Yoga and Naturopathy, Unani, Siddha and Homeopathy
BALM	Banyan Academy of Leadership in Mental Health
BMC	Brihanmumbai Municipal Corporation
BT	Business and Technology
CCD	Cultural Concepts of Distress
CCL	Children in Conflict with Law
CEHAT	Centre for Enquiry into Health and Allied Themes
CGH	Clustered Group Homes
CHC	Caring for the Caregiver
CHMU	Community Mental Health Unit
CIL	Citizens For Inclusive Living
CMHC	Community Mental Health Centre
CRHT	Crisis Resolution and Home-Based Treatment
CSP	Care and Support Programme
CT	Computed Tomography
CTI	Critical Time Intervention
DMHP	District Mental Health Programme
DNA	Deoxyribonucleic Acid
DrInC	Drinker Inventory of Consequences
DSM	Diagnostic and Statistical Manual of Mental Disorders
DZ	Dizygotic

ECRC	Emergency Care and Recovery Centre
ECT	Electroconvulsive Therapy
ENRICH	Empowering Families to Fulfill Their Needs and Rebuild Families Through Information, and Skills of Caregiving Toward the Holistic Development of Families
GMCH	Government Medical College and Hospital
GWAS	Genome-Wide Association Studies
HA	Home Again
HIV	Human Immunodeficiency Virus
HPA	Hypothalamic–Pituitary–Adrenal
ICD	International Classification of Diseases
ID	Intellectual Disability
IDEAS	Indian Disability Evaluation and Assessment Scale
IPH	Institute for Psychological Health
IPM	Institute of Palliative Medicine
IT	Information and Technology
LGBTQI+	Lesbian, Gay, Bisexual, Transgender, Queer, Intersex
LGBTQIA+	Lesbian, Gay, Bisexual, Transgender, Intersex, Queer/ Questioning, Asexual
LMIC	Low- or Middle-Income Country
MAST	Michigan Alcohol Screening Test
MCM	Mohalla Committee Movement
MHA	Mental Healthcare Act
MHAT	Mental Health Action Trust
MHCA	Mental Health Care Act
MI	Motivational Interviewing
MIDC	Maharashtra Industrial Development Corporation
MZ	Monozygotic
NER	North-East Region
NGO	Non Government Organization
NIMHANS	National Institute of Mental Health and Neurosciences
NMHP	National Mental Health Programme
NRI	Non Resident Indian
OARS	Open Questions, Affirming, Reflecting and Summarizing
OPD	Out Patient Department
OSCC	One Stop Crisis Centre
OYA	Open Your Arms Foundation
PA	Personal Assistant
PET	Positron Emission Tomography
PHC	Primary Health Centre
PHFI	Paul Hamlyn Foundation
PMI	Persons with Mental Illness
POCSO	Protection of Children from Sexual Offences Act
PORT	Patient Outcomes Research Team
PTSD	Post Traumatic Stress Disorder

PWDVA	Protection of Women from Domestic Violence Act
PwMI	Person with Mental Illness
RASHMI	Research Advocacy, Support, and Help for Mentally Ill
RPD	Rights of Persons with Disabilities
SAA	Schizophrenia Awareness Association
SCARF	Schizophrenia Research Foundation
SMI	Seriously Mentally Ill
SO	Significant Others
SSCH	Sri Shankara Cancer Hospital
SST	Social Skills Training
TA	Therapeutic Alliance
Tele-MANAS	Tele Mental Health Assistance and Networking Across States
TISS	Tata Institute of Social Sciences
UDHR	Universal Declaration of Human Rights
UHC	Universal Health Coverage
UN	United Nations
UNCRPD	United Nations Conventions on the Rights of Persons with Disabilities
USA	United States of America
WGRC	Women's Grievance Redressal Cells
WHO	World Health Organization
WPA	World Psychiatric Association
YLD	Years Lived with Disability

List of Figures

Fig. 2.1	Overview of the World mental health report: Transforming mental health for all	31
Fig. 2.2	Key shifts to transform mental health for all	32
Fig. 2.3	Three transformative paths towards better mental health	33
Fig. 3.1	https://www.news18.com/news/india/india-lost-more-people-to-suicide-than-coronavirus-in-2020-shows-ncrb-data-4388651.html	61
Fig. 4.1	Risk factors for mental health	76
Fig. 5.1	The biopsychosocial model of mental health	92
Fig. 14.1	ECRC locations (2022)	235
Fig. 14.2	ECRC locations in Tamil Nadu (2022)	236
Fig. 14.3	Active aftercare service users (2022)	239
Fig. 14.4	Active HA locations (2022)	242

List of Tables

Table 2.1	Importance and challenges in the area of mental health	27
Table 2.2	Origins of mental disorders, mental health and well-being	37
Table 2.3	Multidimensional nature of mental health, mental disorders and mental health interventions	38
Table 2.4	Approaches to develop practice of spirituality and evaluate its impact (Murthy & Banerjee, 2021)	45
Table 2.5	Recommendations for research on 988 crisis lines (Miller et al., 2022)	45
Table 5.1	Limitations of the biomedical model for mental illness	91
Table 5.2	Psychosocial treatment recommendations for schizophrenia as per updated PORT Guidelines (2009)	96
Table 10.1	Decisional balance sheet	168
Table 10.2	Adopted from Miller and Rollnick (1995)	168
Table 11.1	Learning-based procedures used in social skills training	181
Table 11.2	Types of social skills as target behaviours for social skills training	181
Table 13.1	Religion, spirituality and health (Koenig et al., 2012) summary of evidence	208
Table 13.2	Approaches to develop practice of spirituality and evaluate its impact	220
Table 13.3	Spiritual assessment (Chaturvedi, 2022a, b)	221
Table 13.4	Priority areas for action to bring spirituality in social work practice	223
Table 14.1	ECRC phases and processes	234
Table 14.2	Steps involved in reintegration	237
Table 14.3	Client transition to HA	240
Table 14.4	The Banyan's reach in the three models of care	247

Part I
Overarching Conceptual Foundations

Chapter 1
Introduction

Meenu Anand

Abstract The introductory chapter of the *Mental Health Care Resource Book: Concepts and Praxis for Social Workers and Mental Health Professionals* sets its contextual foundation. Covering the intricacies and ambiguity around the very notion of mental health, it locates the notion of normality and melancholia through the centuries. Reiterating the inextricable link between physical and mental health, the chapter shoves on the socio-cultural determinants of mental health. Problematizing the hegemony of normative and the hierarchical as well as pervasive dominance of medicalized lexis, it dwells on the experience of epistemic injustice in the mental health care system and exclusion of the *person* and his/ her subjective experience. Embedding the scholarship of Mad Studies, it expounds on the scuffle against the biomedical model thereby echoing the need to highlight issues related to intersectionality across gender, race, disability, social class, culture, and generation. The chapter envisions the critical and leadership role of the social work profession in the field of mental health while acknowledging the contribution of other Psy professionals. It highlights the unique forte of social work viz. strong theoretical insights, practice skills, unique methods of working with individuals, groups and communities and how these get translated into their professional service at the grassroots. As a protuberant feature, the chapter offers a transient preview into the entire resource book, which is indeed an unambiguous annulment from the biomedical model and the related exclusive medical supremacy. It highlights the adoption of a strengths-based and emancipatory approach and integration of innovative, psychosocial, and spiritual voices/experiences by speckled mental health professionals. It illustrates the integration of an array of erudite as well as experiential reflections covered in the book while aiming to draw attention to the imperative need for the unification of academic as well as grassroots realities on the subject. Travelling through each of the three parts of the resource book, the chapter highlights how each section précises the intricate entwining of mental disorders and socio-cultural veracities while endeavouring to syndicate theoretical treatise along with the success stories as well as challenges from the field.

M. Anand (✉)
Department of Social Work, University of Delhi, Delhi, India
e-mail: meenuanand75@rediffmail.com

M. Anand (ed.), *Mental Health Care Resource Book*,
https://doi.org/10.1007/978-981-97-1203-8_1

Keywords Mental health · Cultural · Grassroots · Praxis · Experience

> It is not easy to understand people, who is mad and who is wise. God help us all from being seen through (Hamsun, 1909).

How can we intellectualise mental health; what is the relationship between mental health and normality? What precisely constitutes mental health? Vacillating on an intricate continuum, experienced distinctly from one individual to another, mental health seems to be a more complex concept than mental illness (Zachrisson, 2019). Unique to each person with altering grades of struggles and distress, the notion varies potentially across different socio-cultural contexts with significantly distinct clinical outcomes. Since much less attention is devoted to mental health (than to mental illness), there is not a *rich vocabulary to talk about it*. Oblivious to the very nature of mental health that encompasses thriving, flourishing, handling relationships, managing stress, feelings of well-being and gratification; most scholars describe and render it to mere symptoms/ names of disorders. While the discourse on mental health might have taken centerstage or even become somewhat decorative in the post-pandemic world, framing what we think and observe, what is 'inside' the frame and what falls 'outside' it; or comprehending the symptoms of wellness is indeed an arduous mission.

Mental health *has intrinsic and instrumental value*, helping people to *connect, function, cope and thrive* (WHO, 2022a). Embracing emotional, psychological and social well-being, impacts how one reflects, feels and acts. It also enables an individual to govern dealing with challenging life situations, relating to people around and making decisions. Jahoda (1958) identified six concepts associated with positive mental health: attitudes towards the self, development of self-actualization, integration of psychological functions, autonomy, accurate perception of reality, and environmental mastery. Furthermore, it is indeed significant to understand and appreciate mental health from a life course approach spanning through its different stages starting from childhood and adolescence through adulthood and senescence (Mignon, 2019).

World Health Organization (2022a) explicates:

> Mental health is an integral part of our general health and well-being and a basic human right. Having good mental health means we are better able to connect, function, cope and thrive. Mental health exists on a complex continuum, with experiences ranging from an optimal state of well-being to debilitating states of great suffering and emotional pain (p.xiv).

Mental health is not a binary state as one is not either mentally healthy or mentally ill. Rather, it exists on a complex continuum with experiences ranging from an optimal state of well-being to debilitating states of great suffering and emotional pain. Having undergone various highs and lows in my own life especially during challenging and transit phases, having strongly felt being drifting towards the languishing end of the continuum, I have wondered numerous times about what quite is mental health! Since mental disorders, just like mental health, affect one's thoughts, feelings, dispositions and actions, mental conditions for some individuals can be enduring and may continue throughout their lifetime. Many other persons may have sporadic incidents of mental illness while being able to function effectively most of the time. People with mental health conditions are more likely to experience lower levels of mental well-being even though it may not always happen.

Mental and physical health have a bidirectional relationship as they are inextricably intertwined and thus cannot be dispersed from each other. There is also often an underestimation and a failure to appreciate the association between mental disorders and other health ailments (Prince et al., 2007). Mental disorders upsurge peril for communicable and non-communicable ailments. Elaborating the nature of this duple relationship, Rosado (2018) expounds that poor mental health is a risk factor for chronic physical conditions; persons with serious mental health conditions are at high risk of experiencing chronic physical conditions, and persons with chronic physical conditions are at risk of developing poor mental health. Furthermore, mental disorders in every culture are often associated with enduring ailments linked with lifestyle influences including inadequate diet, smoking, obesity and cardiovascular ailments.

Mapping the Prevalence of Mental Disorders

WHO (2022b) estimated that in all countries, mental health conditions are highly prevalent. About one in eight people in the world live with a mental disorder. In 2019, 970 million people around the world were living with a mental disorder, with anxiety and depressive disorders being the most common. In 2020, the number of people living with anxiety and depressive disorders rose significantly because of the COVID-19 pandemic. Initial estimates showed a 26% and 28% increase respectively for anxiety and major depressive disorders in just one year (WHO, 2022b). Mental disorders are also the leading cause of Years Lived with Disability (YLDs), accounting for one in every six YLDs globally. Schizophrenia, which occurs in approximately 1 in 200 adults, is a chief concern: in its acute states, it is the most impairing of all health conditions. People with schizophrenia or other severe mental health conditions die on average 10–20 years earlier than the general population, often of preventable physical diseases. Estimates show approximately 300 million people worldwide suffer from depression (WHO,) and bipolar disorder affects approximately 60 million people (WHO,).

Even the most updated epidemiological data, however, may not reflect the real burden of mental health problems with accuracy. Mental disorders are commonly under-diagnosed and only less than 50% of those meeting criteria for a common mental health problem are detected or identified. In addition, many people do not have access to a mental health professional for diagnosis. For this reason, lifetime prevalence rates for mental problems may be higher than previously thought and could potentially affect even nearly half of the world's population (Artal, 2019). Mood and psychotic syndromes (including anxiety, depression, bipolar disorder and psychosis) are one of the most sombre public health challenges in the contemporary world impacting central facets of human life viz. capacity to work, function and develop valuable social affiliations. Young people in specific at more at-risk, with over 75% of adult mental disorders emerging before the onset of 25 years (McGorry, 2007; Hickie et al., 2013) and over 45% of the total illness burden being seen among persons belonging to the age group of 10–24 years (Sullivan et al., 2012).

At the home front, as per the National Mental Health Survey 2015–2016 by NIMHANS, one or more mental health conditions require active intervention for close to 15% of Indians. In addition, since 1990, the proportion of mental disorders in India's overall illness burden has nearly doubled. The survey also indicated that among the mental illnesses that develop primarily during adulthood, depression and anxiety disorders had the highest mental disorder burden in India, followed by schizophrenia and bipolar disorder. In 2017, the prevalence rate of depressive disorders was more than 3750 per 100,000 people, and the prevalence rate of anxiety disorders was 3200–3399 per 100,000 population (Anand, 2022a; Dandona et al., 2020). According to a Lancet study conducted across Indian states spanning from 1990 to 2017, there were 197.3 million persons affected by mental disorders, covering 14.3% of the total population of the country. Furthermore, mental disorders were found to the leading cause of YLDs in India, contributing to 14·5% of YLDs.

Social Determinants of Mental Health

Social inequality is a major determinant of health and is configured in ways that reflect local histories that are normalised, justified or rendered invisible through cultural frameworks of identity. The social determinants of health are based on universal processes but take unique forms in each society based on its cultural history, politics and economy (Kirmayer, 2012). These not only include individual attributes such as the ability to manage one's thoughts, emotions, behaviours and interface with others, but also social, cultural, economic, political and environmental factors such as national policies, social protection, living standards, working conditions, and community social supports (WHO, 2013). Gender as a social construct, differentially affects the power and control men and women have over the socio-economic determinants, their status, roles, and treatment in society. Women experience the impact of gender-based socialisation through the patriarchal structures in their day-to-day lives. Their subservience takes diverse forms including discernment, disdain, abuse, control, explanation, violence, and subjugation within the family, at work and in society at large (Anand, 2022b).. From a gendered standpoint, mental health concerns of women, men as well as LGBTQIA + necessitate due attention within the context of their social position and from a human rights perspective (Srivastava & Anand, 2020). Furthermore, since the determinants of mental health traverse with other relegated positions and challenges, in particular, those clustered around structures of racialization and class, factors such as gender, poverty, education, employment, homelessness, isolation, inequality, social constraints and violence; they become significant areas of analysis from the mental health perspective.

Normality and Melancholia Through the Centuries

Madness has occurred since the existence of documented history with the prepotency of supernatural perception and attribution of symptoms of mental distress to the forces relating to evil spirits or black magic. In all cultures and in all times, the acuity of madness, possession or mental disorder has generated a skirmish between fear and compassion (Porter, 1993). It was however only with the arrival of the psychiatric profession in the eighteenth century that these were medicalized and retitled as mental illness (Foucault, 1988; Leblanc & Kinsella, 2016; LeFrancois, Menzies & Reaume, 2013). The notion of normality is polyvalent and relative and is primarily based on the socio-historical milieu in which it is conceptualised. Zachrisson (2019) explicates the complex relationship between mental health and normality and questions the very notion of normalcy:

> It depends on which concepts we chose for mental health and normality. If we mean an ideal state of health, with total freedom from neurotic symptoms and inhibitions, the answer is no!….. Most people manage every morning to restore their sense of reality and the relation to themselves and others, after they have spent the night in the labyrinths of their dreams, filled with delight, chaos and dread. This is really the triumph of the ego over obscure forces of the mind. It deserves our respect and admiration (Zachrisson, 2019, p. 5).

Normality has become a contested term influenced profoundly by the dual continuum model. The notion of 'abnormal' has become so hegemonic that most people use it without reluctance, halt to reflect on it while labelling anyone who deviates from 'normal' as outlandish and suspicious. Thus, an individual who does not 'fit-in' is considered 'abnormal' or 'mentally unstable/mad'. Therefore, if 'mental disorder' means any disability or disorder of mind, this implies that there is some sort of mental 'order', an internal state where there is tranquillity and consistency. The boundary between mental health and mental disorder is therefore concerned with the controversial idea of normality and what society regards as 'normal' (Anand, 2020; Coppock & Hopton, 2000). The boundaries between the *other* and the *rest* have become distinct and compartmentalised into discrete worlds that never amalgamate.

The Medicalized Dominion of DSM

In the province of mental health, psychiatry draws on an ever-growing theoretical body of knowledge about mental illness based on biomedical model guidelines of epidemiology (Johnstone, 2021). The diagnostic and Statistical Manual of Mental Disorders (DSM) considered as the 'bible' of psychiatry, continues to exert an overarching power and a dominant discourse over psychiatric diagnosis and considered as a result of psychiatry's endeavour to 'own the contemporary meaning of madness', to exert its 'area of responsibility and control' although psychiatry 'has had serious trouble maintaining agreements about the meaning of madness and the methods for recognising it' (Kirk et al., 2013; Venkatesan & Suresh, 2023).

Psychiatry as what Dorothy Smith (2005) calls *'a regime of ruling'*, mostly relies on the use of psychotropic medications as the primary means to treat mental health conditions thereby reflecting the medicalization of mental disorders. However, despite the advances of medication, serious mental illnesses like schizophrenia often have chronic and disabling effects, and 'symptomatic remissions do not predict functional recovery' (Harvey et al., 2012, p. 6). Research on the lived experiences of medication users also reflects complex experiences with medication, side effects, and medication expectations. While on one hand, persons using psychotropic medication have expressed positive impacts including symptom relief, higher functioning, and a positive long-term outlook (Lee et al., 2020), many have also described the experience of using medication as feeling 'like a zombie', 'cloudy' or 'dazed' (Murphy et al., 2015; Werremeyer et al., 2017).

Banton et al. (1985) believe that the medical discourse creates a gap between the personal experience of pain/suffering and the broader social context supporting that experience. This is due to the fact that attempts are made to treat the individual instead of dealing with the social circumstances underlying the distress. By reducing the network of social, moral, political and economic factors which cause distress leading to pathology in an individual, the latter becomes appropriate for treatment. All other non-medical professions involved in the process of providing help to people who have had a psychiatric diagnosis are exposed to the situation where the medical diagnosis becomes one of the central points of attention.

Problematizing the Hegemony of Normative

Johnstone (2021) reiterates the hegemony of a psychiatric diagnosis that in itself is open to subjectivity and expounds the nexus across the players in the lucrative Mental Health-Medical-Industrial Complex which partners the pharmaceutical industry with the DSM thereby implying that expanding the available diagnoses benefits the pharma industry's expansionist agenda. Since the mental health advocacy groups and mental health research are heavily funded by the pharma industry (Burstow, 2015), there is sparse discourse and scarce funding for psychosocial treatments. Heavily dominated by the hegemonic bio-medicalized model, alternative models including psychotherapy, peer intervention, family-based interventions and novel recovery approaches hardly find takers.

Owing to the hierarchical and pervasive dominance of medicalized lexis, the voice as well as the experience of the person is excluded as he/she is viewed as needing help and not having any useful knowledge to contribute to finding a solution. Capponi (2003) who identifies as 'Mad' describes the experience of epistemic injustice in the mental health system:

> ..every individual is different, in spite of similar backgrounds and diagnoses, in terms of potential, character, insight, interests and abilities. These differences might be obscured by labels and behaviours, by homelessness and poverty, but they are there. And they need to be expressed in order for us to find out what makes us special, what makes us unique. The

failure to see us as people, not as pathologies, continues to wear us down (Capponi, 2003, p. 150 as cited by Johnstone, 2021).

Thus, while psychiatry is patently regarded as a formidable regime of ruling with its own arbitrary criteria, the impact is seen in the loss of focus on the 'person' in distress along with the socio-cultural aspects of his/her life. There is indeed de-contextualising of person's problem in order to re-contextualise the symptoms to align with an invented concept called a 'disorder.' As pointed by Szasz (1961), illnesses are conditions of the body and, as such, only a body or one of its organs can have an illness. The mind (thinking) is neither a body nor an organ. It is rather an activity of the body much like running and jumping and, as such, it can no more have a disease than running or jumping can—hence Szasz's (1961) identification of 'mental illness' as a metaphor (cited Burstow, 2018).

The Socio-Cultural Context of Suffering

The social constructivist theory of mental illness thrusts that '*mental illness is socially constructed, produced and distributed'* (White, 2018, p. 29). The labelling process operates inside a social system characterised by inequalities prevalent within the society based on class, gender and ethnicity. In this social system, mental illness follows the social gradient of disease where the lower one is in the social order, greater the chances of mental illness. Medicalization of symptoms based on ever pervasive psychiatry can individualise (and thus, de-politicise) issues by dislocating them from structural causes (Zola, 1972). Biomedical approach and pharmaceutical interventions often neglect the social context and cross-cultural differences thereby diminishing social problems to mere labelling based on bodily symptoms, prognosis and treatment, much in contrast to the subjective experience of the individual and his/her suffering. By turning attention and responsibility towards the individual, attention is often deflected from socio-cultural, political and economic determinants of health (Lock, 2001).

Capponi (2003) in her memoir 'Beyond the Crazy House', documents personal insider experiences with several DSM categories of mental illness including her own experiences with self-harm. She contrasts her own insider account of self-harm behaviour with the official abbreviated psychiatric description which regards the behaviour as a destructive symptom serving no purpose and needing to be stopped. She narrates various 'first voice accounts of self-harm and common themes emerge of countering the numbness from psychoactive medication, relieving emotional despair through visible physical wounding and regaining a sense of personal agency' (as cited by Johnstone, 2021). Sharma (2023) too reveals her own journey from being a 'patient' to being 'emancipated and empowered' after recovering and healing from bipolar disorder after eighteen years of struggle. The loss of intellectual courage or confidence in one's own abilities owing to a psychiatric label and understanding of the world can be corrosive as it can undermine personal resiliency and coping.

Mad Studies: Mapping the Marginal Voices

The last few decades have witnessed the increasing visibility of scholarship proposing alternative and positive approaches to madness, outside of the definitions of psychiatry. In the incarnation as Mad Studies, madness is approached not as an illness or disorder, but a source of creativity and identity (Rashed, 2019). Beresford and Russo (2022) alludes:

> We live in a world that generates madness and distress, fails frequently to address them adequately or appropriately and often can even make them worse (pp.1).

Mad Studies as a counter-discourse to psychiatry and psychiatric discourses is an emerging field that explores 'the various ways to take up the matters of "psychiatrization", "madness", the oppression and agency of Mad subjects (Menzies et al., 2013, p. 1). In other words, Mad Studies devotes in the radical reclamation of *'psychic spaces of resistance against the psychiatric domination of Mad people as a collection of chemical imbalances needing to be corrected in a capitalist system that prizes bourgeois conformity and medical model "fixes" above all'*. In its critical treatise, the term 'mad' is redefined as 'a critical alternative to represent 'mental illness' or 'disorder' as a way of naming and responding to emotional, spiritual, and neuro-diversity' (Menzie et al. 2013, p. 10). Extenuating its mission, Mad Studies, which initiated from consumer/survivor crusades in Canada, divulging the systemic and symbolic violence which is fundamental to the psychiatric system; rejects the biomedical model of psychiatry that involves involuntary incarceration and many medicalized psychiatric interventions. As an emerging academic field of study, the Mad movement links the scuffle against the medical model with other movements surrounding around gender, race, disability, social class, culture, and generation. Offering effective opposition to the marginalisation and oppression of experiencing madness and distress; Mad studies is an evolving field that scrutinises society's structural aspects which lead people to having breakdowns, the way they become psychiatric subjects (Eromosele, 2020; Sharma, 2023). Sharma (2023) while 'inaugurating' Mad Studies in the Indian context through her book 'Barriers to recovery from psychosis', questions the very *unequal social world that damages a majority of people and ecology due to inherent injustice, greed, power imbalances and imposition of hegemonic epistemic regimes on people with lesser power to create counter epistemologies* (Sharma, 2023, p. 6). She also indicates the '*massive ignorance about psychiatry's oppressive role in society*' with people envisaging it '*as a benign saviour*' (Sharma, 2023, p. 9).

Mad Studies considers psychiatric verdict not as an impartial, inert tool of scientification but to quote Datta (2014), *'as a social act' which engenders 'social consequences' and underscores the 'wider social, political and economic forces more than scientific advancement' that determine the concept and nature of mental disorders* (2014, p. 1). Predominantly, numerous diagnostic systems in psychiatry such as DSM progressively pathologize day-to-day behaviour in a manner that echoes the academic and ethical corruption of contributing medical professionals and institutions associated with corporate pharmacological companies. One of the objectives of Mad Studies' is to contest the hegemonic and profitable practices extensively disseminated through psychiatry including explicit medicalization (Venkatesan & Suresh, 2023).

Appraising psychiatry, Sharma (2023) claims:

...the promise with which psychiatry enters our lives does not match up to reality; it does not relieve suffering. Instead 'treatments' worsen health condition over time, or produce comorbidities at the very least. In a nutshell, psychiatric 'treatments' far from healing push one towards disability! (Sharma, 2023, 11).

The Mad Studies scholarship includes *'all that is critical of psychiatry from a radically socially progressive foundation in which the medical model is dispensed with as biologically reductionist whilst alternative forms of helping people experiencing mental anguish are based on humanitarian, holistic perspectives where people are not reduced to symptoms but understood within the social and economic context of the society in which they live'* (Venkatesan & Suresh, 2023). Disentangling the fundamental empiricism of the biomedical model, it robustly condemns immoral and insensitive treatment practices in addition to legitimising the thrust on the 'person' thereby adopting an eclectic approach in mental health care.

Revulsions of Dishonour and Stigma: Subjugation into the Oblivion

Mental disorders are associated with varied notions, misconceptions, distressing images and stereotypes. The lack of knowledge and awareness renders mental disorders as among the most denounced conditions. Conventionally defined as a *'mark of disgrace or disapproval with a person, a particular context or a set of circumstances'* (Stevenson, 2010), stigma in the context of mental health, refers to a group of factors conniving together within an authority-based system leading to the discernment of persons with mental disorders (Buchter & Messer, 2017). Moreover, stigma is not confined to the person and his/her familial level and infiltrates deeper at the structural as well as institutional levels (Hatzenbuehler, 2016). It is also one of the core reasons impeding persons with mental disorders to seek care. As a social process connected to dominance and exclusion, it affects the prospects of tangible opportunities, indents the self-esteem, and influences service delivery. Labelling of a psychiatric disorder also leads to discrimination, withering of social relationships, and social exclusion of persons with mental disorders who are kept away from mainstream social life (Anand, 2021; Goffman, 1963). Persons with mental disorders also face discrimination on a daily basis including in the fields of education, employment and housing and are socially excluded (Anand, 2021; Thornicraft, 2006; Thornicraft et al., 2007). They are pilloried, mainly as a result of 'ignorance, prejudice or discrimination' by others. Such persons, therefore, may not only be discriminated against but may also be socially vetoed, disregarded and 'shunned' as mental health problems constitute 'the forgotten millions'. (Agarwal, 1998).

The discriminatory treatment at the institutional level finds evidence in the reports by the National Human Rights Commission (2016) that reflected on the inhuman conditions in which persons with mental disorders within the institutional settings were cared for, the gross deficiencies in the physical structure and functioning of the hospitals, severe staff shortages and violations of patients' rights. In addition, the shame of mental illness can aggravate the challenges associated with determining its incidence (Baumann, 2007; Jackowska, 2009). Stigma can therefore be understood as an obstruction to recovery among persons with mental disorders (Sarkar & Punnoose, 2016) as they continue to be abjured and banished.

Davar (2022) recounts both her personal experience and the progress made by survivors against the background of a subcontinent that was the subject of psychiatrisation under British imperial and colonising power. Describing mother's forced incarceration, of her being tied up, treated inhumanly, tightly tied down in ropes or cloth, given electric shock (ECT without anaesthesia), and deserted by her own family; she writes about the impact of these memories on her as a young child and the enduring impacts in the subsequent decades.

When a person is labelled as having a mental disorder, it is tough for them to get cleared of the docket (Rosenhan, 1975) that is taken as a finality to their very being and also abridges the quality of life. It is an arduous task for people to really understand the *human* behind the medical label, with the distresses and dreams; strengths and susceptibilities; insurgencies and subjugations. The theory of labelling draws attention to the fact that classifying people as mentally unstable also establishes the ways in which people understand themselves and confines them as being 'incompetent'. The distressing and enervating impact of a psychiatric diagnosis on the social value of a person is echoed in the individual's loss of integrity within systems of support, whether they are medical or social systems owing to their mental disorder (Foucault, 1975; Lamovec, 1998). Perceived as perilous, incurable or unintelligible, there is fear mongering about them in the larger society and final verdicts are passed on lives of the affected persons as making them the *permanent travellers through 'the system of help'* (Kvaternik & Grebenc, 2009). The impacted persons and their emotional turmoil diagnosed as a specific mental disorder become irrefutable proof by oratorical tautology far from attempting to understand the *real* causes of their distress.

Mental health is viewed as a site of grave power inequity, marginalisation and epistemic injustice. Addressing the root causes of mental distress requires skills to reach out beyond the medical services provided by the health care system. It requires knowledge about those underlying factors that have a critical influence on people's mental health and well-being (Krech, 2019). The need for diverse mental health professionals therefore arises to address the needs of the persons with mental health difficulties, systemic structures of subjugation and hegemonic oppression and power inequalities that create conditions leading to such challenges.

Envisioning the Role of Social Work in Mental Health

Amalgamation of theoretical insights with grassroots practice has always been the forte of social work. In the field of mental health along with the critical players from the disciplines of psychiatry and psychology with their unique traditional interdisciplinary boundaries, social work has a unique forte that necessitates a rethinking of their utmost significance as irreplicable professionals.

Professional social workers, in this context, have a diverse arena of expertise, including clinical evaluation, individual and family counselling, treatment and psychosocial rehabilitation of the client. With the person-in-environment approach, they can effectively work at micro, mezzo and macro systems to create an enabling environment in the community. Moving beyond the biomedical diagnosis as moral categories, professional social workers can understand the day-to-day lives of people with diverse conditions of distress and adopt professional methods and skills that will enable them to understand people's lives. Adopting a person-in-environment approach, the client is placed in his/ her wider social context and enabled to gain full realisation of the psychosocial condition. Listening to the socio-cultural narratives by the clients, their unique experiences related to their suffering can help them to understand and position their clients' suffering at the micro, mezzo and macro levels.

I strongly feel, especially in the post-pandemic scenario, that social workers can and must take up the mantle of leadership in this field with their stout belief in the significance of having robust and caring families and communities. With their training in social work methods and practice-based skills and competencies, they can work at the level of legislation and carry out the much-needed advocacy for the clients from a rights-based approach.

Adopting a strengths-based perspective, social workers as experts, can adopt a vocabulary that can facilitate the process of normalisation and de-stigmatisation of people with diverse mental health needs. With a focus on 'describing' situations which are challenging rather than 'classifying' the symptoms, social workers can put the 'person' at the centerstage. Employing a participatory approach with a strong belief in the power of survival (Kvaternik & Grebenc, 2009), they can effectively use their practice skills to seek specific information from the clients including their feelings, desires, changes sought in life, perceived threats and obstacles, need for help and how they wish to receive it, sources of support (if any) with thrust on catharsis and giving due dignity to the person.

Another chief area where the contribution of social workers is unparalleled is community mental health. Trained in community organisation as a method of practice, with the skills and techniques of group work, they can effectively execute their preventive and promotive roles in the prevention of mental disorders, working with community structures with due acknowledgement to contextual, transactional, cultural, and relational forces operating in the communities. In the coming decades, I do anticipate the incredible contribution of social work in educational institutions, psychosocial rehabilitation of clients in schools/colleges/communities, occupational/

professional settings, skills and capacity building trainings with numerous stakeholders, workplace mental health, etc. I also envision a management role for social workers in policy and programme development keeping in mind their expertise to navigate through the rights and choices of clients, thereby playing a decisive role in changing public mental health policy towards a rights-based perspective. Identifying the potential of social workers, they can strongly advocate for epistemic justice for the persons with mental health conditions, initiating and strengthening anti-stigma work across the national and global terrains.

Role of Diverse Psy Professionals

With the enduring challenged nature of biomedical discourse and the work of psy-professionals, there is an urgent need to bring about diverse specialities from varied mental health professionals to provide mental healthcare services. They may strive to offer a gamut of mental health services as there is indeed a bulging scope as well as the need to recognise the varied interventions by a diverse set of mental health practitioners. Currently psychiatrists are leading the field as psychopharmacologists as their training is largely based on prescribing medications to treat mental disorders. Psychologists possess the proficiency to provide psychological testing that can assist in determining diagnoses in addition to providing psychotherapy and individual as well as group counselling. Psychiatric nurses working in medical settings to provide care and treatment to persons with mental disorders (Sawyer et al., 2016) and can be trained further towards developing empathy and developing a holistic perspective.

In the contemporary disempowerment and the relentless erosion of community, there is a need to thrust on building connections among people across societal structures while grappling together with the challenges. Through participatory (not simply representative) governing, expansion of the commons (co-ownerships), and equalitarian professional relationships, Psy professionals can work towards eliminating systemic coercion while allowing each discipline to contribute in their own exclusive manner (Burstow, 2018) with respect for collectivity and egalitarianism.

Why This Book?

The foremost resolve of this resource book on Mental Health Care is to provide a one-stop foundation valuable for students, researchers, academicians and diverse mental health professionals to plausibly comprehend and appreciate the arena of mental health, and develop knowledge about practice-based skills while connecting to voices from the field. This book is a concise compendium of the basic concepts and actions required to effectively promote positive and strengths-based mental health. The principal motive for producing this resource book is to address the contemporary absence of a single volume that packs together concepts, skills as well as praxis woven together by methodical thinking about the knowledge base on mental health, skill-set and grassroots realities that are indeed formulated as well as practiced by mixt mental health professionals. It also focuses on survivors' and caregivers' experiences, lives, viewpoints and optimism surrounding mental health.

Another unique aspect of this resource book is its unambiguous annulment from the biomedical model and the related theoretical and treatment premises allied with it. Rebuffing the exclusive medical supremacy in the field of mental health, it adopts the strengths-based approach thereby integrating innovative, psychosocial, spiritual voices/experiences by speckled mental health professionals.

Organisation and Contents of the Book

The book brings together an array of erudite as well as experiential reflections on the subject of mental health. It aims to draw attention to the imperative need for unification of academic as well as grassroots realities on the subject. It seeks to reconnoitre and essay the inclusion of practice-based interpositions, which is actually the 'need of the hour'. It précises the intricate entwining of mental disorders and socio-cultural veracities while endeavouring to syndicate theoretical treatise along with the success stories as well as challenges from the field.

The book is divided into three parts. The First part 'Overarching Conceptual Foundations' has seven chapters that bring together a theoretical understanding on mental health thereby laying a contextual backdrop to understand its intricacies. After this introductory chapter authored by me that lays the critical backdrop for this resource book on mental health care, the second chapter by R. Srinivasa Murthy essays a critical foundation for understanding the very ideas of mental health and mental disorders. His chapter *Understanding Mental Disorders, Mental Health and Well-Being* locates the recent developments on the subject. Tracing the trajectory of mixt discourses on mental health in the last five decades, Murthy reveals through personal as well as professional experiences, the evolution of various models including the mounting crusade from mental illness towards mental health. His chapter seeks to convey newer understandings on the theme and explicates the augmentation of perception regarding persons with mental disorder from the mere biological perspective towards the more eclectic bio-psycho-social-spiritual lens. Citing various international and national policies, programmes and reports, he holistically covers both challenges as well as newer opportunities for professional social workers in India. Placing social work as a specialty and professional social workers as a unique professional group, Murthy uniquely envisions the scope for action by social workers in the field of mental health.

Vibhuti Patel in her chapter *Social and Cultural Determinants of Mental Health* accentuates an understanding of the interplay of social, cultural, emotional, psychological and biological factors that determine mental health and illness. Describing the risk factors impacting the vulnerable groups of population, she highlights the nature and impact of intersectional vulnerabilities with regard to diverse groups including Dalits, ethnic-religious-sexual minorities, survivors of sexual violence, persons with disabilities, poor and unemployed, etc. Through her exhaustive narration, Patel illustrates the successful initiative by the Women's Grievance Redressal Cells (WGRC), a project by Mohalla Committee Movement, Mumbai. Expounding the holistic approach and collective efforts by women and various stakeholders, she elaborates and makes eclectic micro, mezzo and macro suggestions to ensure inclusive family and community-based structures and creation of systems that promote intersection justice through gender inclusive mental health legislations, evidence-based policy, affirmative action backed by adequate funds and competent/ empathetic functionaries.

The fourth chapter *Interrogating the gendered terrain of mental health Women's mental health: The unchartered terrain* helmed by me, highlights gender oppression as a dominant factor that impacts the development of and recovery from mental disorders. Locating the provenance of mental health differences between men and women to sex and gender distinctions, I put forth my argument regarding understanding the role of culture and development in order to gain a better understanding of mental health and illness. Unfolding the intricate entwining of individual, socio-cultural as well as structural factors in society and their impact on psychiatric labelling, I seek to levy a deeper understanding of socio-cultural factors in the aetiology of mental distress, epidemiological inequalities in the diagnosis of mental disorders and opportunities available for treatment as well as remission. In my narration, I also attempt to elucidate significant multi-layered protective factors to promote mental health and well-being among diverse sections of populations.

Integration and interaction of biological, psychological, and social determinants and processes in understanding the pathogenesis of illnesses and their impact on the recovery and well-being of an individual is highlighted in *A Biopsychosocial Approach to Mental Health*. Ananya Mahapatra and Prerna Sharma abridge the theoretical underpinnings of the Biopsychosocial Model and elaborate on its significance in conceptualising mental disorders. They formulate practical strategies which can be implemented in clinical assessment, patient care, service delivery, research and policymaking. Mahapatra and Sharma also highlight the benefits of adopting a holistic approach in integrating humanistic perspectives in service delivery thereby fostering therapeutic relationships that take into account the lived experience of clients while acknowledging their role in the treatment process.

One of the most pertinent discourses on *Community Mental Health: Evolution, Current Status, and Future Perspectives* is narrated by Anish K. R. and Ginu George P. They unravel the past, present, and future of community mental health at the national as well as international levels. This chapter sets the tone for understanding the context of community mental health which is particularly relevant for intervention by mental health professionals. Anish and Ginu trace the evolution of community mental health through the diverse government policies and programmes and cite models and human resources for community mental health practice with a futuristic perspective.

The right to a standard of living adequate for health and well-being has been proclaimed as a human right by the Universal Declaration of Human Rights. In the concluding chapter of the first part of the book, *Contextualizing law and policy framework on mental health*, Saumya Uma, illustrates how mental health law provides normative standards of behaviour and treatment, which enable individuals and communities with mental illnesses to assert their human rights. She alludes that it is the convergence of law and policy on mental health that contributes to the accessibility of mental health care and augment the quality of the health services provided. Uma discusses the components of mental health as a human right and provides an overview of the present law and policy framework pertaining to mental health in India and also critiques the national law and policy framework vis-à-vis established international human rights standards. She also identifies gaps in law and policy that ought to be addressed through advocacy, practice-based skills and field-based actions.

Second part of the book 'Practice Skills in Mental Health' encompasses six chapters that translate the theoretical discourses into practice-based skills. Each chapter, unique with its own peerless kind, seeks to demonstrate the application of theoretical insights into practice-based skills through detailed chronicles located in institutional as well as non-institutional settings.

Smita N. Deshpande, Mary E. Hawk and Vishwajit L. Nimgaonkar bring together the much-needed and a fresh treatise titled *Skill Sets and Novel Approaches for Rehabilitation of Persons with Mental Disorders*. Going beyond the traditional biomedical approach, they accentuate the significance of innovative methods to integrate persons with mental disorders into society and creating conditions whereby the benefits of existing treatment and policies can be fully realised. Focusing on the socio-ecological model, they focus on the individual, community and policy-level approaches to rehabilitate persons with mental disorders. They describe the Proximal approaches that involve treating the individual experiencing mental illness directly, cognitive remediation using yoga and meditation. Furthermore, 'Palliative care for severely disabling mental illnesses' at the individual level and 'Homelessness and mental disorders: Housing and supported living services', *The* 'Housing First' *model* at the community level are some of the innovative therapies highlighted by them.

An overarching theme, which emanates from the core values of social work, is the significance of the 'therapeutic relationship' in a helping profession. M. Manjula and Reshma Antony expound on the very concept of therapeutic relationship, its various dimensions, principles and skills in the chapter *Therapeutic alliance in psychotherapy: Clinical significance and skills training*. They also encompass desirable personal attributes of the therapist that can contribute positively to the professional alliance. They also exemplify the methods of professional training to strengthen the therapeutic alliance-building skills of the therapist.

The two subsequent chapters encapsulate crucial key skills-based techniques for providing mental health care to persons with mental disorders. *Motivational interviewing: Walking towards change* essayed by Prerna Srivastava and Kannappa V Shetty highlights the approach as an evidence-based counselling and a collaborative technique adopted effectively by mental health practitioners. Through case illustrations, the authors feature its application as a skilful clinical method useful in various fields including healthcare, rehabilitation, dentistry, public health, education, information technology, etc. *Practicing Social Skill Training in Mental Health* helmed by

Pravin Yannavar elucidates the very nature of this technique thereby demonstrating it as an essential and viable alternative to pharmacological treatment. He signifies its usage in the treatment and rehabilitation of persons who often have deficits of social skills, viz., inability to express thoughts, feelings and emotions that may have arisen either as part of the illness or due to restriction of learning new opportunities to acquire. Through case illustrations, Yannavar elaborates on the practice of this technique and its holistic attempts to enable the client to gain new skills and confidence.

Group Therapy: Basic Concepts and Skills by Sangeetha Reddy Duvvur contributes yet another exclusive homily necessitating mental health care services in groups. Recognising the distinctive importance of working in groups for persons with mental health challenges, Duvvur introduces with conciseness, a comprehensive body of text emphasising the interpersonal and interactional underpinnings of group therapy. Striving to achieve a feat at different points through tangible and practical illustrations and case examples, she brings together key ideas in group therapy. Duvvur focuses on the hands-on constituents of group therapy including group content and processes, group dynamics, and stages in addition to enlightening the readers about leadership, process-oriented and facilitation skills applicable to numerous group work settings, viz., task, psychoeducational, crisis-intervention, therapy groups, etc.

Part Two of the book concludes with one of the most significant and popular contemporary discourses in mental health care, viz., Spirituality. R. Srinivasa Murthy in yet another authoritative chapter *Integrating 'Spirituality' in Social Work- Challenges and Opportunities,* argues about the existence of spirituality throughout human history and the growing recognition of religious and spiritual factors contributing to the mental health of individuals, families and communities. He centres this chapter on the importance of spirituality in mental health and its implications for social work practice. Citing illustrations from his own battle with cancer and his professional experiences spanning more than five decades, Murthy alludes how people with spiritual practices are known to live longer and respond to adverse life situations with greater resilience and the overall advantages of spirituality. Relating these with social work practice, he provides detailed research evidence regarding the relationship between spirituality and health/mental health, serious medical illnesses, suicide, HIV/AIDS, loneliness, etc. Last but not the least, he expounds the implications of these developments for training and practice by social workers.

The Third and the final part of the book 'Experiential Insights from Praxis' is all-encompassing of field-based narratives that reflect multifaceted challenges, efforts towards treatment of mental illness and inclusion. The six chapters included in the concluding part entail the promotion of positive mental health through the embellishment of success stories in diverse settings in India. The first chapter *The BANYAN Journey: A continuum in community mental health care* highlights the story of The Banyan, one of the leading mental health service organisations of India. The Banyan offers comprehensive mental health and social care solutions for persons who are homeless, living in poverty and having severe mental disorders. The authors M. Namrata Rao, Lakshmi Ravikanth, Lakshmi Sankaran, Palaakshee Bansal and Rima

Chowdhury explore the organization's flagship programmes including hospital-based services (Emergency Care and Recovery Centres), inclusive living options (Home Again) and mental health and social care units (NALAM). They demonstrate the adoption of person-centred, cross-sectoral and transdisciplinary approach in line with variegated socio-political and cultural contexts.

No manuscript on mental health care, especially in the indigenous context, can be complete without the discussion on family caregivers. Known to the substratum of caregiving, the contribution of family caregivers indeed needs to be recognised for its immense value and strength. Amrit Bakhshy in the chapter *Indian Family Caregivers of Mentally Ill: Larger Canvas, beyond Family Caregiving* signifies the role of family caregivers who formulate the critical link between the person with mental disorders and mental health professionals. Remarkably, he elaborates on this unique honorary workforce that provides selfless service, out of sheer love and bonding, mostly at the cost of their own health and well-being. He argues that it is the altruistic and ardent service by the family members which can be attributed as the reason behind the higher rate of recovery for persons with mental disorders in India as compared to those in the developed countries. One of the most unrivalled aspects of Bakhshy's chapter is the coverage of exclusive countrywide initiatives by some of the caregivers who have come forward to start their NGOs, making efforts towards creating awareness, promoting of peer support groups, running residential and day rehabilitation centres and providing wide-ranging services.

Another significant contribution from the praxis comes from Anuradha Sovani who shares the unique journey of Institute for Psychological Health in providing mental health care by focusing on disability, distress and development. As a founding member of IPH, she traces its journey through *Three decades of a journey towards Mental Health for All: The story of IPH*. With the vision beyond the confines of psychopharmacology, the adoption of a widely encompassing team, Sovani successfully highlights various unique practices at IPH and dwells on important lessons learned in its thirty-two-year journey, also delineating the challenging areas where much work is still needed.

The predicament of the destitute persons is brought to the forefront by Mohd. Tarique critically analyses the State mechanism to address homeless persons with mental illness, which he argues, is about first turning them invisible and then punishing them under Beggary laws. His chapter *Destitution, Mental Illness & Law: Issues, Challenges & Possibilities* elaborates on Koshish, initiated by Tata Institute of Social Sciences, Mumbai as its field action project as a response to the criminalization of destitution happening in the form of Beggary Prevention Legislations. He documents two crucial intervention models developed by Koshish over the years. Both models are based on the fundamental need and capacity of every human being; the need to be loved and accepted and compassion and empathy to understand other person's suffering and pain. In addition to sharing experiential reflections about key community-based interventions and investment in youth, Tarique calls for the need for empathy and compassion in order to trigger the change.

Raheen Jummani brings together her reflections on the journey of learning and experimenting that began with the thought of repaying to society the warmth it has bestowed in abundance. In her chapter *Embrace All.... No Labels Attached: Reflections by OYA Foundation*, she traverses the insights gained through the organisation 'Open Your Arms Foundation' (OYA). She traces the initial journey of OYA when the main challenge was to mitigate the taboo against mental health and familiarise everyone with the concept of mental well-being. Through case vignettes, Jummani endeavours to illustrate a few success stories about OYA's creative approaches that had an enormous impact on the lives of the clients.

The concluding chapter of the book helmed by me summarises mental health as a flourishing, strengthening and empowering experience. It paves the way for the futurist vision on the subject entailing recognition of the significance of peer support, reduction of stigma, evidence-based research with thrust on survivor research, mental health activism, role of diverse Psy professionals and the scope for leadership role for professional social workers in the province of mental health.

References

Agarwal, A. K. (1998). The forgotten millions. *Indian Journal of Psychiatry, 40*, 103–119.

Anand, M. (2020). *Gender and mental health: Combining theory and practice*. Springer.

Anand, M. (2021). Mental health and human rights: An Indian inquiry. *Indian Journal of Social Psychiatry, 37*, 235–241. https://doi.org/10.4103/ijsp.ijsp_187_20

Anand, M. (2022a). Supporting social work students facing mental health challenges: Reflective experiences by faculty from University of Delhi. *Social Work Education*. https://doi.org/10.1080/02615479.2022.2098943

Anand, M. (2022b). Gender and mental health: Traversing treatise. *Indian Journal of Social Psychiatry, 38*, 108–113. https://doi.org/10.4103/ijsp.ijsp_158_20

Artal, F.J.C. (2019). Differences in Prevalence of Mental Health with the Inclusion of Diversity, Gender and Lifespan. In S. Bährer-Kohler, & B. Bolea-Alamanac (Eds.) *Diversity in global mental health*, Springer briefs in psychology (pp.7–17). Springer. https://doi.org/10.1007/978-3-030-29112-9_2

Banton, R., et al. (1985). *The politics of mental health*. Macmillan Press.

Baumann, A. E. (2007). Stigmatization, social distance and exclusion because of mental illness: The individual with mental illness as a "stranger." *International Review of Psychiatry, 19*(2), 131–135. https://doi.org/10.1080/09540260701278739

Beresford, P., & Russo, J. (2022). *The Rutledge international handbook of mad studies*. Taylor and Francis.

Buchter, R. B., & Messer, M. (2017). Interventions for reducing self-stigma in people with mental illnesses: A systematic review of randomized controlled trials. *German Medical Science: GMS e-Journal, 15*.

Burstow, B. (2015). *Psychiatry and the business of madness: An ethical and epistemological accounting*. Palgrave Macmillan

Burstow, B. (2018). Mental health' praxis—not the answer A constructive antipsychiatry position. In B. M. Z. Cohen (Ed.) *Routledge international handbook of critical mental health* (pp. 31–38). Rutledge

Capponi, P. (2003). *Beyond the crazy house: Changing the future of madness*. Penguin.

Coppock, V., & Hopton, J. (2000). *Critical perspectives on mental health*. Routledge.

Dandona, R., et al. (2020). The burden of mental disorders across the states of India: The global burden of disease study 1990–2017. *Lancet Psychiatry, 7*(2), 148–161. https://doi.org/10.1016/S2215-0366(19)30475-4

Datta, V. (2014). When Homosexuality Came Out (Of the DSM). *Mad in America* (online). https://www.madinamerica.com/2014/12/homosexuality-came-dsm

Davar, B. (2022). Shifting identities as reflective personal responses to political changes. In P. Beresford & J. Russo (Eds.), *Routledge International handbook of mad studies* (pp. 34–40). Rutledge.

Eromosele, F. (2020). Frantz fanon in the time of mad studies. *World Futures, 76*(3), 167–187. https://doi.org/10.1080/02604027.2020.1730737

Foucault, M. (1975). *The birth of clinic: An archaeology of medical perception.* Vintage Books.

Foucault, M. (1988). Madness and civilization: A history of insanity in the age of reason (R. Howard, Trans.). Vintage Books.

Goffman, E. (1963). *Stigma.* Simon and Schuster.

Hamsun, K. (1909). *En vandrer spiller med sordin.* Gyldendal

Harvey, P. D., Heaton, R. K., Carpenter, W. T., Green, M. F., Gold, J. M., & Schoenbaum, M. (2012). Functional impairment in people with schizophrenia: Focus on employability and eligibility for disability compensation. *Schizophrenia Research, 140*(1–3), 1–8. https://doi.org/10.1016/j.schres.2012.03.025

Hatzenbuehler, M. L. (2016). Structural stigma: Research evidence and implications for psychological science. *The American Psychologist, 71*(8), 742–751.

Hickie, I. B., Scott, E. M., Hermens, D. F., et al. (2013). Applying clinical staging to young people who present for mental health care. *Early Interventions in Psychiatry, 7*, 31–43.

Jackowska, E. (2009). Stigma and discrimination towards people with schizophrenia: A survey of studies and psychological mechanisms. *Psychiatria Polska, 43*(6), 655–670.

Jahoda, M. (1958). *Current concepts of positive mental health.* Basic books.

Johnstone, M. (2021). Centering social justice in mental health practice: Epistemic justice and social work practice. *Research on Social Work Practice, 31*(6), 634–643. https://doi.org/10.1177/10497315211010957

Kirk, S. A., Gomory, T., & Cohen, D. (2013). *Mad science: The disorders of American psychiatry.* Transaction Publishers.

Kirmayer, L. (2012). Rethinking cultural competence. *Transcultural Psychiatry, 49*(2), 149–164. Sage. https://doi.org/10.1177/1363461512444673

Krech, R. (2019). Foreward. In S. Bährer-Kohler, & B. Bolea-Alamanac (Eds.) *Diversity in global mental health*, Springer briefs in psychology (pp. ix–xii). Springer. https://doi.org/10.1007/978-3-030-29112-9_2

Kvaternik, I., & Grebenc, V. (2009). The role of social work in the field of mental health: Dual diagnoses as a challenge for social workers. *European Journal of Social Work, 12*(4), 509–521. https://doi.org/10.1080/13691450902981426

Lamovec, T. (1998). Psihosocialna pomocˇ v dusˇevni stiski [Psychosocial help in mental distress]. College for Social Work (Visoka sˇola za socialno delo).

Leblanc, S., & Kinsella, E. (2016). Toward epistemic justice: A critically reflexive examination of "sanism" and implications for knowledge generation. *Studies in Social Justice, 10*(1), 59–78.

Lee, M. Y., Eads, R., Yates, N., Liu, C., & Wang, C. (2020). Revisiting medication: Listening to lived experiences from persons in mental health recovery without ongoing medication use. *Social Work in Mental Health, 18*(3), 285–301. https://doi.org/10.1080/15332985.2020.1742849

LeFrancois, B., Menzies, R., & Reaume, G. (2013). *Mad matters: A critical reader in Canadian mad studies.* Canadian Scholars Press.

Lock, M. (2001). Medicalisation: Cultural concerns. In N. J. Smelser & P. B. Baltes (Eds.), *International encyclopedia of the social and behavioral sciences* (pp. 9534–9539). Kluwer Academic.

McGorry, P. (2007). Issues for DSM-V: Clinical staging. A heuristic pathway to valid nosology and safer, more effective treatment in psychiatry. *American Journal of Psychiatry, 164*, 859–860.

Menzies, R., LeFrançois, B. A., & Reaume, G. (2013). *Mad matters: A critical reader in Canadian mad studies.* Canadian Scholars' Press.

Mignon, S. I. (2019). *Social work and mental health: Evidence-based policy and practice.* Springer.

Murphy, A. L., Gardner, D. M., Kisely, S., Cooke, C., Kutcher, S. P., & Hughes, J. (2015). A qualitative study of antipsychotic medication experiences of youth. *Journal of the Canadian Academy of Child and Adolescent Psychiatry, 24*(1), 61–69.

National Human Rights Commission. (2016). *Report of the technical committee on mental health.* In P. Murthy, S. Kumar, N. Desai & B. K. Teja (Eds.). http://nhrc.nic.in/Documents/Mental_Health_report_vol_I_10_06_2016.pdf

Prince, M., Patel, V., Saxena, S., Maj, M., Maselko, J., Phillips, M. R., & Rahman, A. (2007). No health without mental health. *Lancet, 370*, 859–877. https://doi.org/10.1016/S0140-6736(07)61238-0

Porter, R. (1993). *The Faber book of madness.* Faber.

Rashed, M. A. (2019). *Madness and the demand for recognition: A philosophical inquiry into identity and mental health activism.* Oxford University Press.

Rosado, J. (2018). *The relationship between mental health and physical health.* Lecture Delivered at Migrant Clinicians Network, Webinar. https://www.migrantclinician.org/files/staff/MCNFSU%20-%20%20Physical%20and%20Mental%20Health%20%28Converted%20PPT%20Slides%29.pdf

Rosenhan, D. L. (1975). On being sane in insane places. In T. J. Scheff (Ed.), *Labeling madness* (p. 5474). Prentice-Hall.

Sarkar, S., & Punnoose, V. P. (2016). Stigma toward psychiatric disorders: What can we do about it? *Indian Journal of Social Psychiatry, 32*, 81–82.

Sawyer, A.-M., Stanford, S., & Campbell, J. (2016). Mental health social work: Perspectives on risk, regulation, and therapeutic interventions. *Australian Social Work, 69*(2), 129–132. https://doi.org/10.1080/0312407X.2015.1129428

Sharma, P. (2023). *Barriers to recovery from 'Psychosis': A peer investigation of psychiatric subjectivation.* Rutledge.

Smith, D. (2005). *Institutional ethnography: A sociology of the people.* Altamira Press.

Srivastava, N., & Anand, M. (2020). Understanding gender and mental health. In M. Anand (Ed.), *Gender and mental health: Combining theory and practice* (pp. 3–18). Springer.

Stevenson, A. (2010). Oxford Dictionary of English.

Sullivan, P. F., Daly, M. J., & O'Donovan, M. (2012). Genetic architectures of psychiatric disorders: The emerging picture and its implications. *Nature Reviews Genetics, 13*, 537–551.

Szasz, T. (1961). *The myth of mental illness.* Paul B. Hoeber.

Thornicraft, G. (2006). *Shunned: Discrimination against people with mental illness.* Oxford University Press.

Thornicraft, G., Rose D., Kassam, A., & Sartorius, N. (2007). *Stigma: Ignorance, prejudice or discrimination?.* https://www.kcl.ac.uk/aboutkings/principal/dean/akc/archivedandouts/trs/trsdocs07/08/Spring/SupplementaryarticleforLecture5.pdf

Venkatesan, S., & Suresh, A. (2023). Critique of DSM, medicalisation and graphic medicine. *Journal of Graphic Novels and Comics, 14*(2), 233–247. https://doi.org/10.1080/21504857.2022.2053558

Werremeyer, A., Skoy, E., & Aalgaard Kelly, G. (2017). Use of photovoice to understand the experience of taking psychotropic medications. *Qualitative Health Research, 27*(13), 1959–1969. https://doi.org/10.1177/1049732317693221

White, K. (2018). The social construction of mental illness. In B. Kohen (Ed.), *The Routledge international handbook of critical mental health* (pp. 24–30). Routledge.

World Health Organization. (2013). *Social determinants of health?* World Health Organization. https://www.who.int/news-room/questions-and-answers/item/social-determinants-of-health-key-concepts

World Health Organization. (2018a). *Mental health included in the UN sustainable development goals.* http://www.who.int/mental_health/SDGs/en

World Health Organization. (2018b, March 30). *Mental health: Strengthening our response.* http://www.who.int/news-room/fact-sheets/detail/mental-health-strengthening-our-response

World Health Organization. (2022a). *World mental health report: Transforming mental health for all.* https://www.who.int/publications/i/item/9789240049338

World Health Organization. (2022b). *Mental Health and COVID-19: Early evidence of the pandemic's impact.* https://www.who.int/publications-detail-redirect/WHO-2019-nCoV-Sci_Brief-Mental_health-2022.1

Zachrisson, A. (2019). Mental health—A normal state? *The Scandinavian Psychoanalytic Review.* https://doi.org/10.1080/01062301.2019.1693197

Zola, I. K. (1972). Medicine as an Institution of Social Control. *Sociological Review, 20*(4), 487–504.

Chapter 2
Understanding Mental Disorders, Mental Health and Well-Being

R. Srinivasa Murthy

Abstract Significant advances in the understanding of mental disorders, mental health and well-being have occurred in recent decades. Tracing the trajectory of diverse discourses on mental health over the previous five decades, author, through his personal and professional experiences, covers the growth of multiple frameworks in the broad context of mental health. The chapter seeks to bring newer understandings on the theme and explain the augmentation of perception regarding persons with mental disorders from the mere biological perspective towards the more eclectic 'bio-psycho-social-spiritual' lens. Citing various international and national polices, programmes and reports, it holistically covers both challenges (converting new knowledge into practice) as well as new opportunities (greater scope for work, wider impact) for professional social workers in India. This chapter emphasises the significance of engaging with individuals, families, communities and the Government, on mental health and analyses implications of these developments for the profession of social work. Recognising social work as a speciality and social workers as a professional group having a special position in India towards mental health and well-being of the population, the chapter envisions the scope for action by social workers in the field of mental health in India.

Keywords Mental health · Well-being · Mental disorders · Social work · Individuals · Families · Communities

Introduction

Understanding of mental disorders, mental health and well-being is at a crucial point in human history, due to a number of developments in the last century and more specifically during the last two decades. This is a very good time for humanity and indeed a unique opportunity for social workers to 'make a difference'. Currently, there is a better understanding of the origins of mental disorders, mental health and

R. Srinivasa Murthy (✉)
Professor of Psychiatry, NIMHANS (Retired), Bangaluru, India
e-mail: smurthy030@gmail.com

M. Anand (ed.), *Mental Health Care Resource Book*,
https://doi.org/10.1007/978-981-97-1203-8_2

well-being from both bio-psycho-socio-spiritual dimensions as well as the climate and environment. There is a shift from considering persons diagnosed with mental disorders as 'bad', 'mad', or 'sad' towards being perceived as 'individuals' and as 'equal' members of the society. The place of care has shifted totally from custodial institutions to the community viz. 'asylums as community to community as asylum' (Scull, 1989). The last three years of the COVID-19 epidemic has brought to the forefront, the importance of the health of the total population and social determinants of health in general and mental health in particular. The recognition of the health impact of chronic stresses like discrimination and marginalisation referred to as 'weathering' (Geronimus, 2023) calls for societal level interventions. Along with the new understanding, there is a bigger picture of biological aspects of mental health, from thinking of a single molecule like 'dopamine' to 'psychoneuroimmunology' (Littrell, 2019). There have also been several important recent international publications namely The Lancet Commission on Mental Health and Sustainable Development (Patel et al., 2018), Lancet-World Psychiatric Association Commission: Time for united action on depression (Herman et al., 2022), the World Mental Health Report 2022 by the World Health Organisation in June 2022, (WHO, 2022; Cuipers et al., 2023), the Lancet Commission on Stigma and Discrimination in October 2022 (Thornicroft et al., 2022), the Mental State of the World in 2022 (Sapiens Lab, 2023), the Countdown initiative of Global Mental Health Network (GMHN) to monitor the mental health of nations and the Surgeon General Report on 'Our Epidemic of Loneliness and Isolation' released in May 2023 (Office of the Surgeon General, 2023). All these initiatives present a modern view of mental disorders, mental health and well-being which is based on the psychological, social, spiritual and environmental dimensions of mental health. These developments are especially relevant to the practice of social work.

Table 2.1 presented below seeks to present the following as the representative views:

One of my longstanding colleagues, Ms. Gupta (2023), a Psychiatric Social Worker, from Chandigarh, in a recent discussion about the importance of social work, aptly placed the relevance of social work to mental health and well-being, in the current times as follows:

> I feel proud to be a Psychiatric Social Worker because our horizon is broader. We reach out to communities, we are well informed about the social services availability and we go a step ahead to help the clients, families and communities

Personal Journey (1972–2023)

At a personal level, since the time I entered psychiatry in 1972, I have witnessed a revolution in the way mental health, mental disorders and mental health care are understood and responded to. Let me explain. In 1972, it was the practice to categorise mental disorders under 'functional psychosis' (to include schizophrenia, manic depressive illness etc.) and 'organic psychosis'. At that point of time, cognitive

Table 2.1 Importance and challenges in the area of mental health

'Suicide is an individual action with social origins' (Durkheim, 1897)
'Mental Health is the defining public health challenge of our times….I think of mental health, as the fuel that allows us to show up for our communities, our friends, our family and our lives. And when that fuel tank is low, it compromises our ability to be who we can be in our best moments and to show up at work or in school' (Murthy, 2022)
'The moral failure of humanity in the past does not mean we must tolerate this failure any longer' (Klineman, 2009)
'When I started this journey to resolve the mental health crisis, I believed that technology and science would provide the answers we need. A new drug, a killer app, a breakthrough would make the difference. Years of listening to families and touring homeless shelters and clubhouses, clinics and hospitals, left me convinced that the problems are more complex and the solutions far simpler than most of us realise. We must summon the will to enact them, because we have for too long asked individuals and families to bear this crisis of care alone' (Insel, 2022)
'We know so much about the physical world and so little about mental life. This isn't because physicists are smart and psychologists are stupid. It is because my chosen domain of study is so much harder than Barrow's. The mysteries of space and time is so much easier than our minds to grasp than those of consciousness and choice' (Bloom, 2023)
'The dimension of 'Social Self' is the most challenged across the world followed by Mood and Outlook, and has the largest drop from older to younger generations…… Family relationships are increasingly disintegrating across the globe…….The fraying of adult family relationships may have its origins in changing childhood experiences……Friendships too, are deteriorating…..The risk of mental health challenges is ten times higher among those who lack close family relationships and friendships compared to those with many with close family and friends.' (The Mental State of the World in 2022, Sapien Labs, March 1, 2023)
'Whole Health Centres around, what matters to you, not what is the matter with you'. (Achieving Whole Health: A New Approach for Veterans and the Nation, 2023)
'Humans are social: we live longer when we have meaningful relationships and see others, and we have numerous studies showing that social isolation, especially for certain groups, has negative consequences. Understanding that should be our starting point for the future' (Devi Sridhar, The Guardian, March 2023)
'There aren't enough therapists to go around—but there are plenty of smartphones' (Khullar D, New Yorker, 2023)
'When we move away from a focus on psychological problems and toward "mental health" more broadly, clinicians stumble into terrain that extends beyond our expertise' (Green H, 2022)

disturbances were not recognised as part of functional psychosis or treatment, while in 2023, cognitive aspects of psychosis are a vital part of understanding of all psychosis, as well as interventions. Another example is the identification of 'expressed emotion', in the 1970s (Leff & Vaughn, 1980, 1981; Leff et al., 1982, 1985, 1987). The finding of the family members' reaction to the person with a diagnosis of schizophrenia, as being a vital contributor to the course and outcome of the illness moved the understanding from purely 'psychogenic origin' to the larger psychosocial aspects of life. Similarly, advances in psychological therapies like the behaviour therapy and cognitive behaviour therapy, yoga/meditation, during the last fifty years, created space for the efforts of the individual as an essential part of the therapy. In the last decade, the central role of the individual, in the control of even severe symptoms like hallucinations in the 'Avtar Therapy' has moved the focus back to the individual as the central focus of mental health and well-being.

In a dramatic way, the deviancy model that dominated mental health is getting slowly replaced by the normalcy model. At the level of mental health, the recognition of the value of exercise, sleep, nutrition, mindfulness, social connectedness and spirituality has enlarged the scope of mental health from a purely clinical discipline to one of public health. Similarly emerging issues of loneliness is moving the focus of mental health from illnesses to wellness. A good reflection of these changes is the recent flagship programme of the Government of India, 'Tele-MANAS' focussing on 'reaching the unreached' utilising both the information technology and largely psychosocial interventions (NIMHANS, 2022a, b, c, d).

This chapter will cover (i) recent developments in the understanding of mental disorders, mental health and wellbeing; (ii) newer understanding of origins of mental health and well-being; (iii) current approaches to mental health care; (iv) importance of the person, family, community for mental health and (v) implications of all these developments for the profession of social work.

1. Recent Developments in Mental Health and Well-Being

Scope of Health

In the year 1948, the World Health Organization (WHO) defined health as "a state of complete physical, mental and social well-being and not merely the absence of disease and infirmity". Some professionals criticise this definition as being excessively broad, vague, and unmeasurable. Health care focused more on a biomedical reductionist model than on achieving the more holistic vision of health. In the year1984, the WHO revisited and updated the definition of health, shifting it from a desirable state of being to a dynamic set of resources for living well "*the extent to which an individual or group is able to realize aspirations and satisfy needs to change or cope with the environment... health is a resource for everyday life, not the objective*"—that emphasized the social and personal resources as well as physical capabilities that are a part of health (NASEM, 2023).

WHO Action Plan for 2013–2030

The WHO Action Plan for Mental Health, 2013–2030 (WHO, 2013), has the following six priorities: universal health coverage, human rights, evidence-based practice, life course approach, multisectoral approach and empowerment of persons with mental disorders and psychosocial disabilities. This new understanding is presented in the World Mental Health Report 2022 (WHO, 2001, 2022) and reflected in the global focus to depression in the last few years by making it the theme of depression for the World Health Day in 2013, increased emphasis on universal coverage for mental health, approaches to empower individuals for mental health like the developing caregiver materials for persons with developmental disorders and initiating suicide prevention programmes.

The Mental Health Atlas (WHO, 2020).

The Mental Health Atlas released by the World Health Organisation every three years is a compilation of data provided by the countries around the world on mental health policies related to legislations, financing, human resources, availability and utilization of services and data collection systems. Progress up to 2020 indicates that the targets committed to by WHO Member States have not been achieved. There are massive inequalities in the availability of mental health resources and their allocation between 'High- and Low-income countries' and across regions. While guidelines for the integration of mental health into primary health care exist and have been adopted by most countries, with ongoing activities for training and supervision, the integration of interventions for service delivery, such as pharmacological and psychosocial interventions for mental health conditions, remains limited. The Mental Health Atlas 2020 also shows significant limitations in the capacity of countries' mental health information systems to report on specific indicators such as service utilization. WHO notes, that the global targets can be reached in 2030 only if there is a collective global commitment over the next ten years across all Member States to make massive investments and expanded efforts at the country level relating to mental health policies, laws, programmes and services. In another report of the mental health policies in the Commonwealth countries, Bhugra et al. (2019) surveyed 52 member countries and found that less than half of the countries had a mental health policy. Furthermore, deinstitutionalization was not seen as a priority in many countries and there was no equity between physical and mental health funding.

WHO World Mental Health Report (WMHR) 2022 (WHO, 2022; Cuiper et al., 2023)

The WMHR 2022, titled '**Transforming Mental Health for all**' released on June 17, 2022, is a milestone in the development of mental health in the world. This has come after two decades of publication of the World Health Report 2001(WHO, 2001), which had focused on organization of mental health at the level of primary health care.

There are seven important reasons to consider this report as significant. Firstly, this is the Report from the World Health Organization, where the Ministries of Health of all countries of the world, contribute to policy development and WHO is the lead organization for health in the world. Secondly, this Report is coming 21 years after the last report of October 2001(WHO, 2001). Thirdly, unlike the 2001 Report which was a World Health Report with special focus on Mental Health, this report is a standalone full report on mental health (this Report is twice the size of the 2001 Report). Fourthly, the report reflects the developments of the last two decades in understanding of mental disorders and mental health, especially about the plasticity of the brain, social determinants of health and rights of persons with mental disorders.

Fifthly, the COVID 19 pandemic has sensitized the general population, politicians, planners and the population to the importance of mental health as part of life. Sixthly, the report presents mental health in an engaging and easy to read non-technical language suitable for reading of professionals and non-professionals (there are more than 70 case studies) (innovations, country reports, personal narratives, graphics etc.) which is a feature of the report. Lastly, the report is a treat to read from the design point of view, with excellent graphics and photographs. The World Mental Health Report 2022 is designed to **'inspire and inform the indisputable and urgent transformation required to ensure better mental health for all'**. While promoting a multisectoral approach, this report is especially written for decision-makers in the health sector.

The WMHR2022 is organized on three overarching themes, namely, (i) principles and drivers of public mental health; (ii) the case for transformation and (iii) mental health reform. The Report is presented in eight chapters, namely, introduction, principles and drivers in public mental health, world mental health today, benefits of change, foundations for change, promotion and prevention for change, restructuring and scaling up care for impact, and conclusion. These are summarized in Figs. 2.1, 2.2 and 2.3. There is hope for new beginnings in mental health and well-being.

Global Action on Depression

Global launch of the Lancet-World Psychiatric Association Commission: Time for united action on depression, on 16th February 2022, reflects on the importance of the pandemic as follows:

> Our task has never felt more urgent. The potentiation by the COVID-19 pandemic of adverse societal factors such as deep-rooted structural inequalities and personal impacts such as social isolation, bereavement, sickness, uncertainty, impoverishment, and poor access to health care has had negative impacts on the mental health of millions of people. It has generated a so-called perfect storm that requires responses at multiple levels. The consequences of the pandemic thus emphasise the need to make the prevention, recognition, and treatment of depression an immediate global priority, which we address through a number of key messages and recommendations (Herman et al., 2022).

The recommendations of the Commission call for action at four levels viz. (i) the community and people living with depression; (ii) health-care practitioners; (iii) researchers, research funders; and (iv) decision makers and policy makers.

Equally important is the report of the Lancet Commission on Stigma and Discrimination in Mental Health, released in October 2022. This report recognises the importance of the lived-in experiences of persons diagnosed with mental disorders to fight stigma and discrimination, in addition to public mental health education (Thornicroft et al., 2022).

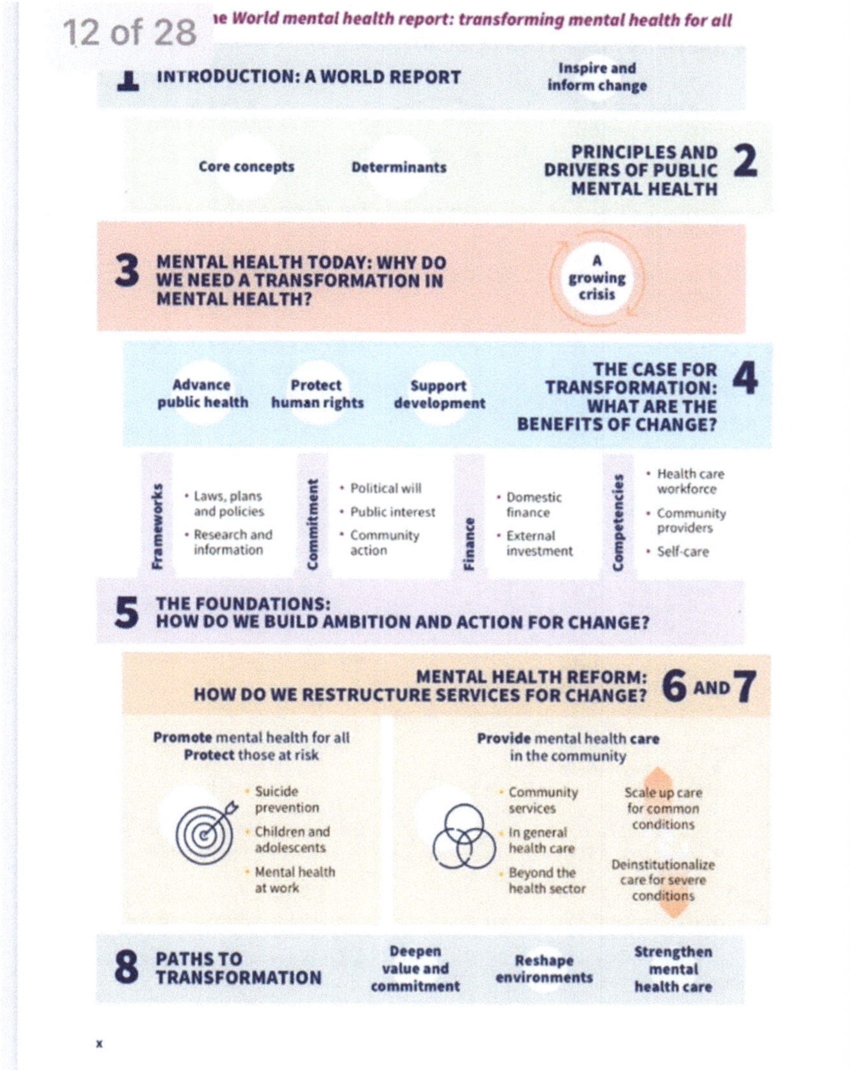

Fig. 2.1 Overview of the World mental health report: Transforming mental health for all. *Source* World Mental Health Report 2022, pp. xii. Available at https://www.who.int/publications/i/item/9789240049338

Universal Health Care Policy, 2022

Universal Health Coverage (UHC) is the concept that everyone, everywhere should be able to access good quality health (including mental health) services they need without suffering financial hardships. There is an increasing acknowledgement of the importance of integrating mental health care into PHC (United For Global Mental

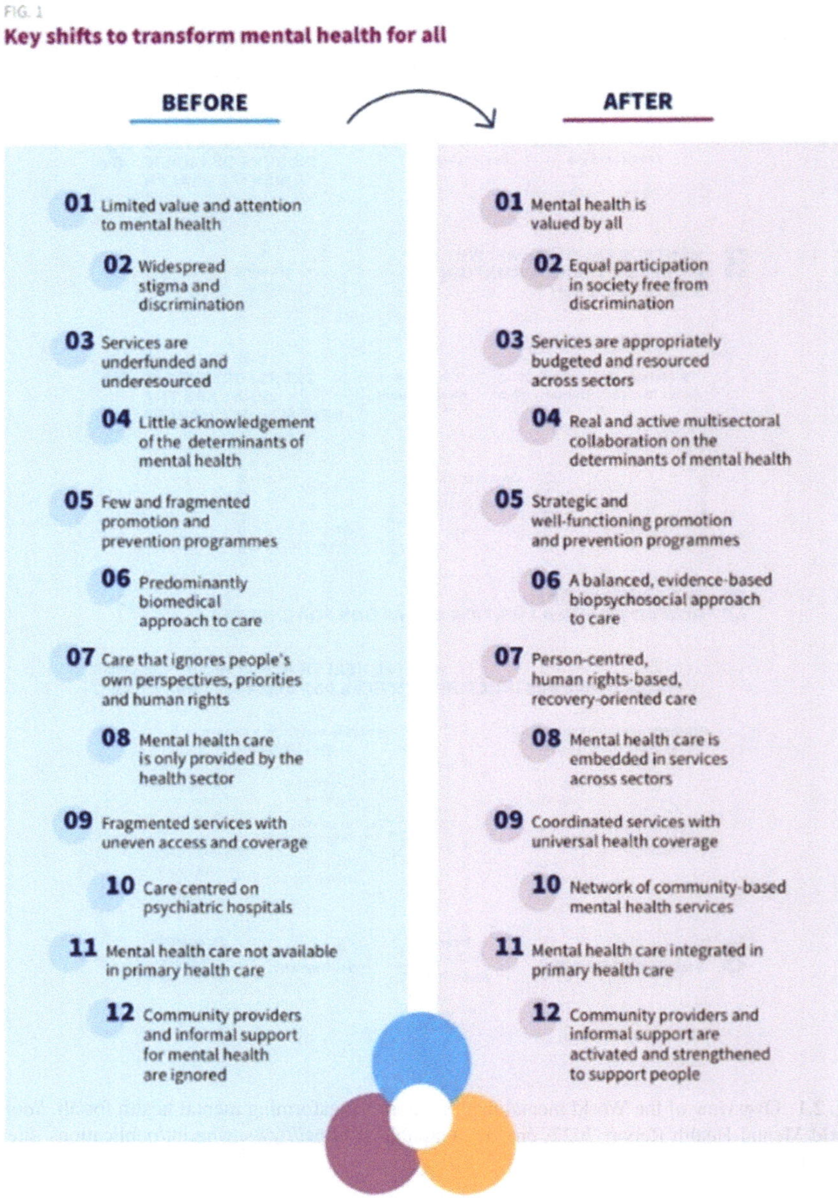
FIG. 1
Key shifts to transform mental health for all
BEFORE
AFTER
01 Limited value and attention to mental health
02 Widespread stigma and discrimination
03 Services are underfunded and underesourced
04 Little acknowledgement of the determinants of mental health
05 Few and fragmented promotion and prevention programmes
06 Predominantly biomedical approach to care
07 Care that ignores people's own perspectives, priorities and human rights
08 Mental health care is only provided by the health sector
09 Fragmented services with uneven access and coverage
10 Care centred on psychiatric hospitals
11 Mental health care not available in primary health care
12 Community providers and informal support for mental health are ignored
01 Mental health is valued by all
02 Equal participation in society free from discrimination
03 Services are appropriately budgeted and resourced across sectors
04 Real and active multisectoral collaboration on the determinants of mental health
05 Strategic and well-functioning promotion and prevention programmes
06 A balanced, evidence-based biopsychosocial approach to care
07 Person-centred, human rights-based, recovery-oriented care
08 Mental health care is embedded in services across sectors
09 Coordinated services with universal health coverage
10 Network of community-based mental health services
11 Mental health care integrated in primary health care
12 Community providers and informal support are activated and strengthened to support people

Fig. 2.2 Key shifts to transform mental health for all. *Source* World Mental Health Report 2022, pp. 254. Available at https://www.who.int/publications/i/item/9789240049338

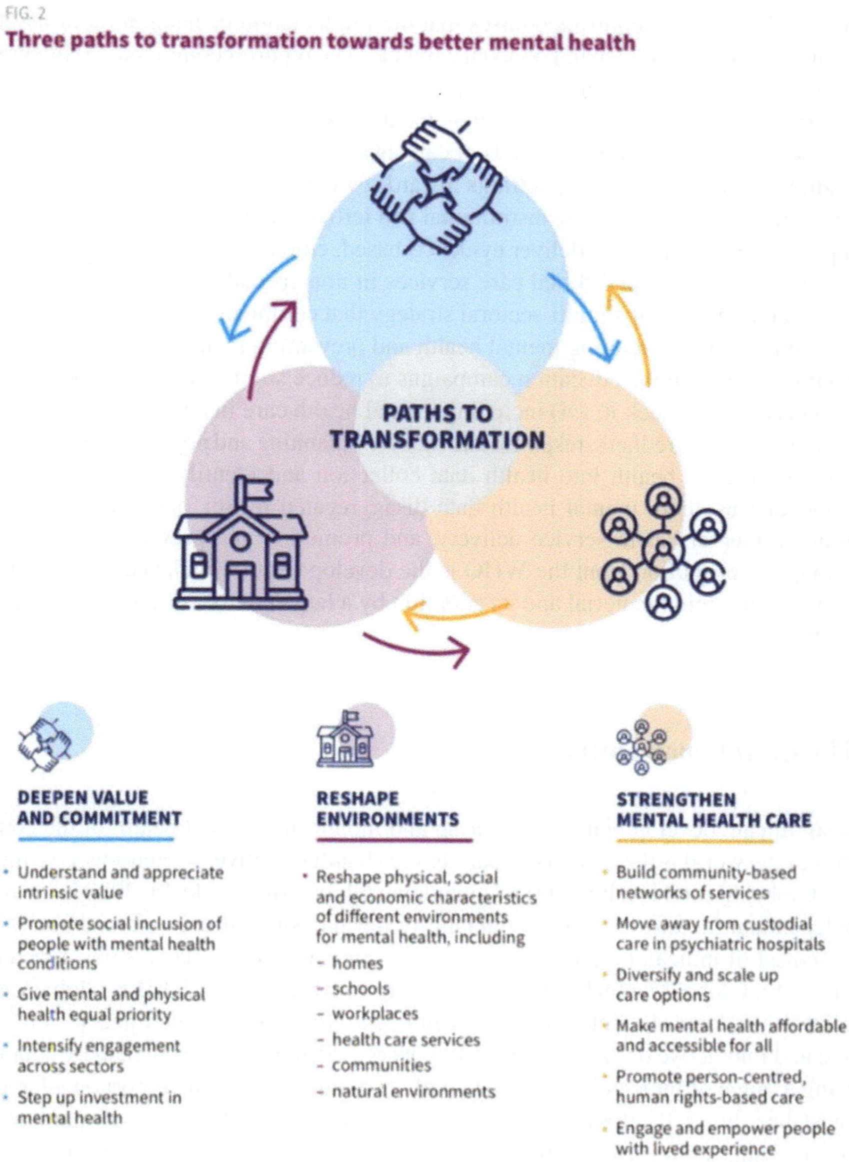

Fig. 2.3 Three transformative paths towards better mental health. *Source* World Mental Health Report 2022, pp. 250. Available at https://www.who.int/publications/i/item/9789240049338

Health, 2022). The report recognises that the implantation of integration of mental health with UHC will depend on local contexts. The report recommends (i) integrate mental health into UHC policies and programmes, keeping people with lived experience at the core of planning and implementation; (ii) expand coverage for mental health services by shifting the focus of care away from an almost exclusive focus on institutional and tertiary care settings towards evidence based primary and community care that is supported by institutional and tertiary care; (iii) train, supervise and support health workers to deliver evidence-based, culturally appropriate and rights-based mental health and social care services in non-specialised settings; (iv) coordinate and implement a multi-sectoral strategy that combines universal and targeted interventions for promoting mental health and preventing mental health conditions; (v) investing in public education campaigns to reduce stigma and encourage people who need help to seek it; (vi) including mental health care in emergency (including pandemics) preparedness, response and recovery planning and programmes; and (vii) integrate mental health into health data collection and identify, collate, routinely report and use core mental health data disaggregated by sex and age in order to improve mental health service delivery, and promotion and prevention strategies. A major contribution from the WHO is the development of evidence based mental health intervention material and its adoption by a large number of countries (WHO, 2006).

The *Countdown* Initiative

A significant development in measuring and monitoring mental health of the countries of the world is the United Global Mental Health Initiative, 'Countdown' (United For Global Mental Health, 2021). Countdown Global Mental Health 2030 is the first independent monitoring and accountability mechanism that uses a broad and integrated set of indicators to monitor progress for mental health. This is developed by United for Global Mental Health in partnership with the WHO, UNICEF, GlobalMentalHealth@Harvard, Global Mental Health Peer Network and The Lancet. This is a free and interactive dashboard which lets users search mental health data by country using a range of indicators, combined with an annual monitoring report on what the latest data shows. It helps to monitor action to campaign, to advocate, to communicate and to change policy and practice so that everyone everywhere is able to exercise their right to the highest attainable level of mental health. The data collection is clustered around three themes viz. (i) determinants of mental health; (ii) factors supporting the demand for mental health care and (iii) factors shaping the strength of the mental health system. These indicators go beyond traditionally-defined health indicators and span the entire spectrum of the Sustainable Development Goals (SDGs).

Pandemic and Mental Health

The COVID-19 pandemic, 2019–2023, has brought to focus on the importance of population mental health. There is both a threat and an opportunity to rethink mental health. A recent book described the impact of the COVID-19 pandemic as follows:

> The pandemic has, in this sense, given us an opportunity to make a decisive break from the ethos that has governed our work and caused out burnout over the past fifty years. It's a chance to remake work and reimagine its place in our lives. If we don't take this opportunity, we will slip back into patterns that created the burnout culture in the first place (Malesic, 2022).

Similar is the observation by Taylor (2020, 2022).

> The pandemic changed everything about our lives: how we worked, socialised, travelled. Dealing with so many changes at once was a mental challenge for us all ..... The pandemic has also taught us the importance of developing resilience – the ability to manage the stressors, large and small, in our lives. Resilience may be one positive legacy of a very tough couple of years.

The above developments have brought mental health and well-being to the centre of public health.

2. Newer understandings of mental disorders, mental health and well-being

The evolution of the concepts of mental health and mental illnesses has been comprehensively covered in the earlier book 'Mental Health in India-Issues and concerns' by Mane and Gandevia (1993) from the Tata Institute of Social Sciences, Mumbai. There are three initial chapters focusing on 'Evolution of the concept of mental health (Murthy, 1993); 'Concepts and trends in mental health' (Viswanathan & Wetzel, 1993) and 'Social work response to mental illness and mental health' (Nadkarni & Das, 1993).

Mental Health and Well-being is an essential component of all religious traditions. Verhagen et al. (2010) have brought together the way an interface of psychiatry and mental health occurs in the major religions of the world. Their book contains chapters on Hinduism (Murthy, 2010), Judaism (Uri et al., 2010), Christianity (Peteet, 2010), Islam (Okasha, 2010), Buddhism (Udomran, 2010, Shinfuku & Kitanishi, 2010) and in African religions (Njenga et al., 2010). These historical and cultural resources are vital as they are widely used by the general population, and they can be a valuable resource in understanding pain, suffering, losses and also to promote resilience. A number of Indian psychiatrists have addressed this subject (Neki, 1977; Rao, 1997; Wig, 1990, 1999, 2006; Shamsunder, 2008; Sharma, 2009; Murthy, 2010). A good example of such a use is the wide acceptance of mindfulness, gratitude, forgiving, kindness etc. as mental health promoting practices in the last two decades (Jeste, 2020).

Recent Developments

During the last two decades, there has been a revival of the understanding of social factors and mental health. The most recent review of mental health by the Lancet -WPA Future of Psychiatry (2017) summarises the challenges as follows:

> A large body of evidence shows the importance of social determinants for mental disorders. Societal factors such as social inequality, crime, poverty, poor housing, adverse upbringing conditions, poor education, unemployment, and social isolation are related to increased rates of mental disorders. The relevance of some social determinants varies across the world. Examples are substantial urbanisation in LMICs; increasing social isolation in high-income countries; the changing flow of refugees in some regions; and different levels of economic instability, civil unrest, and inequality between rich and poor people. Most of these social determinants influence physical health problems too, but they can be seen as particularly relevant to psychiatry (Bhugra et al., 2017a, b).

Further, the group recognised psychiatry in the first quarter of the twenty-first century to be at the cusp of major changes as follows:

> Increased emphasis on social interventions and engagement with societal expectations might be an important area for psychiatry's development. This could encompass advocacy for the rights of individuals living with mental illnesses, political involvement concerning the social risk factors for mental illness, and, on a smaller scale, work with families and local social networks and communities. Psychiatrists should therefore possess communication skills and knowledge of the social sciences as well as the basic biological sciences (Bhugra et al., 2017a, b).

A recent review of 'Screening and Interventions for Social Risk Factors 'by the US Preventive Services Task Force (Eder et al., 2021) noted that of all the interventions studied, 73 addressed multiple social risk domains. The most frequently addressed domains were food insecurity, financial strain, and housing instability. The authors concluded that there is need for more randomized clinical trials that report health outcomes from social risk screening and interventions.

The major developments in the understanding of origins of mental disorders, mental health and well-being have been the recognition of the importance of the biology, psychology, social life, economics, environment and spirituality. Presented below are the major ideas in this context (Tables 2.2 and 2.3).

COVID-19 and Social Determinants (Murthy, 2020)

The importance of social determinants of mental disorders and mental health has received support from the country level experiences of the impact of the pandemic during the last five years (2019–2023). The most recent study aimed to quantify the impact of the COVID-19 pandemic on the prevalence and burden of major depressive disorder and anxiety disorders globally in 2020 (COVID-19 collaborators, 2021). The study reported nearly 30% increase in both the disorders. Further, increases in the prevalence of major depressive disorder and anxiety disorders during 2020 were

Table 2.2 Origins of mental disorders, mental health and well-being

Evidence of the value of daily exercise, adequate restful sleep, nutrition, connectedness, yoga, meditation, wisdom towards promoting mental health of the population is growing (Firth et al., 2020; Gupta, 2020; Lam and Riba, 2016; Varambally & Gangadhar, 2016; Murthy, 2016, 2021, 2022; Jeste, 2020)
For non-syndromal 'distress' associated with stresses of various life situations and associated with chronic medical conditions, benefits can be provided by sharing of feeling, journaling (Pennebaker and Evans, 2014), music/art, thinking differently (WHO, 2020) and spirituality (Koenig, 2012)
Social networks are vital for mental health: In a longitudinal study, researchers from Harvard and Peking universities analyzed 12 years' worth of data from men and women aged 65 years or older and found that loneliness and depressive symptoms appeared to be related risk factors of worsening cognition (Dickens et al., 2013). At the beginning stages of readjustment of relationships, there is likely to be greater confrontation and reduced cohesion;
A number of environmental interventions like individual exposure to exposure to nature or greening of the residential areas and increasing cohesion in the community are beneficial from the mental health of the population (Murthy, 2020)
Loneliness of old age can be addressed by the use of cultural and spiritual resources (Murthy and Banerjee, 2021)
Measures that promote resilience and post-traumatic growth can mitigate the negative effects of adverse situations like exposure to disasters/conflicts, severe life-threatening situations like cancer, and result in positive growth of individuals. (Murthy, 2016; Southwick & Charney, 2012, 2018)
Changes and stresses of all types are associated with mental health implications (Murthy, 2017)
Childhood trauma of any type is associated with negative mental health consequences throughout life (Murthy, 2014)
Domestic violence is associated with higher levels of mental disorders (Begum et al., 2015) and suicide
Inequality of all types are associated with increased mental disorders. Wilkinson and Pickett (2010, 2018a, b) present international research studies showing associations with drug abuse, teenage pregnancies, violence, imprisonment, and quality of life. As the movement makes progresses, we can expect less inequalities between sexes and this raise the possibility of reduction of inequality as a contributor to wellbeing of the total population;
A new area of study is coming to the forefront is the impact of the 'unjust society', called 'Weathering', and the extraordinary stress of the ordinary life in populations like Blacks in America, the marginalised populations in India (Geronimus, 2023). This is an area in which social workers in India can make an impact
Urbanisation, slums: Mobility of populations and urbanisation affects mental health through the influence of increased stressors and factors such as an overcrowded and polluted environment, high levels of violence, access to illicit drugs, and reduced social support. In most developing countries, over 10% of the population living in urban areas live in slums. For example, low-paid urban workers often live in crowded spaces with poor basic sanitation, food supplies, and shelter, as well as few—if any—basic governmental and social support services (Murthy, 2018)
Loneliness: A number of longitudinal studies indicate that loneliness proceeds depression, sleep difficulties, high blood pressure, physical inactivity, functional decline, cognitive impairment and increased mortality. Physical and mental health components of quality of life were significantly reduced by loneliness. Severe loneliness was associated with reduced patient satisfaction. (Musich et al., 2015; Office of the Surgeon General, 2023)

Table 2.3 Multidimensional nature of mental health, mental disorders and mental health interventions

A. Impact of child trauma
– Longitudinal study (Atkinson et al., 2023)
– Adolescent mental illness and adult disorders (Thomson et al., 2023)
– 20 years follow up (Oncioin et al., 2023)
– Non-affective psychosis (Hjern et al., 2023)
– Depression and chronic inflammation (Iob et al, 2023)
B. Brain-body interactions
– Synergetic effects of childhood adversity and polygenic risk (Aas et al., 2023)
– HPA Axis (Marquis-Feixa et al., 2023)
– Reduced frontal grey matter in childhood trauma (Begemann et al., 2023)
– Neurophysiological effects of mindfulness (Garland et al., 2023)
– Low status and schizophrenia (Selten & Ormel, 2023)
– Preterm birth band brain impact (Gilchrist et al., 2023)
– Cortical thickness and child trauma (Yang et al., 2023)
C. Psychosocial factors and mental disorders
– Negative parenting (Dotterer et al, 2023)
– Moral injury in soldiers
– Social capital and psychosis (Totenberg et al., 2023)
– Suicidality and neighborhood (Dykxhoorn et al, 2023)
– Intergenerational trans suicides (Stallman 2023)
– Social activity and risk of depression in elders (Ryu et al., 2023)
– Socio-economic status and bipolar disorder (Sletved et al., 2023)
– Covid-19 risk of depression (Alzueta et al., 2023)
D. Non-pharmacological interventions
– CBT and CBT plus medicines (Hudson et al., 2023)
– Mindfulness and negative symptoms of schizophrenia (Shen et al., 2023)
– Journalling in cancer (Wu et al., 2023)
– Smartphone based treatment for depression (Chan et al., 2023)
– Internet therapy after trauma (Bragesjo et al., 2023)

both associated with increasing SARS-CoV-2 infection rates and decreasing human mobility. In another study, from the America, longitudinal study of a nationally representative group of U.S. adults ages 18 years and older surveyed in March 2020 and April 2021 in the 'COVID-19 and Life Stressors Impact on Mental Health and Well-being' (CLIMB). The prevalence of elevated depressive symptoms persisted from 27.8% in 2020 to 32.8% in 2021. Importantly the central drivers of depressive symptoms were low household income, not being married, and experiencing multiple stressors during the COVID-19 pandemic. Authors conclude, 'Mental health gaps grew between populations with different assets and stressor experiences during the COVID-19 pandemic' (Ettman et al., 2021) American Indian or Alaska Native, Latino, Black, and Asian or Pacific Islander persons were more likely than White persons to have a COVID-19–associated hospitalization, ICU admission, or in-hospital death during the first year of the US COVID-19 pandemic (Acosta et al., 2021). Health care workers (HCW) from nine Eastern Mediterranean Regional (EMR) countries, working with the pandemic, 57.5% had depression, 42.0% had stress, and 59.1% had anxiety. Considering the severity, 19.2%, 16.1%, 26.6% of patients had severe to extremely severe depression, stress, and anxiety, respectively. Depression, stress, anxiety, and distress scores were significantly associated with participants' residency, having children, preexisting psychiatric illness, and being isolated for COVID-19. In addition, females, those working in a teaching hospital, and specialists had significantly higher depression and stress scores. Married status, current smoking, diabetes mellitus, having a friend who died with COVID-19 and high COVID-19 worry scores were significantly associated with higher distress scores. Authors urge for immediate implementation of 'special interventions to promote mental well-being among HCWs responding to COVID-19' (Ghaleb et al., 2021).

Another area of growing concern embraces the mental health needs of newer groups of personnel like health personnel reporting high levels of burnout (Hurt, 2021), and the caregivers who are becoming the alternate mental health workforce (Murthy, 2016).

On the positive side, there have been revisions of the legislation relating to mental health care in a number of countries like India in 2017, higher use of information technology, tele-mental health and growth of private psychiatry, resulting in increased availability of services (Khullar, 2023).

The changing understanding of mental disorders, mental health and well-being and the multi-dimensional nature of mental health is also illustrated by the articles in the recent issues of 2023 in one of the leading psychiatry journals, namely the Psychological Medicine (Table 2.3).

There are also books addressing the changing understanding of mental disorders, mental health and mental health care. Three of them are considered here to illustrate the trend. The book, 'Healing: Our Path from Mental Illness to Mental Health' by Thomas Insel (2022), is an important book in understanding the concept of mental and wellbeing, as well as mental health care for many reasons. Firstly, the recognition that for too long we have focussed on mental illnesses affecting a small proportion of the population, at any one point of time, to the mental health of the total population. Secondly, Insel was the Director of the National Institute of Mental Health for 14 years with billions of dollars of research investment in a wide range of subjects related to mental illnesses. Thirdly, it describes the need to shift from mental illness to mental health in United States of America, (with one of the highest mental health resources) where the mental health situation is described as being unsatisfactory. Fourthly, he synthesises the problem as 'for too long we have asked individuals and families to bear this crisis of care alone'. He shares his own learning as follows:

> When I started this journey to resolve the mental health crisis, I believed that technology and science would provide the answers we need. A new drug, a killer app, a breakthrough would make the difference. Years of listening to families and touring homeless shelters and clubhouses, clinics and hospitals, left me convinced that the problems are more complex and the solutions far simpler than most of us realise. We must summon the will to enact them, because we have for too long asked individuals and families to bear this crisis of care alone.

Fifthly, the books bring together the best of research to argue for a shift in focus, as seen from the concluding paragraph:

> "The problems are indeed complex, but we have solutions that are effective. For most problems, we don't need to know more to deliver. We know what works. We simply need to find the will and way to deliver to people, place and purpose. Recall Kennedy's vision in 1963, that people with mental illness would "no longer be alien to our affections". They need be alien no longer. Recovery is, after all, not just an outcome for those with an illness. Recovery is a measure of who we are".

There is much that can be achieved by reframing the focus of our work on mental health and not mental illness and from shifting from patients to the total population. Similar is the observation of Vivek Murthy, Surgeon General of United State of America in the May 2023 report of 'Our Epidemic of Loneliness and Isolation'. He observes:

> When taken together, this evidence consistently shows that wider social networks and more frequent social engagements with friends and family are associated with better cognitive function and may protect against the risk of dementia. This suggests that investments in social connection may be an important public health response to cognitive decline.

The multi-dimensional understanding of addiction in India is brought out in a recent book, 'Most of what you know about addiction is wrong' by Kala (2023). This book provides a comprehensive way of understanding the role of history, culture, religion, social changes, economy, politics (local, national and international) in the prevalence of drug addiction and its treatment, as applicable to India in general and Punjab in particular. Following an analysis of the wide range of forces contributing to addiction in India, author recommends the following eight areas for action: (i) decriminalisation the use and possession of small quantities of drugs; (ii) regulate and make available certain THC content cannabis; (iii) legalise mild plant based opiates like poppy husk; (iv) persons using drugs in public should be mandatorily referred to social workers and psychologists for counselling for safe use of drugs and assessment; (v) drugs awareness programmes should be essential part of school curriculum; (vi) syringes/needle exchange programme to prevent the spread of HIV/ Hepatitis C; (vii) programmes for deaddiction should be expanded to reach people addicted to drugs; and (viii) expert committee for consideration and development of substitution therapies. My own addition to these excellent set of recommendations is to include (ix) promotion of mental health sat the level of individuals, families and communities, to decrease the need for drugs and (x) to address the cultural, religious, social change, economic, political (local, national and international) factors associated with addiction. This book should be an essential reading for all social workers in India, to both understand the multiple dimensions of mental health, well-being and addiction and more importantly, the wide range of interventions where social workers can make a vital contribution.

At the turn of the last century, Murthy (1998) foresaw the changing scope of mental health and mental health care as follows: (i) mental health professionals should be advocates of mental health; (ii) research studies should focus on the issues of social change, development and mental health; (iii) efforts should be essentially multi-disciplinary, including law, architecture, sociology, anthropology, economics, industry, education, welfare, religion and philosophy; (iv) mental health interventions should be aimed at the general population and social institutions; (v) mental health professionals should become active partners in social policy development; and (vi) professional training of mental health professionals should include training in skills and methods of promoting mental health along with the care/support of persons with mental disorders.

However, it is appropriate to recognise that there are challenges. There are concerns of merging mental health and mental disorders. For example, Hugh (2022) notes, as a psychologist:

> I am heartened by the increase in our attention on mental health. But I see it as one way of looking at our lives among others. Mental health professionals are understandably interested in mental health - but we need to remain interested in how people lead lives that are good, happy or meaningful without ever spending much time with clinicians'. He goes on to observe, 'When we move away from a focus on psychological problems and toward "mental health" more broadly, clinicians stumble into terrain that extends beyond our expertise. We ought to be appropriately humble. We need to be mindful of the perennial difficulty of defining the boundary between sanity and madness, or of deciding what constitutes a good and valuable life.

This is also a viewpoint needing consideration as we develop the scope of mental health and well-being.

3. Current approaches to mental health care

This year is an important time in the history of mental health services in the low and middle-income (LAMI) countries. It was nearly 50 years back, in 1974, the World Health organization (WHO) held the first meeting on 'Organisation of Mental Health Services in Developing Countries' at Addis Ababa, Ethiopia (WHO, 1975; Giel & Harding, 1976). The 1975 initiative to outline the need for national level thinking in developing policies, to integrate mental health with general health care, involve non-specialists in mental health care as measures to develop mental health care in developing countries was path breaking. What was interesting is that the WHO put these ideas to practice as part of 6 year international, 7 country project, 'Strategies for Extending Mental Health Care' (1975–1981) (Harding et al., 1980; Sartorius et al., 1983; Wig et al., 1984; Murthy and Wig, 1983). This project is important as a demonstration of the feasibility of integrating mental health care in primary health care in LAMI countries. The multicentric, eleven country project 'Mental Illness in general health Care' (Ustun & Sartorius, 1995) was another attempt at demonstrating both the need and feasibility of addressing the common mental disorders at PHC level. This period was followed by the focus on developing national mental health plans in a number of countries of Asia, Middle East, Africa and South America during the next two decades. India was one of the first to develop the National Mental Health Programme (NMHP) in August 1982 (Wig and Murthy, 2018). WHO initiated a number of pilot innovative programmes under, 'Nations for Mental Health'. The publication of the World Health Report 2001with the subject of 'Mental Health- New Understanding, New Hope' was the next milestone. (WHO,

2001) This document boldly presented 10 recommendations namely: provide treatment in primary care, make psychotropic drugs available, give care in the community, educate the public, involve communities, families and consumers, establish national policies, programmes and legislation, develop human resources, link with other sectors, monitor community mental health and support more research.

Recent Mental Health Initiative in India

February 1, 2022, was an important day in the history of mental health care in India. On that day, the Finance Minister of Government of India, Mrs. Nirmala Seetharaman, as part of the annual budget speech, for the first time in the history of budget presentation in Independent India, referred to mental health and allotted funds for the same as follows: "the pandemic has accentuated mental health problems in people of all ages. Several factors have contributed to a steep rise in depression and anxiety, including restrictions on social contact, lockdowns, economic insecurity, and school and business closures." Further, she outlined the intervention "To better the access to quality mental health counselling and care services, a National Tele Mental Health program will be launched–51 nodal centres for telemedical mental health will be operated, with NIMHANS serving as the nodal centre. The International Institute of Information Technology, Bengaluru will provide technical support". The Government India viewed this commitment, important initiative, was seen in the daylong meeting to launch tele mental health on February 26, 2022 and develop action plans in the coming months (The Hindu, Feb 3, 2022). This development is significant for a number of reasons. Firstly, recognition of the impact of the pandemic as a mental health event and not only a physical health event. Secondly, the focus on the social determinants as contributors to mental health. Thirdly, the recognition of the total need of the total population for mental health and focus on population level interventions. Fourthly, focus on coverage of the total population by a decentralised approach to care rather than a clinic-based interventions. Fifthly, the utilisation of information technology to reach the unreached population. In the early part of 2023, TELE-MANAS programme has been launched through 5 coordinating centres and 51 services centres connected by the internet and mobile phone network. This is one of the biggest initiatives of the last 50 years in India. What is significant, for the discussions in this chapter, is the high importance provided in the programme for non-medical professionals (psychologists, social workers, nurses etc.) and non-pharmacological interventions. The results of this initiative can shape the future of mental health in the country (NIMHANS, 2022a, b, c, d).

Similarly, in a number of developing countries innovative approaches like 'Friendship Bench' where the resources of community is utilised to provided care within the community (Thornicroft et al., 2011; Murthy, 2011; Chibanda et al., 2015, 2016, Fernando et al., 2021; Gureje et al., 2020; Doukain et al.,2021).

Lessons from Mental Health Care in Developed Countries

The pandemic has presented challenges of meeting the mental health needs of the population even in economically rich countries, in spite of the much better resources for mental health care (Murthy, 2020). There is a continuing epidemic of depression and suicide. The need for innovation to reach all those who need the care is in all countries. For example, the launch of the 'Mentally Healthy Nation' by the American Psychiatric Association (APA). The goal of the APA initiative is significant for the scope of the activity to reach the general public through podcasts to engage the public in conversations about the current mental health crisis. Each episode of Mentally Healthy Nation will be centred around an aspect of mental health that impacts the community, where people live, learn, work and worship. The goal is to help ease the stigma of mental illness and to reach a more mentally healthy nation. It can be expected that there will be many innovations mental health care in the coming decade. Another initiative of United States of America, launched in June 2022, is the 988 helpline. This is a 24-hour helpline to link people in distress with immediate help and professional services. The results of this innovation can influence mental health development in countries (Miller et al., 2022).

4. Importance of the person, family, community for mental health

This section of the chapter illustrates the way individual, family, community, national and international level interventions are needed to address many of the issues of mental disorders, mental health and well-being. As noted in the earlier section, the concept of mental health currently involves the biology, psychology, social determinants, spirituality and climate/environment. Both the understanding and interventions have to encompass all of these aspects of mental health and well-being.

Following is an illustration of how this can be done in practice. Disasters have impact on the mental health of the population. (Murthy, 2014; Christodolou et al., 2016; Murthy, 2016, Murthy 2020). From the many disasters, it is known that the greater the impact of the disaster, higher the rates of emotional distress and disorders. Women, elderly and children are more at risk of developing emotional problems after disasters. Persons with losses of family members, property, displaced and those with physical health problems are at greater risk. Self-care, adequate medical care, social supports and rehabilitation minimises the impact.

This is well illustrated by the three years follow up study after the 2015 earthquake in Nepal. A cross-sectional descriptive design was used where 1076 adults within the age range of 19–65 were randomly selected and interviewed from four adversely affected districts due to the 2015 Nepal earthquake. The prevalence of PTSD among earthquake survivors was 18.9%. Odds of having PTSD was 1.6 times higher among females and nearly 2 times higher amongst illiterate survivors. Participants from the *Janajati* ethnic group and those who had a business occupation had a 50% lower risk of having PTSD. Around 39% of the participants had moderate social support and had 60% lower odds of having PTSD compared to those with poor social support. Participants with medium and very high-level damage to personal property were more likely to have PTSD. Authors conclude: 'Post-traumatic stress disorder is prevalent amongst survivors three years after the 2015 Nepal Earthquake. It is important to provide psychological and social support for survivors to decrease the health burden from PTSD. Socio-demographic characteristics such as females, farmers, those survivors who endured significant personal property damage were at higher risk' (Pandey et al., 2023).

The lesson of the last 40 years of work, following the Bhopal Gas tragedy in December 1984 illustrate both the long-term needs and the scope for psycho-social-spiritual interventions (Murthy and Issac, 1987; Murthy et al., 1987; Murthy, 2014a, b, 2016a, b, c). At the time of disaster, in 1984, none of the 5 medical colleges had psychiatry departments. Following the field visit by Prof. B. B. Sethi of K. G. Medical College, Lucknow and Prof. R. Srinivasa Murthy of NIMHANS, Bangalore, population was described to be having 'Wounded bodies and Wounded minds'. Immediate mental health care was initiated by shifting a team of mental health professionals from Lucknow and the Bangalore team training the medical officers in essentials of mental health care, using a special manual (Sethi et al., 1987; Murthy & Issac, 1987; Murthy et al., 1987). The needs were reviewed in 2014 (after thirty years of the disaster and a new manual of mental health care was developed to meet the continuing needs (Murthy, 2017). Similarly, the next major disaster was the 'Super cyclone of Orissa' that occurred in 1999 killing more than 20,000 people. Recognising the large population needing emotional support and the multi-dimensional nature of the needs, a programme of trained community volunteers (*Snehakarmis*) was adopted to spread the mental health messages and skills of self-care to the total population. The approach was taken to the next higher level during the Gujarat riots of 2002. Four manuals for self-care, for women, for children/teachers and community volunteers were utilised to reach emotional support to the disaster survivors. This approach has been utilised in the subsequent disasters like the tsunami of 2004. In the national disaster service, emotional health care has now become an integral part of the interventions. Along with these initiatives in the mental health area, there were other psycho-social interventions like early warning to population, building of disaster shelters, public education, early relocation of people to safe places have become essential part of disaster response, resulting in drastic reduction of deaths in disasters (Lakshminaraya et al., 2004). There has been similar focus on innovations to meet the mental health needs of refugees (Vijayakumar, 2016), farmers suicide (Murthy, 2012). The utilisation of the cultural resources of spirituality, with examples from cancer care and support to caregivers of special children is described later in this book (Chapter number thirteen by Prof. R. Srinivasa Murthy).

The range of initiatives of care, both needed and feasible to be undertaken to address are public health problems like child trauma, domestic violence, drug dependence, homelessness, suicide prevention, migrant mental health, working women, loneliness etc. In addressing all of these and related social issues there is need for systematic efforts (Tables 2.4 and 2.5).

Table 2.4 Approaches to develop practice of spirituality and evaluate its impact (Murthy & Banerjee, 2021)

• Examination of the concept of spirituality in different religions • Adaptation of the concepts/practices to modern societal realities in rural, urban, and other settings and different population groups • The development of case studies of persons utilizing these measures and finding meaning of life Preparing people, as they age, (from 50 years on) to include this in the overall life plans • Case control studies of people in society with varying degrees of spirituality • Longitudinal studies in the elderly, to understand the value of spirituality in promoting QOL, mental wellness, preventing depression, dementia, etc., and coping better with adverse life situations of disease, grief, etc • Standardization of spiritual practices as applicable to all groups, for wider dissemination in the society QOL: Quality of life

Table 2.5 Recommendations for research on 988 crisis lines (Miller et al., 2022)

• Conduct observational and randomized, controlled trials that examine how crisis line training increases positive counsellor behaviours and reduces negative counsellor behaviours • Conduct randomized, controlled trials to identify suicide risk assessment practices in crisis contexts that are most effective at reducing suicide risk in the moment and in the future • Evaluate which components of evidence-based interventions, such as dialectical behaviour therapy, may be feasibly adapted for crisis contexts • Follow up with callers after the crisis conversation to investigate whether they were connected to services and the impact these services had on reducing suicide risk • Gather information on the individuals who contact crisis lines • Conduct studies with callers and counsellors to assess how the quality of the therapeutic alliance between counsellors and callers impacts the callers' suicide risk at follow-up • Conduct observational studies to examine how counsellor qualifications and certifications are associated with crisis line effectiveness

5. Implications of these developments for the profession of social work

The aforementioned review presents both challenges for mental health and well-being, as well as opportunities for future. With the current understanding of mental disorders, mental health and well-being, the boundaries for interventions are widened, barriers broken and opportunities for interventions enlarge. Especially relevant to social work is the focus on the individual efforts, strengthening of family and social institutions and interventions at the level of societal and environmental factors. These are all areas of activity for professional social workers (Gupta, 2023).

This new situation is presented in a recent book of psychotherapy (Hill & Dahlitz, 2022),

> 'the twenty-first-century psychotherapist can no longer be constrained by specific schools of practice or limited reservoirs of knowledge. From basic neuroscience to body-brain systems and genetic processes, therapists will discover how to become more "response-able" to their clients". Further they note "this new "era of information" needs to be integrated and made manageable for every practitioner".

Similarly, Littrell (2019) links social work to psychoneuroimmunology as follows:

> A wealth of information regarding how the immune system can influence the brain and result in changes in mood and behavior has accumulated. Inflammation is a causal factor in some cases of major depression and psychotic disorders and predicts whether trauma will result in Posttraumatic Stress Disorder (PTSD). Fortunately, studies in the area of psychoneuroimmunology have also suggested ways to decrease inflammation. Knowledge of this information is vital for social workers so that the impact of their interventions can be maximized. Moreover, for macropractice social workers, the information underscores the importance of access to nutritional food, access to safe places for exercise, and the time for food preparation and exercise, which should be considered as social justice issues. Keywords psychoneuroimmunology, inflammation in depression, inflammation in psychosis, microbiome, vaccinating against PTSD, yoga and distress.

Conclusion

The following are the areas relevant for future action:

1. The emerging understanding of mental disorders, mental health and well-being will be influenced by advances in knowledge in the fields of biology, psychology, sociology, economy, spirituality and environmental studies.
2. There is need to understand and document the social (individual, family, community, external world) dimensions of mental disorders, mental health and well-being. This has to occur both globally and locally.
3. The scope of mental health has moved from 'deviancy' model to 'normalcy' model. Mental health is no more seen in terms of clinical disorders and persons with mental disorders as persons to be cared/ controlled. The personhood of the persons with mental disorders has come to the forefront. In addition, Mental Health and Well-being are seen as TOTAL POPULATION issue rather that of a limited section of population with mental illnesses.
4. The increasing understanding of social determinants, opens up avenues for wide range of interventions and professional role of social workers at the level of individuals, families and communities become central.
5. There is a wide range of social interventions that can address the mental disorders, mental health and well-being of individuals that brings social workers into 'therapeutic' role, much more than it was till recent times.
6. There is need to build mental health and well-being programmes on the existing beliefs, practices of individuals and communities.
7. The training of social workers should include skills relating to address all these areas.
8. There is need to develop legal and administrative frameworks for social workers to work both as individuals and as part of teams.
9. Research: Interventions should be rigorously evaluated both globally and locally, as the local situations (history, culture, religion, economy, etc.) will define the scope for interventions. Two areas are detailed to illustrate the type of work that needs to be undertaken in all of the issues and interventions (Tables 2.4 and 2.5). As noted earlier, the new initiative to address suicide prevention, in

USA, 988 telephone based support was launched last year. It is recognised that this initiative should be rigorously evaluated.

10. All of these activities should be initiated as multisectoral and multidisciplinary activities, which requires collaboration and leadership skills. Mechanisms and systems should be created to both document and disseminate all the emerging information/ skills to all stakeholders.

A good model (for social workers) would be to think of the needed changes in the society. In the recent Surgeon General Report on 'Our Epidemic of Loneliness and Isolation' (2023), twelve broad areas are identified for specific action. These include (i) National, Territory, State, Local, and Tribal Governments, (ii) Health Workers, Health Care Systems, and Insurers, (iii) Public Health Professionals and Public Health Departments; (iv) Researchers and Research Institutions; (v) Philanthropy; (vi) Schools and Education Departments; (vii) Workplaces (viii) Community-Based Organizations; (ix) Technology Companies; (x) Media and Entertainment Industries; (xi) Parents and Caregivers and (xii) Individuals (Office of Surgeon General, 2023). This approach of looking at mental health from a multidimensional and multidisciplinary view is applicable to child trauma, domestic violence, drug dependence, homelessness, suicide prevention, migrant mental health, working women, loneliness etc.

Development of innovative interventions rooted in the cultural resources would be an important contribution of Indian social workers to the rest of the world. As noted earlier, social workers are eminently equipped to act at all of these levels. What is required is to understand the issues in the 'Local' context and develop culturally relevant solutions and demonstrate their effectiveness. This is the challenge of the 21st Century and an opportunity for all mental health professionals in general and Indian social workers in particular.

Acknowledgements My sincere thanks to Dr. Meenu Anand, Delhi School of Social Work, Editor of the book, for the opportunity to bring my five decades of experiences in this chapter. My thanks to Prof. Subhasish Bhadra, Ajmer School of Social Work, Ajmer and Ms. Suman Gupta, Psychiatric Social Worker, Chandigarh, Ms. Anuradha, Bangalore, for their critical comments and insights.

References

Aas, M., Alameda, L., Forti, M. D., et al. (2023). Synergistic effects of childhood adversity and polygenic risk in first-episode psychosis: The EU-GEI study. *Psychological Medicine, 53*, 1970–1978.

Acosta, A. M., Garg, S., Pham, H., et al. (2021). Racial and ethnic disparities in rates of COVID-19–associated hospitalization, intensive care unit admission, and in-hospital death in the United States from March 2020 to February 2021. *JAMA Network Open, 4*(10), e2130479. https://doi.org/10.1001/jamanetworkopen.2021.30479.

Alzueta, E., Podhajsky, S., Zhao, Q., et al. (2023). Risk for depression tripled during the COVID-19 pandemic in emerging adults followed for the last 8 years. *Psychological Medicine, 53*, 2156–2163.

American Psychiatric Association. (2021). *Mentally healthy nation.* APA.

American Psychological Association. (2009). *Psychology and global climate change: Addressing a multi-faceted phenomenon and set of challenges.* APA.

Atkinson, L., Joshi, D., Raina, P., et al. (2023). Social engagement and allostatic load mediate between adverse childhood experiences and multimorbidity in mid to late adulthood: The Canadian longitudinal study on aging. *Psychological Medicine, 53*, 1437–1347.

Beck, M. (2016). The risk implications of globalisations: An exploratory analysis of 105 major industrial incidents (1971–2010). *International Journal of Environment Research and Public Health,* 13(3), pii: E309.

Begemann, M. J. H., Schutte, M. J. L., Dellen, E., et al. (2023). Childhood trauma is associated with reduced frontal gray matter volume: A large transdiagnostic structural MRI study. *Psychological Medicine, 53*, 741–749.

Begum, S., Donta, B., Nair, S., & Prakasamm, C. P. (2015). Socio-demographioc factors associated with domestic violence in urban slums, Mumbai, Maharashtra. *Indian Journal of Medical Research, 141*, 783–788.

Bhugra, D., Tasman, A., Pathare, S., et al. (2017a). The WPA-lancet psychiatry commission on the future of psychiatry. *Lancet Psychiatry, 4*, 775–818.

Bhugra, D., Tasman, A., Pathare, S., et al. (2017b). The WPA-lancet psychiatry commission on the future of psychiatry. *The Lancet Psychiatry, 4*, 775–818.

Bhugra, D., Pathare, S., Joshi, R., Kalra, G., Torales, J., & Ventriglio, A. (2019). A review of mental health policies from Commonwealth countries. *International Journal of Social Psychiatry, 64*, 3–8.

Bloom, P. (2023). *Psych: The story of the human mind*. Harper Collins. ECCO Press.

Bragesjö, M., Arnberg, F. K., Lauri, K. O., et al. (2023). Condensed Internet-delivered prolonged exposure provided soon after trauma: A randomised trial. *Psychological Medicine, 53*, 1989–1998.

Chan, C. S., Wong, C. Y. F., Yu, B. Y. M., et al. (2023). Treating depression with a smartphone-delivered self-help cognitive behavioral therapy for insomnia: A parallel-group randomized controlled trial. *Psychological Medicine, 53*, 1799–1813.

Chibanda, D., Bowers, T., Verhey, R., et al. (2015). The Friendship Bench programme: A cluster randomised controlled trial of a brief psychological intervention for common mental disorders delivered by lay health workers in Zimbabwe. *International Journal of Mental Health Systems, 9*, 21. https://doi.org/10.1186/s13033-015-0013-y.

Chibanda, D., Weiss, H. A., Verhey, R., Simms, V., Munjoma, R., Rusakaniko, S., Chingono, A., Munetsi, E., Bere, T., Manda, E., Abas, M., & Araya, R. (2016). Effect of a primary care–based psychological intervention on symptoms of common mental disorders in Zimbabwe. *JAMA, 316*, 2618.

Christodoulou, G. N., Mezzich, J. E., Christodoulou, N. G., et al. (2016). *Disasters-mental health context and responses.* Cambridge Scholars Publishing.

COVID-19 Mental Disorders Collaborators. (2021). Global prevalence and burden of depressive and anxiety disorders in 204 countries and territories in 2020 due to the COVID-19 pandemic. *Lancet*.https://doi.org/10.1016/S0140-6736(21)02143-7.2021.

Cuijpers, P., Javed, A., & Bhiui, K. (2023). The WHO world mental health report: A call for action. *The British Journal of Psychiatry, 222*, 227–229.

Devi, S. (2023). Was the Covid pandemic bad for mental health? It depends who you ask. *The Guardian.*

De Silva et al. (2016). Evaluation of district mental healthcare plans: The PRIME consortium methodology, 208 (Suppl 56), pp. s63–s70.https://doi.org/10.1192/bjp.bp.114.153858:10.1192/bjp.bp.114.153858.

Dickens, A. P., Richards, S. H., Greaves, C. J., et al. (2013). Interventions targeting social isolation in older people: A systematic review. *BMC Public Health, 11*, 647.

Dotterer, H. L., Vazquez, A. Y., Hyde, L. W., et al. (2023). Elucidating the role of negative parenting in the genetic v. environmental influences on adult psychopathic traits. *Psychological Medicine, 53*, 897–907.
Doukani, A., et al. (2021). A community health volunteer delivered problem-solving therapy mobile application based on the friendship bench 'Inuka Coaching' in Kenya: A pilot cohort study. *Global Mental Health (camb), 8*, e9. https://doi.org/10.1017/gmh.2021.3.
Durkheim, E. (1897). *Suicide*. Routledge.
Dykxhoorn, J., Ashok, K., Sörberg Wallin, A., & Dalman, C. (2023). Objective and subjective neighbourhood characteristics and suicidality: A multilevel analysis. *Psychological Medicine, 53*, 1166–1175.
Eder, M., Henninger, M., Durbin, S., et al. (2021). Screening and interventions for social risk factors. Technical brief to support the US preventive services task force. *JAMA, 326*(14), 1416–1428. https://doi.org/10.1001/jama.2021.12825.
Ettman, C. K., Cohen, G. H., Abdalla, S. M. et al. (2021). Persistent depressive symptoms during COVID-19: A national, population-representative, longitudinal study of U.S. adults. *The Lancer regional Health-the Americas*. https://doi.org/10.1016/j.lana.2021.100091.
Fernando, S., et al. (2021). The friendship bench as a brief psychological intervention with peer support in rural Zimbabwean women: A mixed methods pilot evaluation. *Global Mental Health (camb), 2021*(8), e31. https://doi.org/10.1017/gmh.2021.32.
Firth, J., et al. (2020). A meta-review of "Lifestyle psychiatry": The role of exercise, smoking, diet and sleep in the prevention and treatment of mental disorders. *World Psychiatry, 19*, 360–380.
Garland, E.L., Fix, S.T., Hudak, J.P. et al (2023). Mindfulness-Oriented Recovery Enhancement remediates anhedonia in chronic opioid use by enhancing neurophysiological responses during savouring of natural rewards. *Psychological Medicine, 53*, 2085–2094
Geronimus, A. T. (2023). *Weathering: The extraordinary stress of ordinary life in an unjust society*. Virago Press.
Ghaleb, Y., Lami, F., Nsour, A. I., et al. (2021), Mental health impacts of COVID-19 on healthcare workers in the Eastern Mediterranean Region: A multi-country study. *Journal of Public Health*, 1–9.https://doi.org/10.1093/pubmed/fdab321.
Giel, R., & Harding, T. W. (1976). Psychiatric priorities in developing countries. *The British Journal of Psychiatry, 128*, 513–522.
Gilchrist, C.P., Thompson, D.K., Alexander B. et al (2023). Growth of prefrontal and limbic brain regions and anxiety disorders in children born very preterm. *Psychological Medicine, 53*, 759–770.
Gupta, S. (2020). *Keep sharp: Build a better brain at any age*. Hachette.
Gupta, S. (2023). Personal communication.
Gureje, O., et al. (2020). The effect of collaborative care between traditional/faith healers and primary health care workers to improve psychosis outcome in Nigeria and Ghana (COSIMPO)–a cluster randomized controlled trial. *Lancet, 396*(10251), 612–622. https://doi.org/10.1016/S0140-6736(20)30634-6.
Harding, T. W., Climent, C. E., Diop, M., Giel, R., Ibrahim, H. H. A., Ignacio, L. L., et al. (1980). The WHO collaborative study on the strategies for extending mental health care, II: The development of new research methods. *American Journal of Psychiatry, 140*, 1474–1480.
Herman, H., Patel, V., Kieling, C., & Berk, M. (2022). *Time for United Action on Depression: A Lancet-World Psychiatric Association Commission*. https://doi.org/10.1016/S0140-6736(21)02141-3.
Hill, R., & Dahlitz, M. (2022). *The practitioners guide to the science of psychotherapy*. Norton.
Hjern, A, Palacios, J, Vinnerljung, B. (2023). Early childhood adversity and non-affective psychosis: a study of refugees and international adoptees in Sweden. *Psychological Medicine, 53*, 1914–1923.
Hudson, J.L., McLellan, L.F., Eapen, V. et al (2023). Combining CBT and sertraline does not enhance outcomes for anxious youth: a double-blind randomised controlled trial. *Psychological Medicine, 53*, 1741–1749.

Hurt, A. (2021). Physician burnout, depression compounded by COVID: Survey – Medscape.
Hurt, A. (2022). Physician burnout, depression compounded by COVID: Survey. Medscape - Jan 21, 2022.
Insel, T. (2022). *Healing: Out path from mental illness to mental health.* Penguin Press.
Iob, E., Ajnakina, O., & Steptoe, A. (2023). The interactive association of adverse childhood experiences and polygenic susceptibility with depressive symptoms and chronic inflammation in older adults: A prospective cohort study. *Psychological Medicine, 53*, 1426–1436.
Jeste, D. (2020). *Wiser: the scientific roots of wisdom, compassion and what makes us good. Sounds True.* Boulder.
Kala, A.K. (2023). Most of what you know about addiction is wrong. *Speaking Tiger*. New Delhi.
Khullar, D. (2023). *Can A.I. treat mental illness*? New Yorker.
Klineman, A. (2009). Global mental health: a failure of humanity. The Lancet, 374, 603–604. DOI: https://doi.org/10.1016/S0140-6736(09)61510-5
Koenig, H. G. (2012). Religion, spirituality, and health: The research and clinical implications. *International Scholarly Research Network Psychiatry*, 1–33.https://doi.org/10.5402/2012/278730
Lakshminarayana, R., Murthy, R.S., & Diaz, J. O. P. (2004). *Disaster mental health in India.* New Delhi: Indian Red Cross.
Lam, L. C. W., & Riba, M. (2016). *Physical exercise interventions for mental health.* Cambridge university Press.
Leff, J., & Vaughn, C. (1980). The interaction of life events and relatives' expressed emotion in schizophrenia and depressive neurosis. *British Journal of Psychiatry, 136*, 146–153.
Leff, J., & Vaughn, C. (1981). The role of maintenance therapy and relatives' expressed emotion in relapse of schizophrenia: A 2-year follow-up. *British Journal of Psychiatry, 139*, 102–104.
Leff, J., & Vaughn, C. (1985). *Expressed emotion in families: Its significance for mental illness.* Guilford Press.
Leff, J., Kuipers, L., Berkowitz, R., et al. (1982). A controlled trial of intervention in the families of schizophrenic patients. *British Journal of Psychiatry, 141*, 121–134.
Leff, J., Kuipers, L., Berkowitz, R., et al. (1985). A controlled trial of social intervention in the families of schizophrenic patients: Two year follow-up. *British Journal of Psychiatry, 146*, 594–600.
Leff, J., Wig, N. N., Ghosh, A., et al. (1987). Influence of relatives' expressed emotion on the course of schizophrenia in Chandigarh. *British Journal of Psychiatry, 151*, 166–173.
Littrell, J. L. (2019). The importance of psychoneuroimmunology for social workers. *Families in Society: The Journal of Contemporary Social Services, 100*, 17–33.
MacKenzie, M. J., Bosk, E., & Zeanah, C. H. (2017). Separating families at the border—consequences for children's health and well-being. *New England Journal of Medicine, 376*, 2314–2315.
Maguen, S., Nichter, B., Norman, S. B., et al. (2023). Moral injury and substance use disorders among US combat veterans: Results from the 2019–2020 National Health and Resilience in Veterans Study. *Psychological Medicine, 53*, 1364–1370.
Malesic, J. (2022). *The end of burnout-why work drains us and how to build better lives.* University of California Press.
Mane, P., & Gandevia, K. Y. (1993). *Mental health in India: Issues and CONCERNS.* Bombay: Tata Institute of Social Sciences.
Marques-Feixa, L., Palma-Gudiel, H., & Romero, S. (2023). Childhood maltreatment disrupts HPA-axis activity under basal and stress conditions in a dose–response relationship in children and adolescents. *Psychological Medicine, 53*, 1060–1073.
Miller, A. B., Oppenheimer, C. W., Glenn, C. R., et al. (2022). Preliminary research priorities for factors influencing individual outcomes for users of the US national suicide prevention lifeline. *JAMA Psychiatry, 79*, 1225–1231.

Murthy, S.R. (1993). Evolution of the concept of mental health: from mental illness to mental health. In P. N. Mane, & K. Y. Gandevia (Eds.), *Mental health in India: Issues and concerns* (pp 17–42). Bombay: Tata Institute of Social Sciences.

Murthy, S.R. (1998). Emerging aspects of psychiatry in India. *Indian Journal of Psychiatry, 40*, 307–310.

Murthy, S.R. (2010). Hinduism and mental health. In P. Verhagen, H. M. Van Praag, J. J. Lopez-Ibor, J. Cox, & D. Moussaoui (Eds.), *Religion and psychiatry: Beyond boundaries* (pp.159–180). Wiley. Oxford.

Murthy, S.R. (2011). Mental health services in low and middle income countries. Chapter 39. In G. Thornicroft & G. Szmukler (Eds.), *Oxford textbook of community psychiatry* (pp. 325–336). Oxford University Press.

Murthy, S.R. (2012). Farmers suicide: Need for mental health interventions. *Indian Journal of Social Psychiatry., 28*, 26–35.

Murthy, S.R. (2014a). Impact of child neglect and abuse on adult mental health. *Institutionalised Children Explorations and Beyond, 1*, 150–162.

Murthy, S.R. (2014b). Mental health of survivors of 1984 Bhopal disaster: A continuing challenge. *Industrial Psychiatry Journal, 23*, 86–93.

Murthy, S.R. (Ed.). (2016a). *Manual of mental health care for medical officers of Bhopal.* Bhopal: National Institute for Research in Environmental Health (ICMR).

Murthy, S.R. (2016b). Conflict situations and mental health care in developing countries. In: G. N. Christodoulou, J. E. Mezzich, N. G. Christodoulou, & D. Lecic-Tosevski (Eds.), *Disasters: Mental health context and responses* (pp. 153–72). Cambridge Scholars Publishing.

Murthy, S.R. (2016c). Caregiving and caregivers: Challenges and opportunities in India. *Indian Journal of Social Psychiatry, 32*, 10–18.

Murthy, S.R. (2016d). Self care for mental health-the new frontier. In G. Saha (Ed.), *Different strokes,* (2nd Edition). Bhopal: Publication of Indian Psychiatric Society.

Murthy, S.R. (2018). Globalization, market economy, and mental health. In R. K. Chadda, V. Kumar, S. Sarkar (Eds.), *Social psychiatry: Principles and clinical perspectives* (pp. 508–520). New Delhi: Jaypee Brothers Medical Publishers.

Murthy, S.R. (2020a). *Taking charge of emotional health during the pandemic: what everyone can do*? Newsletter of LGBRIMH, Tezpur, pp. 2–4. 2.

Murthy, S.R. (2020b). COVID-19 Pandemic and emotional health: Social psychiatry perspective. *Indian Journal of Social Psychiatry, 36*, S24–42.

Murthy, S.R. & Banerjee, D. (2021). Loneliness in older people: From analysis to action. *World Social Psychiatry, 3*, 120–122.

Murthy, S.R. & Issac, M. K. (1987). Mental health needs of Bhopal disaster victims and training of medical officers in mental health aspects. *Indian Journal of Medical Research, 86*(Supplement), 51–58.

Murthy, S.R., Issac M., & Chandrasekar C. R. et al. (1987). *Manual of mental health care for medical officers-Bhopal Disaster.* New Delhi: Indian Council of Medical Research.

Murthy, S.R. & Wig, N. N. (1983). The WHO collaborative study on strategies for extending mental health care, IV: A training approach to enhancing the availability of mental health manpower in a developing country. *American Journal of Psychiatry, 140*, 1486–1490.

Murthy, V. H. (2021). Together: healing power of human connection in a sometimes lonely world. Noida" Harper Collins.

Musich, S., Wang, S. S., & Hawkins, K., et al. (2015). The impact of loneliness on quality of life and patient satisfaction among older, sicker adults. *Gerontology and Geriatric Medicine Journal,* 1–9.

National Academy of Science, Engineering and Medicine (NASEM). (2023). *Achieving whole health: A new approach for veterans and the nation.* Washington: NASEM.

Nadkarni, V. V., & Das, S. (1993). Social work response to mental illness and mental health. In P. N. Mane, & K. Y. Gandevia (Eds.), *Mental health in India: Issues and concerns* (pp. 70–93). Bombay: Tata Institute of Social Sciences.

Neki, J. S. (1977). Psychotherapy in India. *Indian Journal of Psychiatry, 19*, 1–10.
NIMHANS. (2022a). *Course content for tele MANAS counsellors.* NIMHANS, Bangalore. Publication No.239.
NIMHANS. (2022b). *Point of care guide for Tele MANAS counsellors.* NIMHANS, Bangalore. Publication No.240.
NIMHANS. (2022c). *Facilitator's manual for trainers of tele MANAS counsellors.* NIMHANS. Bangalore. Publication No.241.
NIMHANS. (2022D). *Operational guidelines: The digital arm of the national mental health programme.* NIMHANS. Bangalore.
Njenga, F. G., Nguithi, A., & Gatere, S. G. (2010). Psychiatry and african religions. In P. Verhagen, H. M. Van Praag, J. J. Lopez-Ibor, J. Cox, & D. Moussaoui (Eds.) *Religion and psychiatry: Beyond boundaries* (pp.143–158). Wiley: Oxford.
Office of the Surgeon General. (2023). *Our epidemic of loneliness and isolation: U.S. surgeon general's advisory on the healing effects of social connection and community.* Washington: Government of USA.
Okasha, A. (2010). Religion and mental health in Islam. In P. Verhagen, H. M. Van Praag, J. J. Lopez-Ibor, J. Cox, & D. Moussaoui (Eds.), *Religion and psychiatry: Beyond boundaries* (pp. 119–142). Wiley. Oxford.
Oncioiu, S. I., Boivin, M., et al. (2023). Mental health comorbidities following peer victimization across childhood and adolescence: A 20-year longitudinal study. *Psychological Medicine, 53*, 2072–2084.
Pandey, R. A., Chalise, P., Khadka, S., et al. (2023). Post-traumatic stress disorder and its associated factors among survivors of 2005 earthquake in Nepal. *BMC Psychiatry, 23*, 340.
Pennebecker, J. W., & Evans, J. F. (2014). *Expressive writing-words that heal.* Idyll Arbor, Enumclaw.
Peteet, J. R. (2010). Christianity and psychiatry. In P. Verhagen, H. M. Van Praag, J. J. Lopez-Ibor, J. Cox, & D. Moussaoui (Eds.), *Religion and psychiatry: Beyond boundaries* (pp. 105–118). Wiley. Oxford.
Patel, P., Saxena, S., Lund, C., et al. (2018). The Lancet Commission on global mental health and sustainable development. *Lancet, 392*, 1553–1598.
Piketty, T. (2014). *Capital in the twenty first century.* Harvard University.
Rao, A. V. (1997). Culture, philosophy, mental health. Mumbai: Bharatiya Vidya Bhavan.
Ribeiro, W. S., Bauer, A., Andrade, M. C. R., et al. (2017). Income inequality and mental illness-related morbidity and resilience: A systematic review and meta-analysis. *Lancet Psychiatry, 4*, 554–562.
Rotenberg, M., Tuck, A., Anderson, K. K., et al. (2023). Neighbourhood-level social capital, marginalisation, and the incidence of schizophrenia and schizoaffective disorder in Toronto, Canada: A retrospective population-based cohort study. *Psychologic Medicine, 53*, 2643–2651.
Rubin, R. (2017). Loneliness might be a killer, but what's the best way to protect against it? *JAMA, 318*(19), 1853–1855.
Ryu, E., Jenkins, G. D., Wang, Y., et al. (2023). The importance of social activity to risk of major depression in older adults. *Psychological Medicine, 53*, 2634–2642.
Sapiens Lab (2023). *Mental state of the world report 2022.* A publication of the Mental Health Million Project. Retrieved from https://sapienlabs.org/mental-health-million-project.
Sartorius, N., & Harding, T. W. (1983). The WHO collaborative study on strategies for extending mental health care, I: The genesis of the study. *American Journal of Psychiatry, 140*, 1470–1473.
Scull, A. (1989). *Social order/mental disorder: Anglo American psychiatry in historical perspective.* Routledge.
Selten, J. P., & Ormel, J. (2023). Low status, humiliation, dopamine and risk of schizophrenia. *Psychological Medicine, 53*, 609–613.
Sethi, B. B., Sharma, M., Trivedi, J. K., et al. (1987). Psychiatric patients attending clinics in gas affected areas in Bhopal. *Indian Journal of Medical Research, 86*(Supplement), 45–50.

Shamsunder, C. (2008). Relevance of ancient Indian wisdom to modern mental health-a few examples. *Indian Journal of Psychiatry, 50*, 138–143.
Sharma, A. (2009). *Spirituality and mental health.* Indian Psychiatric Society in association with Rajayoga Education and Research Foundation.
Shen, H., Zhang, L., Li, Y., et al. (2023). Mindfulness-based intervention improves residual negative symptoms and cognitive impairment in schizophrenia: A randomized controlled follow-up study. *Psychological Medicine, 53*, 1390–1399.
Shinfuku, N., & Kitanishi, K. (2010). Buddhism and psychotherapy in Japan. In P. Verhagen, H. M. Van Praag, J. J. Lopez-Ibor, J. Cox, & D. Moussaoui (Eds.), *Religion and psychiatry: Beyond boundaries* (pp. 181–192). Wiley. Oxford.
Sletved, K. S. O., Ziersen, S. C., Andersen, P. K., et al. (2023). Socio-economic functioning in patients with bipolar disorder and their unaffected siblings–results from a nation-wide population-based longitudinal study. *Psychological Medicine, 53*, 706–713.
Southwick, S. M., & Charney, D. S. (2012). The science of resilience: Implications for the prevention and treatment of depression. *Science, 338*, 79–82. https://doi.org/10.1126/science.1222942.
Southwick, S. M., & Charney, D. S. (2018). *Resilience* (2nd ed.). University Press of Cambridge.
Stallman, H. M. (2023). Intergenerational transmission of suicidality or shared stressors? *Psychological Medicine, 53*, 1126.
Taylor. (2020). *The psychology of pandemic-preparing for the next global outbreak of infectious disease.* Cambridge Scholars Publishing.
Taylor. (2022). *I wrote the book on the pandemic-post covid will take some getting used to.* The Guardian.
The Hindu. (2022). *Mental health in the annual budget: 2022–2023.* The Hindu.
Thompson, E. J., Richards, M., Ploubidis, G. B., et al. (2023). Changes in the adult consequences of adolescent mental ill-health: Findings from the 1958 and 1970 British birth cohorts. *Psychological Medicine, 53*, 1074–1083.
Thornicroft, G., Sunkel, C., Aliev, A. A., et al. (2022). The lancet commission on ending stigma and discrimination in mental health. *The Lancet., 400*, 1438–1480.
Thornicroft, G., Szmukler G., & Muesser K. T. et al. (2011). *Oxford textbook of community mental health.* New York: Oxford.
Udomran, P. (2010). Psychiatry and theravada buddhism. In P. Verhagen, H. M. Van Praag, J. J. Lopez-Ibor, J. Cox, D. Moussaoui (Eds.). *Religion and psychiatry: Beyond boundaries* (pp. 193–208). Wiley. Oxford.
United for Global Mental Health. (2021). *Mental health for all: What can we achieve if we meaningfully integrate mental health into UHC.* UHC Policy Brief series. London: UHC
Uri, A., Navot, N., & Apter A. (2010). Judaism and psychiatry. In P. Verhagen, H. M. Van Praag, J. J. Lopez-Ibor, J. Cox, & D. Moussaoui (Eds.), *Religion and psychiatry: Beyond boundaries* (pp. 89–104). Wiley. Oxford.
Ustun, T. B., & Sartorius, N. (1995). *Mental illness in general health care: An international study.* Wiley.
Varambally, S., & Gangadhar B. N. (2016). Yoga-based interventions for the management of psychiatric disorders. In L. C. W. Lam, & M. Riba (Eds.), *Physical exercise interventions for mental health.* Cambridge: Cambridge University Press.
Verhagen, P. J., van Pragg, H. M., Lopez -Ibor, J. J., Cox, J. L., Moussaoui, D. (2010). *Religion and psychiatry: Beyond boundaries.* Wiley: Oxford.
Vijayakumar, L. (2016). Suicide among refugees-a mockery of humanity. *Crisis, 37*, 1–4.
Viswanathan, N., & Wetzel J. W. (1993). Concepts and trends in mental health: A global overview. In P. N. Mane, K. Y. Gandevia (Eds.), *Mental health in India: Issues and concerns* (pp. 43–69). Bombay: Tata Institute of Social Sciences.
Wig, N. N. (1990). Indian concepts of mental health and their impact on care of the mentally ill. *International Journal of Mental Health., 18*, 71–80.
Wig, N. N. (1999). Mental health and spiritual values. A view from the East. *International Review of Psychiatry, 11*, 92–96.

Wig, N. N. (2006). *The joy of mental health.* Servants of the People Society.
Wig, N. N., & SrinivasaMurthy, R. (2018). The birth of national mental health program for India. *Indian Journal of Psychiatry, 57*, 315–319.
Wig, N. N., Suleiman, M. A., Routledge, R., Srinivasa Murthy, R., Ladrido-Ignacio, L., Ibrahim, H. H., et al. (1983). Community reactions to mental disorders. A key informant study in three developing countries. *Acta Psychiatrica Scandinavica, 61*, 111–126.
Wilkinson, R., & Pickett, K. (2010). *The spirit level—why greater equality makes societies stronger.* Bloomsbury.
Wilkinson, R., & Pickett, K. (2017). Inequality and mental illness. *Lancet Psychiatry, 4*, 512–513.
Wilkinson, R., & Pickett, K. (2018). *The inner level: How more equal societies reduce stress, restore sanity and improve everyone's well-being.* Penguin.
World Health Organisation. (1975). Organisation of mental health in developing countries. TRS 564. Geneva, Switzerland: WHO.
World Health Organisation. (2001). *World health report 2001: Mental health-new understanding, new hope.* WHO.
World Health Organisation. (2006). *MhGap intervention guidelines for mental, neurological and substance use disorders in non-specialised settings.* WHO.
World Health Organization. (2013). *Mental health action plan 2013–2030.* World Health Organization. https://apps.who.int/iris/handle/10665/89966.
World Health Organization. (2016). *mhGAP intervention guide mental health gap action programme version 2.0.* Geneva: WHO.
World Health Organization. (2019). *The WHO special initiative for mental health (2019–20 23): Universal health coverage for mental health.* World Health Organization. https://apps.who.int/iris/handle/10665/310981. License: CC BY-NC-SA 3.0 IGO+.
World Health Organization. (2020). *Doing what matters in times of stress: An illustrated guide.* WHO.
World Health Organization (2021). Mental Health Atlas. (2020). *World health Organisation.* Switzerland.
World Health Organisation. (2022). *World mental health report 2022: Transforming mental health for all.* WHO.
Wu, Y., Yang, D., Jian, B., et al. (2023). Can emotional expressivity and writing content predict beneficial effects of expressive writing among breast cancer patients receiving chemotherapy? A secondary analysis of randomized controlled trial data from China. *Psychological Medicine, 53*, 1527–1541.
Yang, W., Jin, S., Duan, W., et al. (2023). The effects of childhood maltreatment on cortical thickness and gray matter volume: A coordinate-based meta-analysis. *Psychological Medicine, 53*, 1681–1699.

Chapter 3
Social and Cultural Determinants of Mental Health

Vibhuti Patel

Abstract Social determinants of mental health in the industrialised world and in post-colonial societies are found to be directly related to intersectional vulnerabilities of class, caste/race/ethnicity, religion, gender, disability, language, education and geographical location. The chapter highlights the role of family and kinship networks that determine gender norms and socialisation patterns including the role of school, community and societal practices such as gender-based violence in personal and public life, restriction of career choices by parents and after marriage by the husband and in-laws, sexual harassment at workplace, customs and traditions that degrade human beings and make them feel unwanted, children pressurised to perform beyond their willingness and abilities, dehumanising sex stereotypes that promote son preference, aversion to daughters and stigmatisations of the sexual minorities/transgender persons, educated women not allowed self-actualisation by pursuit of knowledge face mental health problems manifesting in depression, loss of interest in life, feeling of hopelessness, suicidal tendency etc. It also covers the issues of populations with intersectional vulnerabilities such as Dalits, ethnic-religious-sexual minorities, survivors of sexual violence, persons with disabilities, poor and unemployed facing discrimination, dehumanisation and exclusion from social spaces that result in acute mental health challenges. The uniqueness of this chapter lies in its extensive mapping of the successful initiative of Women's Grievance Redressal Cells (WGRC), a project by Mohalla Committee Movement, Mumbai. The chapter also makes eclectic suggestions including micro, mezzo and macro interventions to enable respect for gender diversity and plurality in order to ensure inclusive family and community-based structures that promote and ensure overall mental well-being. It thrusts on creation of systems and structures that promote intersection justice through gender inclusive mental health legislations and rules, data driven and evidence-based policy, affirmative action backed by adequate funds, clearly defined functions and competent and empathetic functionaries.

V. Patel (✉)
Distinguished Faculty, Impact and Policy Research Institute, TISS and SNDT Women's University, Mumbai, India
e-mail: vibhuti.np@gmail.com

M. Anand (ed.), *Mental Health Care Resource Book*,
https://doi.org/10.1007/978-981-97-1203-8_3

Keywords Family · Kinship networks · Socialisation pattern · Community · Intersectional vulnerabilities · Mental health law and policy

Introduction

Personal well-being, effective social development and harmonious functioning of the community rest on the foundation of the mental health. This fundamental notion of mental health is unswerving with its extensive and speckled interpretations across diverse tenets and geographies (WHO, 2004). The interplay of social, cultural, emotional, psychological and biological factors determine the mental health and mental illnesses. Socio-cultural elements of mental health in the industrialised world and in the post-colonial societies are found to be directly related to intersectional vulnerabilities of class, caste/race/ethnicity, religion, gender, disability, language, education and geographical location. Now there is an official recognition that *'Mental health problems are both a cause and a consequence of several disorders, non-communicable diseases, addiction problems, injury and violence, social problems and are linked to social determinants of health'*. (Gururaj et al., 2016). The lived experiences of structural and systemic violence, inter-community conflicts, discrimination in the society, economic insecurity and hopelessness generated due to lack of self-actualisation and feelings of self-fulfilment, inability to cope with the swift social-economic change, and the perils of political violence and chronic physical ill-health result in varied forms of mental health challenges leading to social isolation, abandonment by family members and friends. The mental health practitioners have rightly averred, 'No health without mental health'. Mental health is an inseparable part of overall health and contributes to the productivity of an individual, the economy and the functions of society.

Social Determinants of Mental Health

Systems and social structures impact mental health that underwrites both material and immaterial, fundamental values for the individual, society and culture. They impact biological, psychological, social and environmental factors that result in the mental health status and productivity of an individual and society. Structural and systemic aspects include social institutions such as family, kinship network, community life, economic aspects that include the nature of paid and unpaid work, employment status, income, occupational health and safety, labour processes and employer-employee relations, macroeconomic policies and cultural factors that include diversity, customs and traditions. Their responses determine mental health/ill-health and quality of well-being. Safe living environments, secured employment and quality education, constructive leisure-time activities and self-actualisation through channelising of creative potential prove to be supportive of positive mental health that ensures harmonious community life based on the foundation of social solidarity. Community participation resulting in social capital empowers individuals to manage their thoughts and cope with stressors without self-harm, as experienced in the self-help groups of marginalised communities in urban, rural and tribal areas (Patel, 2009).

The social determinants of mental health can be classified as disabling and enabling factors that are connected with the mental health of individuals and population groups. The social workers, counsellors of helplines for children, women and people in distress have revealed that exposure to stressful situations such as illness, deaths, loss of livelihoods and confinement to the home of all family members resulting in massive domestic violence as experienced during the COVID-19 pandemic, post-natal stress for a women especially if a girl is born, caste and communal riots, civil war and cross border wars, natural disasters such as floods, deluge, drought, famine, cyclones, desert storms result in post-traumatic stress disorders. They trigger mental health problems and intensity of long-term illnesses (WHO, 2022).

While enabling factors boost and guard mental health, reduce the likelihood of psychosomatic illnesses and empower both individuals and the community to deal with stressors and enjoy family life as well as community/social life. The interplay of internal protective factors such as individuals' temperament as well as the external factors such as social, economic and environmental eco-system at macro-meso and micro levels determine everyday lives in homes, neighbourhoods, schools and colleges, workspaces and in recreational events (Graham et al., 2008). Thus, the enabling factors for mental health facilitate social, cultural, human and economic capital of every society.

With this perspective in mind, all nation-states have acknowledged the creation of systems, structures and mechanisms to address mental health challenges in the post-pandemic period by allocating funds, functions and functionaries to support helplines for children, young adults, women, sexual minorities, lonely elderly, unemployed men and women forced into domesticity due to increased burden of unpaid care work (Sagar et al., 2020). Acknowledging the spike in mental health problems, the Union Budget of India has allocated Rs. 747 crores for mental health care with a specific focus on the National Tele-mental Health Programme managed by the Indian Institute of Technology, Bangalore, to provide 24 × 7 free counselling and care to people (Tandon, 2022).

Mental health can be considered as a distinct resource, enriching a person's value of life, and can be augmented or reduced by the acts of society. A facet of virtuous mental health is the capacity for reciprocally beneficial and continuing affiliations. There is mounting indication that social unity is significant for the pecuniary bourgeoning of communities and this connection is indeed communal.

Though the idea of mental health is collective, its countenance varies individually, ethnically, and in relation to diverse socio-political contexts. Hence cultural responsiveness is very important to comprehend a specific community's perceptions of mental health prior to making interventions on mental health. The broad nature of mental health also means that it is not only the specialists in the mental health profession but family, community and social networks have an important role to play in the mental well-being of individuals.

Manifestations of Mental Distress

Domestic Violence

Verbal, emotional, psychological physical, economic and sexual violence by the partner and ex-partner, immediate family members, other relatives and family friends can strike a major blow on the mental health. Disparaging condemnation and vocal abuse such as shouting, screaming, mocking, condemning, alleging, name-calling and verbally intimidating can generate mental distress. While counselling the survivors of domestic violence, may they be women, children or elderly; it was reported by them that pressure tactics in the form of sulking, intimidating to deny money, disengaging the phone, taking away the car, committing suicide, separating the children, account them to welfare agencies as 'mentally unstable' unless the victims comply with the tormentors' demands regarding raising the children, misreporting and lying to victims' peers and family, robbing the victims of any decision making power in the day-to-day matters as well as future life. Another major problem encountered in the violent power relations in the domestic arena is disrespect, i.e. persistently putting down the victim in front of family members, guests, neighbours, relatives, colleagues, friends and strangers; not listening or retorting when the victim talks, intruding telephone calls, taking money from victims purse/ bank account without permission, declining to help with housework, childcare and deliberately being disrespectful towards victim's friends, colleagues and relatives. Breaking trust in terms of lying, withholding information, being envious, having other surreptitious relationships, and breaching promises, appointments and shared agreements results in a deep psychological scar. Isolating a victim of domestic violence by monitoring or blocking his/her telephone calls, forcing restrictions on movement and meetings and preventing from seeing friends, colleagues and relatives forces the victim into silence. Stalking/following, opening e-mail/WhatsApp/letters, recurrently spying on calls, and disconcerting the victim in public by the family member is other humiliating form of harassment that results in anxiety and loss of self-esteem among the survivors of domestic violence. The family members threaten the victim by making fuming gesticulations, using corporeal size to coerce, uproar the victim down, damaging the belongings, breaking items, perforating walls, using a knife or a gun, bullying to kill or damaging the victim and the children makes the survivor loose self-confidence and get overpowered by fear-psychosis. The research of the women survivors of sexual violence at the One Stop Crisis centre located in the public hospital in Mumbai revealed that their partners were using strength, threats or coercion to make them perform sexual acts, had sex with them against their will and were intimidated by any degrading treatment based on their sexual orientation (Bhate-Deosthali et al., 2022). Along with rape they also faced physical violence in terms of smacking, hammering, biting, punching, pinching, pushing, kicking, pulling hair out, pushing, burning and asphyxiation. On top of this, when the survivors somehow managed to approach the neighbour/relative/police, doctor, the tormentor denied that the abuse happened and resorted to victim blaming. Display of split personality by the tormentors-cruel in private and gentle in public or guilt-tripping the victim by crying and pleading for mercy, saying it will never happen again were commonly found in domestic violence by the counsellors (CEHAT, 2017).

As per the Protection of Women from Domestic Violence Act, 2005 the criminal justice system of India recognises ‘cruelty’ as starving the victim by denial of food, persistent demand of willful sexual conduct, continually locking a woman out of the house, not allowing access to children thereby leading to psychological agony, physical violence, provoking, demoralising instigating mental anguish, constraining the woman at home and not consenting for her to have her routine interactions with others around, abusing children in their mother’s presence with the intent of causing her mental torture, repudiating the paternity of the children with the goal of imposing mental agony upon the mother, and intimidating divorce unless dowry is given. Continuous gender sensitisation has made some dent in countering misogyny and toxic masculinity and their implications for the mental health of the aggrieved party in the judgements of the Family Courts, Session Courts, High Courts and the Supreme Court of India but still we have a long way to go.

Mental Stress at the Workplace

Workplace stress due to excessive workload, insensitive colleagues and micro-management by the boss creates a toxic work environment. Suspicion, one-upmanship, spying on each other and mercenary instinct fuelled by a cut-throat competitive eco-system create atomisation of the individual which have adverse effects on the employees’ mental health, with an increased risk of anxiety, burnout, depression, micro-aggression and substance abuse disorders. Individuals-men, women and transgender persons who are stressed at work are more likely to engage in unhealthy behaviours, such as cyberbullying smoking, alcohol and drug abuse, and poor dietary patterns. Cyberbullying via a phone, computer or any electronic device is an unkind peer behaviour done purposely, recurrently and with the intent of hurting the other person. In the case of women, cyberstalking becomes a sexual harassment (Mariwala Health Initiative, 2022). Transgender persons have also reported extremely demeaning forms of sexually aggressive behaviour from men and derogatory and prejudicially attitudes of women colleagues and superiors at the corporate houses. At times, both, aggressors and their targets are in the mentally stressed condition. This situation can also result in verbal or physical violence.

Mental Stress in Schools and Colleges

Educational institutions are workplaces for students. Ragging by seniors, humiliation by teachers, persistent derogatory remarks, casteism, communalism, sexism, ableism, colourism and racism vitiate the environment in the educational institutions. As a result, the mental stress of students is also expressed by self-inflicted injuries and suicidal ideation and in many instances actual suicides. The school and college counsellors and community-based social workers have reported that the survivors of child sexual abuse become anorexic and bulimic and indulge in bodily harm.

Suicide

Rates of suicides are considered important indicators of mental health distress, serious psychological state and psychiatric illness. The recent pandemic has resulted in changes in our lifestyles, daily routines, patterns of social interaction and changes in mindsets about paid and unpaid work, online education and physical distancing resulting in social isolation. This has resulted in feelings of tension, worry, stress, insecurity about the future, anxiety, emotional numbness and chronic sadness. The volunteers running telephonic helplines have reported manifestations of mental distress in terms of feelings of exhaustion, chronic headache, change in appetite, disturbed pattern of sleep, weakened immune system, stomach ache, body ache, procrastination, forgetfulness, disorientation, inability to concentrate, withdrawal from social life, easily agitated/irritated, sense of worthlessness, absenteeism from work culminating in suicide. Avers (Singh, 2021), 'While illness was the most attributed cause behind suicide, daily wage workers made up the largest share of total suicides, shows NCRB data. A total of 37,666 daily wage workers died by suicide in 2020—accounting for one-fourth of total suicides'. Fig. 3.1 shows the year-wise suicides reported in India.

There are studies showing strong associations between social solidity, suicide and anti-social behaviour. Disparities in anti-social and suicidal behaviour have been outlined as strengths or absences of social cohesion (OECD, 2001). Feeble social controls and the interruption of local community organisations have long been conjectured to be features producing augmented rates of suicide (Durkheim, 1897). Not being allowed to choose a career, toxic workplace, ill-treatment of Dalits, menstruating women, widows, and childless women in the name of custom and tradition, pressure to perform/score high ranks, sex stereotypes imposing restrictions on adolescent girls and talented women have resulted in the loss of lives via suicides (Radhakrishana & Andrade, 2012).

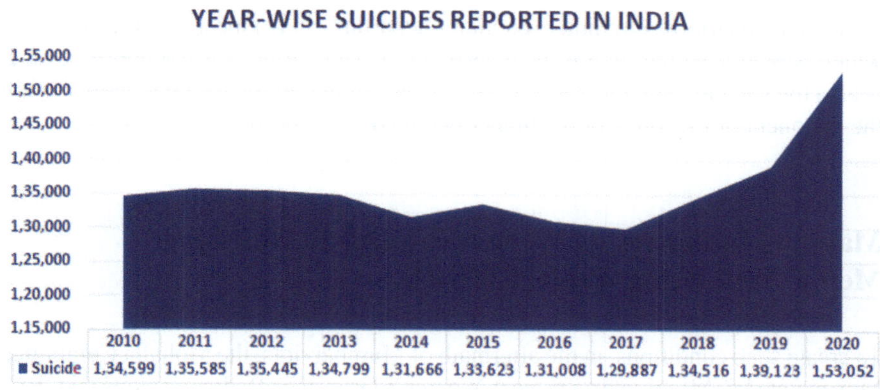

Fig. 3.1 *Source* https://www.news18.com/news/india/india-lost-more-people-to-suicide-than-coronavirus-in-2020-shows-ncrb-data-4388651.html

Mental Distress Due to Conflicts with Neighbours and Clashes in the Community and Commendable Efforts by Women Towards Establishing Mental Well-Being

The vicissitudes have been accelerated by the motion of individuals and the accessibility of instantaneous channels of communication. The swiftly changing world brings innumerable cultures in contact, enabling exchanges and impacts. The inter-mingling and amalgamation of cultures make their understanding important from the perspective of mental health (Sarkar and Varghese, 2017). Mental distress as a result of caste and communal riots has been documented extensively by the UNHRC, NHRC and social scientists.

There are inspiring case studies of women in the communities that have been mainstays of peace-building, peace-making and peace-keeping in the aftermath of the Mumbai riots in 1993. Women's response in the bustees of Mumbai to the proponents of 'World Peace' was *'Peace begins from home'*.

Peace may have dual forms, viz., Public and private. Peace at the level of community goes hand-in-hand with the peace at the level of family and therefore there is an urgent requirement to tackle the issue of domestic violence and women's complaints. There may be an ostensive steadiness and absence of struggle in situations of efficacious intense repression-beating, abuses, and emotional torment wherein all dissension is cruelly, instantly and surgically stifled. This is a state in which only one group (men, in-laws, bully neighbours) governs, in which women's understandings and poise are not permitted to exist.

Another scenario is the one in which egalitarianism and human rights attain acme in each and every core of the community and domestic lives. It is a situation in which there are always paths for settlement of disagreements without breaking the context of mutual respect, acknowledgement of the rights of the other, and credence in good faith of the 'adversary'. It is the situation in which conciliations and coaxing are the techniques for overcoming even major departures in perspectives. It is a state in which people have the right to be diverse and where variance is not deprived of. It is also the state in which variance is not a cause of hierarchy, where the other is not the opponent or the lower or the higher being (Barve, 2003).

Mapping Initiatives by Women Towards Establishing Mental Well-Being: Project WGRC

To create such conditions, in the aftermath of Mumbai riots, the Mohalla Committee Movement (MCM) initiated a project-Women's Grievance Redressal Cells (WGRC) in March 1997, first at the MIDC and on 2 April 1998 in Andheri (E) to enable women of different communities to come together on a common platform.

- **Distressing condition of women in the community**

While working in the community, MCM activists realised that women were doubly oppressed, both socially and economically and hence needed an outlet to voice their grievances. Most of the women-led submissive lives and suffered in silence. Ironically, even though communal harmony prevailed in the area, marital conflicts disturbed the peace and tranquillity of the families. Many of them had to face physical violence in their personal lives.

Even so they were apprehensive of lodging a complaint at the police station, either out of fear of society or due to fear of retaliation/backlash from the family members, especially husbands. It was in this background that the members of MCM along with the police conceived the idea of WGRC in order to help women in distress (Thakkar, 2004).

These Cells made the people aware of a common link between women and the community they live in. As a result, effective outreach programmes were developed, and major extension activities were initiated to promote peace, communal harmony and constructive activities for area development. These Cells, being projects of MCM are working in collaboration with the local police and 3 NGOs function twice a week at the MIDC and Andheri (E) police stations.

Awe inspiring experiences of these two Cells, motivated the members of MCM to start similar Cells in Bandra, Nagpada and Worli.

- **Objectives of Women's Grievance Redressal Cells (WGRC)**
- To work with individual women and men, families, groups and communities to create harmonious gender relations and to promote an ethos of cultural pluralism.
- To give the women a listening ear and to take cognisance of the offences perpetrated on them.
- To coordinate with the police in cases of crimes against women.
- To conduct training programmes/workshops for women as well as their family members on a wide range of issues and themes concerning multicultural existence, developmental problems and skill and capacity enhancing projects.

- To network with women's organisations and other like-minded organisations for collaborative work.
- To facilitate and mediate out-of-court settlements and if needed, to organise legal services for women at affordable rates.
- **Approach of the WGRC**

As the thrust of the Cell is on mediation and reconciliation, all the concerned parties are invited to the Cell and given a fair chance to voice their grievances against each other. Some of the meetings can be very time consuming. However, in some cases, the redressal process is shorter, and cases quickly get resolved.

Due to the consistent activities of MCM in the community, the Women's Cell could get easily established and legitimised as many women who approached the Cell were also members of MCM and attended MCM meetings regularly in their respective beats. The following examples delineate the processual dimension of WGRC's intervention:

a. ***Easing of tension between Hafeeza Shaikh and Vimal Pawar (MIDC)***

For several years, Hafeeza and Vimal were at loggerheads. Even though their fights revolved around issues such as garbage and drainage, their anger and hatred towards each other was immense. Both had lodged complaints and counter complaints against each other at the police station. But to no avail, the animosity between the two continued to prevail. Finally, the duty officer at the police station asked them to visit WGRC.

On visiting the WGRC, both complained bitterly against each other. While Vimal blamed Hafeeza of witchcraft, Hafeeza blamed Vimal for provoking the fights and instigating the neighbours against her. It was evident that both did not want reconciliation. It was a Herculean task for the members of the Cell to bridge the gap between the two as they belonged to two different communities. However, after a continuous dialogue with them at the end of the third session, both agreed to bury the past and forgive each other. The Cell members were jubilant as they were able to resolve the problem that existed for many years and most importantly they were able to bring about peace in the area, especially since Hafeeza's was the only family from the minority community living in a majority dominated area.

b. ***Reformed Swami and relieved Vasanthi (Andheri)***

Vasanthi, a young girl, married C. Swamy in 2003. However, on the very next day of her marriage, her husband demanded money to set up his business. She was shattered. In order to keep her marriage intact, she borrowed a small amount of money from her father and gave it to her husband. Still he continued to harass her mentally and physically for more money. Moreover, he forcibly took her gold ornaments and sold them for a large amount of money. Torture by her husband was so her unbearable that she left her matrimonial home to live with her parents. Her parents felt so cheated by their son-in-law that they decided not to send Vasanthi back and decided to call of the marriage. It was at this point in time that distraught Vasanthi approached the Cell and related her woes to the members. Vasanthi's husband was subsequently called to the Cell and there was a major showdown between the spouses. The members made uphill effort to seek reconciliation between them. But it was only after the second session that Vasanthi's husband agreed to return the money and jewels and do a service job. After the third meeting both the spouses agreed to give their marriage a try and Vasanthi returned to her husband. They are in touch with WGRC and the Cell members have found that Swamy has changed for better.

- **Nature of Grievances**

  a. Marital conflicts (wife-beating, extra-marital relationships, alcoholism, unemployment, financial constraints).
  b. Problems concerning in-laws.
  c. Disputes with neighbours.
  d. Conflicts with kith and kin.
  e. Sexual problems (impotency, violent sexual encounter, pervasive and lustful behaviour).
  f. Love affairs resulting into elopement and marriage.
  g. Divorce, desertion, maintenance, illegal second marriages.

- **Legal Intervention**

The cases that could not be resolved through negotiation were either referred to the family court at Bandra or to individual lawyers. Some women filed their petitions in the family court for maintenance and divorce while others sought the help of their lawyers in connection with illegal marriages, child custody and dowry demand made by their husbands. An advocate from Tata Institute of Social Sciences (TISS) also helped with her legal expertise at the Cell at MIDC.

- **Teamwork between the Police and WGRC members**

In all the Cells, the police constables are a part of the team. Their presence helps WGRC to get a better insight on the problems faced by numerous women and moreover it gives an opportunity to empathise with the victims in need of help. The police also play an important role by visiting the home of the victim and inviting the spouse to the Cell for mediation.

- **Follow-Up Work**

WGRC visits the homes where the conflict is of a serious nature so as to assess the prevailing situation. If the relationship continues to be strained, the spouses are once again invited to the Cell for further mediation.

- **Empowerment of women through Education**

WGRC believes that public education is the major tool for women's empowerment. Hence, it organised five workshops on gender sensitisation at Bandra-Kurla police station for the police personnel of the west region. The team from the legal aid cell of the justice and Peace Commission conducted sessions on The Universal Declaration of Human Rights, laws related to women and crimes against women. The five-day workshop provided legal training to three hundred police personnel that included constables, sub-inspectors, inspectors and assistant commissioners of police. Even women police took an active part in the workshop which was divided into a lecture, a group exercise and a slide show.

WGRC has also organised workshops on women and health, counselling, legal provisions, communication skills and unlearning communalism through creative methods of role play, storytelling, group exercises, street plays, screening of films, vocational training programmes, *haldi kumkum samaroha*, rangoli and poster competitions and teaching precautions like first aid, fire extinguishing skills.

- **Commemoration of International Women's Day**

8 March, International Women's Day, which symbolises solidarity, sisterhood and strength of women, has been a focal point for women from all five Cells to meet at one place and get a feeling of empowerment. For the past seven years, the Cell has been celebrating this day with vigour and enthusiasm reflected in the singing of group song, experience sharing, presentation of annual progress report, speeches of dignitaries and children's stage shows. These events have instilled a feeling of confidence and leadership qualities in women.

- **Pre-emptive measures**

Knitting Communities together has been the most effective tactic for preventing communal conflagration. In 2002, after the communal carnage in Gujarat, there was a lot of tension in the community. Women Grievance Redressal Cell (WGRC) worked with the police and held meetings all across the city through the MCM. WGRC also participated in the MCM-organised painting competitions, cultural programmes on communal harmony, sports like volley ball, gymnastics and athletics, table tennis and 'cricket for peace' as friendly and healthy competitions to inculcate a spirit of recreation to counter cut-throatism and promote peace-making. After these programmes, many participants have expressed their feelings, 'Until now we were very scared and prejudiced about the police and did not feel we could approach them. But these past few days have helped us to overcome this.'

- **Study Rooms**

The other strategy implemented by the Mohalla Committees has been in the setting up of study rooms, as in many slum colonies young students do not have a quiet space where they can study. Often many of them need help with their studies. By using the classrooms of local municipal schools, which are free and unused in the evenings, the Mohalla Committees have been able to provide a much-needed service to their communities.

During the last twelve years of its existence, Women's Grievance Redressal Cells have played an important role in cementing the bonds between communities, spouses, neighbours and enlightened the youth. It is an acknowledged fact that WGRC has played a useful role in forging a meaningful relationship between individuals in the family and also expanded the meaning of family that encompasses the whole community. At the time of communal tension (at times of religious festivals, release of controversial films depicting inter-religious love marriage, during ongoing unsecular episodes happening elsewhere) both police and the Cell members play a proactive role and display courage of conviction to diffuse the tension. This has been possible due to the close and constant co-operation between the police and the Mohalla Committees.

The work of MCM has been successful only in areas where police officers have taken personal interest and have ensured that the right kind of people are inducted into the Committee. After 7 years of functioning of the WGRC, both the communities and the police have realised that the process requires constant vigilance and evaluation. WGRC members are torchbearers of women's dignity, bodily integrity and gender justice. Activities of WGRC have brought women's issues on the agenda of MCM. Now, members in the community accept that women's rights are human rights.

This experience of MCM needs to be replicated throughout the nation to establish mental well-being at the community level.

Promoting Mental Health

Positive mental health is defined as an effectual perception of reality, self-knowledge, exercise of voluntary control over behaviour, self-esteem and self-acceptance, the ability to form mutual and demonstrative associations and effectively contributing towards community and society (Barry, 2009).

A culture-specific method to comprehending and enlightening mental health may be unhelpful, however, if it assumes similarity within cultures and disregards individual variances. Today, most cultures overlap and are heterogeneous. The principles and actions of groups need to be understood in their political, economic, and socio-cultural contexts (Wertsch, 1991).

Stigma is a chief apprehension of people affected by HIV/AIDS and sexual minorities. Attempts to understand this group's concepts of mental health make a major input to evolving pertinent intervention programmes.

Social Capital and Mental Health

For social connectivity and mental health promotion, 'social capital', i.e. a set of shared values that ensures individuals to work as a collective to effectively meet challenges, stand by each other at the time of personal difficulties, economic distress and achieve a common concern. It goes beyond the attributes of 'physical capital' or 'human capital' to enhance individual productivity and focuses on the formation of social organisations such as networks, self-help groups, and associations that can act as their support structures (Bowles & Gintis, 2002). Social capital is determined by economic and social environments and is not an individual perception or resource. It can be exclusionary for non-members and marginal groups, and disproportionate demand on members of social organisations. Higher social capital may defend individuals from social isolation, create social safety, lower crime levels, improve schooling and education, augment community life and expand work consequences (Woolcock, 1998).

Exclusion from Social Space-Caste, Religion, Gender and Disability

While highlighting the pivotal role of intersectoral linkage for mental health promotion, WHO (2004) has rightly observed that the collective action of society, both state and non-state actors is vital for mental health improvement. Both state policies ear-marking government programmes and private institutions in sectors such as education, social justice, labour welfare, transport and communication, environment, housing, and media as well as health care can contribute towards the prevention and treatment of ill health.

Homophobia and Sexual Minorities

Discrimination against and Dehumanisation of the LGBTQIA + community demands serious attention from community-based organisations. At a macro level, collective action for the promotion of gender diversity in all spheres of life depends on consensus building to arrive at collective values as much as the quality of scientific evidence. Hence, the workshops on 'Unlearning Homophobia' that includes exercises such as role play, storytelling, street play, screening of documentaries and personal testimonies of gender-fluid individuals. In terms of action agenda, strong implementation of the National Mental Health Policy of India, 2020, creation of the supportive environment, allocation of funds-functions-functionaries for institutional support to meet the mental health challenges, strengthening community-based mental health care and public education for coping strategies with regards to mental distress of sexual minorities become imperative.

Mental Health Promotion Practices

Over last 40 years, social workers and mental health practitioners have developed many models of positive psychology that promotes interventions aimed at risk and protective factors in a culturally sensitive manner (Keyes, 2002). For example, connectedness to one's culture and land would be classified as a protective factor for Adivasi communities, while people from culturally and linguistically assorted backgrounds may come from societies where a focus on collective well-being is seen as protective for the individual. Macro interventions of creating supportive environments and implementing public policy for social security and social protection of the vulnerable population in terms of safe housing, nutritious means, improving access to education, strengthening community networks in terms of self-help groups, farmers cooperatives, improved infrastructure, workers welfare associations, group insurance can create an atmosphere of social solidarity, community-based efforts in terms of public education campaigns, improved urban infrastructure, and community policing not only prevent violence and promote mental health and well-being of the affected population (WHO, 2004).

Meso and Micro Interventions for Mental Health Promotion

At meso and micro level, successful efforts have been initiated by the feminist movements. One of them is the DILASA Model—A One Stop Crisis Centre (OSCC) for the treatment and counselling of women victims of violence in a public hospital. With the aim to sensitise the public health system to gender and violence issues, CEHAT and the Public Health Department of the Brihanmumbai Municipal Corporation established Dilasa at K. B. Bhabha Hospital, Bandra West. *Dilaasa* means Reassurance and it provides social and psychological support to women survivors of domestic violence. This Centre was set up in a peripheral public hospital in collaboration with Brihanmumbai Municipal Corporation (BMC). CEHAT continues to provide support in terms of counselling and allied services to survivors of domestic violence. The crisis centre model is being replicated in 13 other hospitals in Mumbai and in 6 states of India. In addition, the activities of OIOP focus on prevention of violence against women; community-based support systems for women survivors of violence, action research on violence faced by health care professionals and the violence which exists within the system. It also upscales the training function through regular 'Training of Trainers' programmes and a course for nurses on 'Gender Based Violence and their Role in Responding to the Survivors of Violence' (CEHAT, 2017).

There is a need for an affirmative action to protect girls, young and elderly women from domestic violence and establish human rights for women. The most important tasks in this direction are to improve women's economic capacities, strengthen and expand training and sensitisation programmes and replicate Dilaasa model of one-stop crisis centre housed in the public hospital to facilitate collective intervention of medical staff, police and NGO throughout the country, effectively use of the Media to build Public Awareness, design programmes for the batterers and address domestic violence through Education.

Conclusion

There is a need for an assenting action to shield girl children, young as well as elderly women from domestic violence and affirming the human rights of women. The most imperative tasks in this direction are to advance women's pecuniary capacities, reinforce and expand training and sensitisation programmes, reproduce the Dilaasa model of one-stop crisis centre housed in the public hospital in order to enable joint intervention of medical staff, police and NGO across the country, effectually utilise all forms of media to develop awareness among people, plan events and programmes for the batterers and address domestic violence through education.

Effective public health intervention and community participation can ensure the mental health of individual members. Macro policies regarding drug addiction, tobacco and alcohol consumption, nutritional interventions and advocacy busting the misconceptions about mental health, allocation of funds for mental functionaries-community-based counsellors, psychiatric social workers and doctors through budgetary allocations go a long way to address the mental well-being on a priority basis. The corporate governance also needs to take up the challenge of stress management, anger management and mental illnesses among their managerial cadre and employees seriously and include mental health concerns in their CSR agenda.

References

Barry, M. M. (2009). Addressing the determinants of positive mental health: Concepts, evidence and practice. *International Journal of Mental Health Promotion, 11*(3), 4–17.

Barve, S. (2003). *Healing streams: Bringing back hope in the aftermath of violence*. Penguin Books.

Bhate-Deosthali, P., Rege, S., & Arora, S. (2022). Women's experiences of marital rape and sexual violence within marriage in India: Evidence from service records, UK: *Sexual and Reproductive Health Matters, 29*(2). https://doi.org/10.1080/26410397.2022.2048455

Bowles, S., & Gintis, S. (2002). Social Capital and Community Governance. *The Economic Journal, 112*(483), 419–436. Retrieved August 5, 2022, from https://www.socialcapitalgateway.org/content/paper/bowles-s-gintis-h-2002-social-capital-and-community-governance-economic-journal-112-48

CEHAT. (2017). *Evidence on formal support sought by women facing domestic violence from Dilaasa Case Records*, Mumbai. Centre for Enquiry into Health and Allied Themes. Retrieved from August 2, 2022, from https://www.cehat.org/publications/indexlist/2/Journal%20Articles

Keyes, C. L. M. (2002). The mental health continuum: From languishing to flourishing in life, USA. *Journal of Health and Social Research, 43*, 207–222.

Durkheim, E. (1897). In G. Simpson, J. A. Spaulding, & G. Simpson, (Eds). (1951). *Suicide: A study in sociology.* Free Press.

Graham, T., Michele, T., & Law, A. (2008). Steps, challenges and lessons in developing community mental health care. *World Psychiatry, 7*(2):87–92. Retrieved August 01, 2022, from https://doi.org/10.1002/j.2051-5545.2008.tb00161.x. https://www.ncbi.nlm.nih.gov/pmc/articles/PMC2408397/

Gururaj, G., Varghese, M., Benegal, V., Rao, G. N., Pathak, K., Singh, L. K., Mehta, R. Y., Ram. D., Shibukumar, T. M., Kokane, A., Lenin Singh, R.K., Chavan, B,S,, Sharma, P., Ramasubramanian, C., Dalal, P. K., Saha, P. K. , Deuri, S. P., Giri, A. K., Kavishvar, A. B., Sinha, V. K., Thavody,

J., Chatterji, R., Akoijam, B. S., Das, S., Kashyap, A., Ragavan, V. S., Singh, S.K., Misra, R., & NMHS collaborators group (2016). *National Mental Health Survey of India, 2015-16: Mental Health Systems*. National Institute of Mental Health and Neuro Sciences, NIMHANS Publication No. 130

Mariwala Health Initiative. (2022). Cyber bullying& mental health: a resource. Retrieved August 4, 2022, from https://mhi.org.in/media/insight_files/CYBERBULLYING.pdf

OECD. (2001). *The well-being of nations: The role of human and social capital, education and skills*. OECD Centre for Educational Research and Innovation.

Sagar, R., Dandona, R., & Gururaj, G., et al. (2020). The burden of mental disorders across the states of India: the Global Burden of Disease Study 1990–2017. *The Lancet Psychiatry, 7*(2), 148–161. ISSN 2215-0366. https://doi.org/10.1016/S2215-0366(19)30475-4

Patel, V. (2009). Women's leadership in micro-finance: Issues and challenges. In P. Vibhuti (Ed.) *Discourse on women and empowerment*. The women press.

Sarkar, S., & Varghese, P. (2017). Cultural diversity and mental health. *Indian Journal of Social Psychiatry, 33*(4). https://journals.lww.com/ijsp/Fulltext/2017/33040/Cultural_Diversity_and_Mental_Health.1.aspx

Radhakrishana, R., & Andrade, C. (2012). Suicide: An Indian perspective. *Indian Journal of Psychiatry, 54*(4), 304–319. https://doi.org/10.4103/0019-5545.104793. Retrieved August 4, 2022, from https://journals.lww.com/indianjpsychiatry/Fulltext/2012/54040/Suicide__An_Indian_perspective.2.aspx

Singh, N. (2021). India Lost More People to Suicide than to Coronavirus in 2020 Shows NCRB Data. Retrieved August 4, 2022, from https://www.news18.com/news/india/india-lost-more-people-to-suicide-than-coronavirus-in-2020-shows-ncrb-data-4388651.html

Tandon, A. (2022). Budget 2022–2023: "Thrust on mental healthcare", Chandigarh, *The Tribune*. 1st February, Retrieved July 21, from 2022 https://www.tribuneindia.com/news/business/thrust-on-mental-healthcare-366229

Thakkar, U. (2004). Mohalla Committees of Mumbai: Candles in Ominous Darkness. *Economic and Political Weekly, 39*(6), 580–586. Mumbai.

Wertsch, J. V. (1991). *Voices of the mind: A sociocultural approach to mediated action*. Harvard University Press.

WHO. (2004). *Promoting Mental Health Concepts, Emerging Evidence, Practice*. A Report of the World Health Organization, Department of Mental Health and Substance Abuse in collaboration with the Victorian Health Promotion Foundation and The University of Melbourne. World Health Organisation

WHO. (2022). *World mental health report: Transforming mental health for all*. World Health Organization.

Chapter 4
Women's Mental Health: The Unchartered Terrain

Meenu Anand

Abstract Gender oppression is a dominant factor that impacts the development of and recovery from mental disorder. The current chapter begins by provenance of mental health differences between men and women to sex and gender distinctions and signifies the role of culture and development to gain a better understanding of mental health and illness. Unfolding the intricate entwining of individual, socio-cultural, as well as structural factors in society and its impact on psychiatric labelling, it necessitates a deeper understanding of socio-cultural factors in aetiology of mental distress, epidemiological inequalities in diagnosis of mental disorders and opportunities for treatment as well as remission. The chapter concludes by delineating significant multi-layered protective factors to promote mental health and well-being among varied sections of populations.

Keywords Gender · Mental health · Epidemiology · Treatment and recovery

Introduction

> The myths of gender work at so deep a level in us that it would take more than extraordinary personal awareness to bring them into the light of day… (Roszak in the book, The Gendered Atom, 1999, p. 154).

The interplay between sex and gender is an imperative factor in mental health. Understanding the intersections between gender and mental health, the dynamics of social roles and power has been the subject of scholarly debates in the contemporary socio-cultural milieu. Engrained in inheritances, anatomy and physiology, sex signifies a biological construct, while gender encompasses psychosocial variables that distinguish between women and men expounding societal conditions (Otten et al., 2021). Going beyond the biological distinctions in brains and bodies, an examination of the expanses of culture and development across the lifecycle offers a better comprehension of mental health and illness, and the intricate and sundry social worlds

M. Anand (✉)
Department of Social Work, University of Delhi, Delhi, India
e-mail: meenuanand75@rediffmail.com

M. Anand (ed.), *Mental Health Care Resource Book*,
https://doi.org/10.1007/978-981-97-1203-8_4

that constitute the lives of women and men, families and communities (Andermann, 2010).

The socio-cultural determinants of mental health collectively influence women across the complete life course, expose them to advanced risk factors and abridged access to prospects to protect their mental health (Srivastava & Anand, 2020). Women have historically been assigned roles that are more demanding, horrifying and intended to make them more committed, responsible, less valued and underpaid. They are also prevented from accessing knowledge that comes from exposure to the outside world, making them more vulnerable to exploitation. Since mental health is principally determined by varied socio-cultural constituents of health including gender, social status, employment, education, wealth and social support (Wilkinson & Pickett, 2009), gender profoundly affects socio-economic status, risk for mental illness and the progression of disease. *'Gender determines the differential power and control men and women have over the socioeconomic determinants of their mental health and lives, their social position, status and treatment in society and their susceptibility and exposure to specific mental health risks'* (World Health Organization, 2013).

The World Mental Health Report by the World Health Organization (2022) alludes to the interconnections between gender and mental health:

> Our gender......can affect our chances of developing a mental health condition. Women tend to be more socio-economically disadvantaged than men and are also more likely to be exposed to intimate partner violence and sexual violence in the community, which are strong risk factors for a range of mental health conditions, especially PTSD. Discrimination against a particular group in society increases the risk of social exclusion and economic adversity, both of which undermine mental health (World Health Organization, 2022, p. 22).

It becomes imperative to analyse and understand the individual, socio-cultural and structural factors prevalent in society and how these are inextricably entwined, consequently impacting mental health of people needs to be conceptualized.

Conceptualizing Gender, Mental Illness and the Day-To-Day Negotiations

Social and cultural variables that impact mental health play a vital role in creating power differentials thereby causing women's emotional distress. Pattadath (2018) quotes the feminist scholar Chesler's ground-breaking book titled 'Women and Madness' (1972) where she argues that *women's behaviour is typically devalued, rejected and pathologized—'women, by definition, are viewed as psychiatrically impaired—whether they accept or reject the female role—simply because they are women'* (Chesler, 1972, 115). Writing critically about biomedicine, she contends that the regimes of diagnosis and treatment of mental disorders are inextricably linked to modernity and its regimes of knowledge-construction based on depersonalized data. She investigates the agency of women labelled as mentally ill from a feminist viewpoint, focusing on the *everyday* as a place of experience. The importance of *everyday* is highlighted in the feminist critique of how women's lives are framed in terms of sickness more than men's. By juxtaposing her analysis against both the professionalized language of medicalization and pathologization, as well as the early feminist trope of viewing women's difficulties through the lens of patriarchal oppression, she identifies key lines of enquiry of translations and negotiations engaged in by women who are given a psychiatric labelling.

Ogundare (2019) argues regarding the centrality of culture to the aetiology of mental disorders (as it provides the ideals for defining normalcy), and the characterizations of what institutes a mental disorder (since these are socially and culturally negotiated). Culture impacts the experience, expression, progression and consequence of mental health challenges, help-seeking and the riposte to health promotion, prevention or treatment intercessions (Kirmayer, 2012). Significantly, DSM 5 is acquainted with the term 'cultural concepts of distress' (CCD) which comprehends three expanses, viz. culture syndromes, idioms of distress and cultural, explanations with the intent to rouse further understanding of the constructs and to facilitate its application in clinical practice and research (Lewis-Fernández & Kirmayer, 2019).

The gender perspective on mental disorders is also expounded by Okasha and Chandra (2009):

> ...The view is kaleidoscopic in that it is widened both physically and psychologically—where the disorder is viewed in a much larger context, and the multiple mirrors reflect images on each other. These images are those of the concepts of femininity and masculinity of cultural and social realities, of violence and safety, of social networks and isolation and of motherhood and the nurturing roles of women. A kaleidoscopic view logically reflects the many multi-faceted identities, which women have today and which keep changing based on the interplay of lights and mirrors in the form of roles, relationships, the impact of biology and finally, the state of society (Okasha and Chandra, 2009, p. 2).

Feminist scholars have brought attention to the gender differences and how they significantly affect the prevalence rate of common mental disorders in terms of the age of commencement of symptom, progression of the illness, incidence of symptoms and long-term consequences (Artal, 2019). Gender role stereotype, as hegemonic countenance of socio-cultural dissection of the sexes, has been observed to sturdily impact sex differences in mental health and illness. Women's and men's health-related behaviour and congregation of symptoms advance partly as a consequence of observance to schematized stereotypes about self and others' gender-specific roles (Paykel, 1994). Thus, gender differences gain prime importance with respect to the causation of mental distress/reasons for occurrence and prevalence of mental disorders, access to treatment and rehabilitation of the persons with mental disorders. It is also indeed imperative to bring in *the other* into the discourse on gender and mental health.

Negotiating the Binaries of Gender Scaffolding

Gender identity, or how people define themselves as gendered, is deemed as a recognized effect of the features of the body as role portrayal is governed by normative sex roles (Basu et al., 2018). More often, gender is perceived as a dichotomy based on binary sexes, which are archetypally divided into two discrete categories (male and female) gyrating around sex—which is bestowed at birth—in an embracement of the biological criteria used to classify an individual as male or female (e.g. genitalia, reproductive organs and chromosomes). It is typically related with and considered to fall into two immutable categories of femininity and masculinity and the attitudes, feelings and behaviours associated with a person's sex (Eisend & Rößner, 2022). Such examples of this throughout the larger environment are reiterated by the socializing agents including family, school, media, workplace, etc. The acceptable distinct personality traits and behaviours/mannerisms for men (e.g. being bold, tough, dominating, assertive, aggressive, being emotionally non-expressive, etc.) and women (e.g. being beautiful, nurturing, compromising, polite, being emotionally expressive, etc.) are taught to the children right from an early age. In children, this contradiction is also echoed by connotations between girls and boys through stereotypical activities (encouraging gentle/'light' task allocation for girls, tougher/'heavier' activities for boys), toy choices (dolls/kitchen sets for girls, cars/aeroplanes for boys). In adolescence too, the gender binary categories and constructs are reinforced by the popular culture, peer group and mass media (Leibowitz, 2018).

Judith Butler (1990) abjured the very idea of gender fixity implied in sex–gender division and considered sex as 'embodied gender'—the corporeal incarnation of discursively constituted (performative) gender. Butler argued:

> Sex and, thus, also gender are socially constructed, as a small percentage of the population does not have clearly identifiable sex organs at birth or has chromosomal typing that does not fit patterns associated with the male or female sex (i.e., intersex people). If gender is socially constructed, it can change over time and vary among contexts; thus, it should be considered a nonbinary concept (Butler, 1990, p. 33).

The discourse on non-binary identities has gained traction (Dickey, 2020) within the context of mental health. With increased visibility of transgender people in society, the DSM 5 too uses a language that is moved from the dichotomous classification of gender (binary male and female categories) in preceding versions towards a dimensional comprehension of gender identity and expression, i.e. gender along a spectrum (Leibowitz, 2018). Leibowitz and Janssen (2018) describe the recent/relevant terminologies that describe domains of gender and sexuality and the listing of gender dysphoria as a diagnostic entity in DSM 5. They allude to:

> Historically (and presently), transgender individuals have faced family rejection, high rates of homelessness and victimization and trauma, few opportunities for gainful employment, and significant interpersonal discrimination. Transgender individuals are more likely to receive inadequate health care and historically have been seen by mental health professionals as inherently mentally ill. As a result, particularly in regard to mental health concerns, individuals with negative experiences would be expected to avoid care, even when it could be beneficial (Leibowitz & Janssen, 2018, p. 8).

Research evidence reflects higher degree of mental health concerns among transgender people than in the general population (Dickey, 2020) as many transgender persons may feel hopeless, particularly when their family may not support their identity, which can lead to depression, self-harm and suicide attempts.

Tracing Epidemiological Inequalities in the Manifestation of Mental Disorders

World Health Organization (2022) necessitates the significance of understanding the individual, family and community and structural factors in the context of risk for mental health (Fig. 4.1). Individual characteristics including vulnerability, personality traits, self-concepts, coping strategies, status of education and available resources impact one's mental health. Familial and community-based factors such as structure, engagement in job, responsibilities at home, multifaceted tasks and related expectations, violence and poverty demonstrate the individual factors (Gu, 2006), e.g. women are socialized to be nurturing and adjusting, encouraged to be selfless while ensuring to fulfill and prioritize everyone's needs before own, to be flawless wives, dutiful mothers and colleagues (Sweeny & Taylor, 2022). In addition, the structural elements such as social discrimination, exclusion, health emergencies and climate change contribute to gender inequality in society and enhance the status of one sex's frequency of mental disorders as compared to the others. Women's struggles to provide and survive are aggravated with various socio-economic determinants like poverty, homelessness, lower status, roles and treatment in society.

A significant amount of evidence in psychological research also supports the conclusion that women are more vulnerable than men to have mental disorders (Gu, 2006), have higher rates of psychiatric treatment in mental hospitals, in-patient psychiatric treatment in general hospitals and outpatient care in psychiatric clinics than men (Gove and Tudor, 1973). Furthermore, a high incidence of psychiatric morbidity in women is linked to variables including poverty, domestic seclusion, powerlessness and patriarchal oppression. Maji and Dixit (2018) allude to the self-silencing theory that associates the construction of women's health and well-being with socio-culturally assigned gender roles and relational self of women. Based on their research through narrative analysis, they reiterate the vital affiliation between self-silencing and physical as well as mental disorders like depression, eating disorders, premenstrual dysphoric disorder and even physical conditions like cancer. It is apparent that health-related behaviours, as well as illness experiences of women, are creations of the social doctrine which encourages them to inculcate the feminine identity. Good (1998) cites the epidemiologic and anthropological data analysing distinct forms and groups of psychiatric disorders and psychological anguish among women as compared to men. She expounds:

> The origins of much of the pain and suffering particular to women can be traced to the social circumstances of many women's lives. Depression, hopelessness, exhaustion, anger and

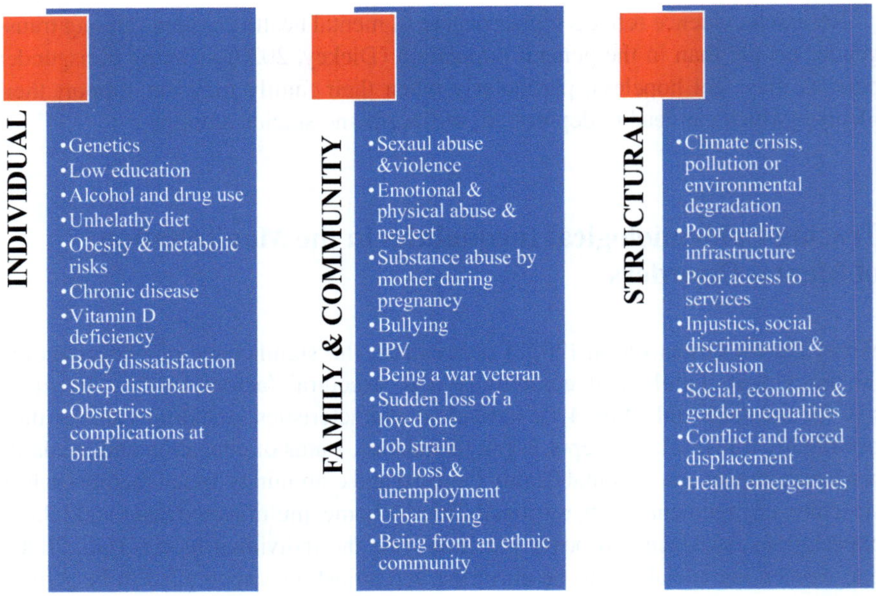

Fig. 4.1 Risk factors for mental health *Source* World Health Organization (2022). World Mental Health Report

> fear grow out of hunger, overwork, domestic and civil violence, entrapment and economic dependence. Understanding the sources of ill health for women means understanding how cultural and economic forces interact to undermine their social status.

Inequity and gender-based violence are perilous for an individual's mental health. Patel (2020) points to the diverse risk factors in terms of the psychosocial stressors that emanate from the external social environment such as women's inferior social status, lack of agency, homelessness, financial adversities, human-made or natural disasters. This produces learned helplessness (women's alleged acceptance or indifference towards predicament such as domestic violence, accidents, etc.) and abridged impetus to lead a vigorous life. Furthermore, strain-causing conditions like illness in the family, death of one's spouse, divorce and accident that might diminish or abolish women's capacity to take up responsibility can be detrimental to mental health and well-being. Furthermore, post-marriage, women get displaced that may lead to cultural loss, loss of social networks and support structures including the acquainted and trusted healing sites.

Chandhok and Anand (2020) further highlight the intricate connection between the effect of violence on women on their mental health based on the research evidence from a qualitative study to recognize numerous relationships between spousal violence and its impact on women's overall health and well-being. They expound the critical relationship between violence and mental health and how patriarchal structures of ascendency and subservience work in equivalence to each other. Comprehending the inherent affiliation between gender, violence and mental health, violence may be considered as the foremost motive for harm and injury against women and the most distinctive cause of depression among women (Zuchoswki, 2014).

Elucidating various factors, World Health Organization (2013) reiterated that *'Depression, anxiety, somatic symptoms and high rates of co-morbidity are significantly related to interconnected and co-occurrent risk factors such as gender-based roles, stressors and negative life experiences and events. Gender specific risk factors for common mental disorders that disproportionately affect women include gender-based violence, socioeconomic disadvantage, low income and income inequality, low or subordinate social status and rank and unremitting responsibility for the care of others. The high prevalence of sexual violence to which women are exposed and the correspondingly high rate of Post-Traumatic Stress Disorder (PTSD) following such violence, renders women the largest single group of people affected by this disorder'.*

Sweeny and Taylor (2022) explicate the pathologizing and biased consequences of clinical construal of maternal distress. Challenging the dominant cultural beliefs of women being the 'natural nurturers', they allude to:

> Motherhood has been characterised by intense and conflicting emotions: of love and loss; exhaustion and elation; guilt and gratitude; fear and fracture; mayhem and monotony; connection and isolation; and, often, of failure. It is a relentless experience of giving and doing what it can feel beyond our resources to give and do, day after day—no matter how exhausted, how desperately in need of respite (Sweeny & Taylor, 2022, p. 167).

Social hierarchies, limited access to resources, lower self-esteem, violence, poverty, lowered access to health care and resources and gendered relations reduce women's mental health and well-being render women 'at risk' for mental health conditions. Several risk factors including physical abuse, trauma, violence, perceived sexism, low self-esteem as well as lack of autonomy and lower income are associated with the onset of mental disorders in women (Zanca et al., 2022).

Translating the Asymmetry in the Prevalence of Mental Disorders

Gender balance in the prevalence of mental disorders is long known to be unequal as women and men are susceptible to diverse kinds of illnesses. According to the World Mental Health Report by the World Health Organization (2022), 13% of the global population is living with mental disorders. In the year 2019, there were 970 million people living with mental disorders out of which 47.6% were men and 52.4% were women. Anxiety disorders and depressive disorders emerged as the two most common mental disorders among women. In 2019, there were 301 million people across the globe living with anxiety disorders, while 280 million were living with depressive disorders (including both major depressive disorder and dysthymia). In 2020, these statistics rose pointedly owing to the COVID-19 pandemic. Globally, there was a greater increase in disorder incidence among females as compared to males. This may also be attributed to the fact that females were more likely to be impacted by the social and economic consequences of the pandemic.

Studies have unswervingly shown that women's experiential universes differ from men's as they are less exposed to external damage and trauma and more subject to chronic and daily challenges and adverse life transitions. Thus, psychosocial stressors and gender roles collectively assume singular significance in mental distress and wellness of women (Basu et al., 2018). There is a female multitude within the internalizing gamut which includes depression, anxiety, eating, post-traumatic stress and somatoform disorders. Men have higher rates of substance dependence, alcohol abuse and antisocial personality disorder (Artal, 2019; Gururaj et al., 2017). Furthermore, research evidence suggests that depressive and anxiety disorders are about 50% more common among women than men throughout the life course. As depressive and anxiety disorders account for most cases of mental disorders, overall, slightly more women (13.5% or 508 million) than men (12.5% or 462 million) live with a mental disorder (Zanca et al., 2022; Vindhya, 2001). Epidemiological studies report a sex ratio (women: men) of 2.1 for lifetime and 1.7 for point occurrence of major depressive disorder in adults. Women have a higher lifetime prevalence of mood and anxiety disorders than men, and a later onset of psychoses (Artal, 2019).

Mental disorders are also common among pregnant women and women immediately post the child birth leading to serious consequences for both mothers and babies. Globally, more than 10% of pregnant women and women who have just given birth experience depression (Khalifeh et al., 2015). In Lower Middle-Income Countries (LMICs), the same is appraised to be significantly higher. Furthermore, women who experience intimate partner violence or sexual violence are predominantly susceptible to mental disorders owing to pertinent interrelatedness between oppression and depression, anxiety, traumatic environments including PTSD and suicidal ideation. Women living with a severe mental disorder are also much more likely to have experienced domestic and sexual violence during their life than other women (Woody et al., 2017).

Overall, women show higher clinical evidence, greater co-morbidity with other mental health conditions and a higher frequency of 'internalising' patterns. Men, on the other hand, show 'externalising' trends along with co-morbidity conditions with conduct and substance use disorders (Zanca et al., 2022). It may also be noted that men have not been the focus of most sociological enquiries related to the diagnosis and treatment of mental disorder in the same way as women. The chief elucidations for the under-representation of men in psychiatric statistics include men not being good at help-seeking behaviour; men being more likely to externalize problems (in crime rather than illness); and being dispirited from conceding distress; male doctors might be unlikely to see male distress as illness; and, finally, men having fewer real-life problems than women (Prior, 1999).

Contesting the 'Diagnosed' Psychiatric Identity

Within the bio-medical paradigm, illness is interpreted strictly according to the biomedical perspective based on the Diagnostic and Statistical Manual or the International Classification of Diseases rather than from a socio-cultural perspective or social interactionism. Pattadath (2018) questions the scrutiny of women's bodies through the psychiatric gaze, where their particular bodily behaviours are used to explain psychiatric diagnosis. For example, the inclusion of premenstrual syndrome (PMS) as a diagnostic category disregards the cultural influences, beliefs and experiences of specific corporeal processes for women. She argues:

> Situating women merely as 'objects' of scientific gaze excludes their voices and subjective embodied experiences. Does the recognition of mood changes during the menstrual period as a medical problem give any legitimacy to women's emotional expressions, or does it merely put their legitimate emotional expressions into a reductive and readily available medical category? (Pattadath, 2018, p. 298).

Contesting the eagerness of medical science to objectify women's suffering and label it as illness, Davar (1999) too questions that '*the defining criterion of PTSD is 'flashbacks' of the victimization episode (mental imaging, nightmares,* etc.*), and reliving the terror associated with that'* (Davar, 1999: 119). She reiterates the significance of understanding the psycho-social contexts within which violence is learned, fostered and sustained, and women in violent situations should not be encumbered with such intangible understandings.

Tactical Challenges of Treatment

When a woman's distress is interpreted as symptomatic of a mental disorder, attention is likely to focus on her body to the neglect of her social circumstances (Stoppard, 2000, p. 101). Women's psychiatric diagnoses are seen as a greater cause of damage to their children than their socio-economic circumstances. Gender norms reinforce their unequal position in relationships, which further reduces their capacities to negotiate their rights (Chandhok & Anand, 2020; Srivastava & Anand, 2020) and seek treatment.

Ogundare (2019) expounds the role of culture and its influence on how individuals manifest symptoms, communicate their symptoms and their willingness to seek treatment. Gender oppression is a dominant factor that impacts the development of and recovery from mental illness. Loganathan and Murthy (2011) in their study of 200 people suffering from schizophrenia, attending urban or rural psychiatry clinics in India explicate the role of gender with respect to stigma. Women described experiences of stigma in relation to marriage, pregnancy and childbirth and described stigma as more devastating, disabling, and life-limiting than the illness itself. Stigma influences not only the individual's anguish from mental disorder but also persons who are closely related to them. Family members and immediate caretakers experience shame, embarrassment, uncertainty about illness, stigma, psychological suffering, poor quality of life and difficult lives, deeply personalized and public stigma, lack of clarity of 'what to do' in times of crises and higher levels of stigma were experienced when expressed emotions are also high (Murthy, 2002). Thara and Srinivasan (2000) describe the associated stigma in the form of struggle in getting marriage proposals for other members of the family, fear of being eschewed away from neighbours and maintaining secrecy about the illness. Raguram et al. (2004) also report regarding the stigma in terms of getting the 'patient' married, difficulties for their relatives to get married and social omission of the caregivers. A qualitative study on families of women with schizophrenia who were separated from their husbands unveiled fears over long-term care of their ill children, (and grandchildren) and who would care for them after they were gone (Raguram et al., 2004; Thara et al., 2003).

Atal and Foster (2021) in their exploratory study to examine low-income women's perceptions of mental illness and its management found that women used the expression 'tension' to talk about mental illness and the same was based on gender-related stressors, particularly surrounding pressures related to motherhood, enduring poverty and domestic conflict. Approaches to handling tension were mixt and engrossed on the resumption of social roles.

Loganathan and Murthy (2011) examine the investigation of the correlation of gender to disability in schizophrenia by Thara and Joseph (1995), which discovered that men tended to be impaired in occupational functioning while women suffered in marital functioning (Shankar et al., 1995; Thara & Srinivasan, 2000). The research evidence by Seeman (1983) related this in terms of gendered educational and occupational expectations of parents' vis-a-vis their sons/daughters with schizophrenia leading to differing implications on the course and conclusion of the illness in men as compared to women. Also, due to the later age of onset of illness in women, parents of daughters with schizophrenia may tend to blame themselves less for their daughter's illness, which usually appears after the daughters have left their parental home. On the contrary, due to the younger age of onset of schizophrenia in men, parents of sons with schizophrenia may tend to blame themselves for contributing to their son's illness (Seeman, 1983).

Intricacies of Remission and Recovery

The colonial assumptions behind psychiatric treatment and the much-cherished recovery create a colossal gap in *'meaning making' of personal experiences within the healing disciplines, also compromises the choices on offer for supporting women who may express a need for such support* (Davar, 2020, p. 19). The diagnosed identity of the women plays a significant role in determining their 'immediate living spaces' thereby severely restricting their connections with the external world. The esteemed idea of living in 'one's own home' probably has its genesis in such contradictions emanating from the diagnosed status of these women. While not all diagnosed women are able to comprehend this valued dream, they slice out a space of their own within the margins of the institutional space 'allotted' to them or attempt to adapt and fit in.

Despite the strides made by the discourse on de-institutionalization in academic sphere, there is escalating institutionalization of persons with mental disorders. There is wariness towards translating the theoretical perspectives of community mental health at the grassroots and reluctance to rehabilitate the persons undergoing treatment in the 'real' world. Maitra and Survase (2020) narrate the experience at *Tarasha* (the field action project initiated by the Centre for Health and Mental Health, School of Social Work, Tata Institute of Social Sciences, Mumbai, India) of working with women living with mental disorders and efforts to enable their recovery and reintegration. They narrate the stigma experienced by women by quoting the statement of a parent while admitting the daughter with the organization *'Melee tar aamchi, Jagli tar tumchi' ('If she dies she is ours, if she lives, she is yours').* The quote eloquently describes the stigma attached to being a woman, mentally ill, single and pregnant! They explicate how the same was not the case when it came to men as they were granted leave of absence. Families awaited the return of the man's return as in most cases he was the breadwinner of the family, a head of the household, husband to his wife and as father to his children. While men's roles were inimitable, the same was not true for women as they could be easily castoff and substituted. More importantly, while families were quick to abandon women with mental disorders; in case of men, their wives continued to care for their husbands and rarely left him despite the mental illness. The same has been corroborated in another study by Schomerus et al (2012) covering 76 women with schizophrenia whose marriages had broken. Most had been abandoned by their husbands and very few received financial support, while others experienced thrashing, domestic violence, psychological agony and desertion. Many felt themselves as a burden to their own parents, and received antagonism from family members and their spouse.

It is clear from the aforesaid that gender plays a significant role in causation/ onset of mental disorders, treatment as well as rehabilitation of persons with mental disorders. Let us enumerate the protective factors for strengthening the mental health of individuals and the prevention of mental disorders.

Looking Ahead: Strengthening the Protective Variables

Mental health is an inherent part of individual and collective health and well-being and focuses on the need to transform attitudes, actions and approaches to promote and protect mental health and to provide and care for those in need (World Health Organization, 2022). At a time when the contemporary world continues to grapple with the disruptive reality of the COVID-19 pandemic, which has in addition to challenging global health systems aggravated the existing gender disparities across the globe. Gendering mental health indeed therefore gains prime significance and makes it imperious to have gender-sensitive and inclusive strategies with the active engagement of multiple stakeholders (Anand, 2022b). While science and technological invent are making newer and stronger strides aided by advancement in pharmacogenomics, psychosocial interventions and models of services should develop in parallel with equal speed and fervour.

Gender perspective in the context of mental health suggests an understanding of a braided entwining of estimated boundaries, with a view to unearth their rich effects on the socialization of a person. As a way of highlighting the complex nature of such a webbing, feminist, non-normative queer perspectives, it is imperative to reiterate how gender is inextricable and impacted by factors such as caste, class, religion, sexuality and their eclectic discernible impact on mental health. Basu et al. (2018) highlights the significance of social empowerment in promoting wellness that needs to be premeditated at the macro level in terms of broader socio-economic and work–family milieu to enable access by women to diverse resources, including autonomy over own body, thoughts and emotions.

Holistic gender-sensitive mental healthcare necessitates that mental healthcare planning, delivery, monitoring and quality improvement activities be apprised by knowledge and understanding of gender variations in men and women and their interrelationship with respect to childhood and adult life experiences (e.g. violence and abuse); day-to-day social, cultural, and family realities; expression and experience of mental ill health and treatment needs and responses. A comprehensive cross-sectoral approach is indeed crucial to address the social determinants of mental health through the realization of the human rights of women and girls (Anand, 2022a) rather than adoption of a biomedical lens towards mental disorders.

The gendered lens also provides a useful reflector for considering a slew of biological and social risk factors, not from the perspective of consolidating notions of women's inferiority, but to see men and women and the *Other* as 'equal but different' and address what factors are shared and their unique contributions to the biological, psychosocial and developmental impacts (Anand, 2022a; Wilhelm, 2014).

Gender disparities, discrimination, negligence and stigma all present challenges and barricades in caring for persons with mental health conditions and thus compromise their right to health. As stigma is universal, and the large number of efforts in different countries have not been able to address fully the stigma of mental illness, there is need to think of different levels of interventions. The same can be done by transforming the environments that impact our mental health and by evolving community-based mental health services capable of achieving universal health coverage for mental health (World Health Organization, 2022) with a specific thrust on the unique and specific needs of varied population groups.

References

Anand, M. (2022a). Gender and mental health: Traversing treatise. *Indian Journal of Social Psychiatry, 38*, 108–113. https://doi.org/10.4103/ijsp.ijsp_158_20

Anand, M. (2022b). Gendering Covid-19: Impact and strategies towards gender inclusive recovery. *Impact and Policy Research Review, 1*(2), 50–62. New Delhi: Impact and Policy Research Institute.

Andermann, L. (2010). Culture and the social construction of gender: Mapping the intersection with mental health. *International Review of Psychiatry, 22*(5), 501–512. Informa Healthcare.

Artal, F. J. C. (2019). Differences in prevalence of mental health with the inclusion of diversity, gender and lifespan. In S. Bährer-Kohler, B. Bolea-Alamanac (Eds.), *Diversity in Global Mental Health* (pp.7–17). Springer Briefs in Psychology: Springer. https://doi.org/10.1007/978-3-030-29112-9_2.

Atal, S., & Foster, J. (2021). "A woman's life is tension": A gendered analysis of women's distress in poor urban India. *Transcultural Psychiatry, 58*(3), 404–413. https://doi.org/10.1177/1363461520947836

Basu, J., et al. (2018). Gender and Mental Health: Masculinity, femininity, modernity and daily hassles as predictors of subjective well-being. In G. Misra (Ed.), *Psychosocial Interventions for Health and Well-Being* (pp. 313–333). Springer.

Butler, J. (1990). *Gender trouble: Feminism and the subversion of identity*. Routledge.

Chandhok, G., & Anand, M. (2020). Practicing strengths-based approach with women survivors of domestic violence. In M. Anand (ed.), *Gender and mental health: Combining theory and practice* (pp. 237–251). Springer Nature

Chesler, P. (1972). *Women and madness*. Avon Books.

Davar, B. (1999). *Mental health of indian women: A feminist agenda*. Sage.

Davar, B. (2020). Gender, depression and emotion: Arguing for a de-colonized psychology. In M. Anand (Ed.), *Gender and Mental Health: Combining theory and practice* (pp 19–32). Springer Nature

Dickey, L. M. (2020). History of gender identity and mental health. In E. D. Rothblum (Ed.) *The oxford handbook of sexual and gender minority mental health*. Oxford University Press.

Eisend, M., & Rößner, A. (2022). Breaking gender binaries. *Journal of Advertising, 51*(5), 557–573. https://doi.org/10.1080/00913367.2022.2109780

Good, M.-J. D. L. (1998). *Gender and mental health*. Retrieved from https://www.un.org/womenwatch/daw/csw/mental.htm

Gove, W., & Tudor, J. (1973). Adult sex roles and mental illness. *American Journal of Sociology, 77*, 812–835.

Gu, C. J. (2006). Rethinking the study of gender and mental health. *Graduate Journal of Social Science,* 3(1). Retrieved from https://gjss.org/sites/default/files/issues/chapters/papers/Journal-03-01--01-Gu.pdf

Gururaj, G., et al (2017). *National mental health survey of India, 2015–16: Mental health systems* (Publication No. 130). National Institute of Mental Health and Neurosciences. Retrieved from http://indianmhs.nimhans.ac.in/Docs/Report1.pdf.

Khalifeh, H., Moran, P., Borschmann, R., Dean, K., Hart, C., Hogg, J., Osborn, D., Johnson, S., & Howard, L. M. (2015). Domestic and sexual violence against patients with severe mental illness. *Psychological Medicine, 45*(4), 875–886. https://doi.org/10.1017/S0033291714001962

Kirmayer, L. (2012). Rethinking cultural competence. *Transcultural Psychiatry, 49*(2), 149–164. Sage. https://doi.org/10.1177/1363461512444673.

Leibowitz, S., & Janssen, A. (2018). Affirming and gender-informed assessment of gender diverse and/or transgender youth across development. In A. Janssen, & S. Leibowitz (Eds.) *Affirmative mental health care for transgender and gender diverse youth*. Springer

Leibowitz, S. (2018). Social gender transition and the psychological interventions. In A. Janssen & S. Leibowitz (Eds.) *Affirmative mental health care for transgender and gender diverse youth*. Springer.

Lewis-Fernández, R., & Kirmayer, L. J. (2019). Cultural concepts of distress and psychiatric disorders: Understanding symptom experience and expression in context. *Transcultural Psychiatry, 56*(4), 786–803. Sage https://doi.org/10.1177/1363461519861795.

Loganathan, S., & Murthy, R. S. (2011). Living with schizophrenia in India: Gender perspectives. *Transcultural Psychiatry, 48*(5), 569–584. Sage.

Maitra, S., & Survase, A. (2020). "Melee tar aamchi, Jagli tar tumchi" ("If she dies she is ours, if she lives, she is yours"): Tarasha's experience of working with women living with mental illness. In M. Anand (Ed.) *Gender and mental health: Combining theory and practice* (pp 193–206). Springer Nature.

Maji, S., & Dixit, S. (2018). Self-silencing and women's health: A review. *International Journal of Social Psychiatry, 65*(1), 3–13. Sage.

Murthy, R. S. (2002). Stigma is universal but experiences are local. *World Psychiatry, 1*(1), 28. Retrieved from https://www.ncbi.nlm.nih.gov/pmc/articles/PMC1489817/.

Ogundare, T. (2019). Culture and mental health: Towards cultural competence in mental health delivery. *Journal of Health and Social Sciences, 5*(1), 23-34. https://doi.org/10.19204/2019/cltr6

Okasha, A., & Chandra, P.S. (2009). Current themes in psychiatric disorders in women: Commentary. In P. S. Chandra et al. (Eds.) *Contemporary topics in women's mental health global perspectives in a changing society.* Wiley-Blackwell.

Otten, D., Tibubos, A. N., Schomerus, G., Brähler, E., Binder, H., Kruse, J., Ladwig, K.-H., Wild, P. S., Grabe, H. J., & Beutel, M. E. (2021). Similarities and differences of mental health in women and men: A systematic review of findings in three large german cohorts. *Frontiers in Public Health, 9*, 553071. https://doi.org/10.3389/fpubh.2021.553071

Patel, V. (2020). Urban women and mental health concerns in India. In M. Anand (Ed.) *Gender and mental health: Combining theory and practice* (pp. 129–142). Springer Nature.

Pattadath, B. (2018). Gender, mental illness and the everyday: Understanding the interface of psychiatry with the lives of women diagnosed as mentally ill. In G. Chadha & M.T. Jospeh (Eds.) *Re-imagining sociology in India: Feminist perspectives* (pp. 289–315). Routledge.

Paykel, E. S. (1994). Life events, social support and depression, ActaPsychiatra Scandinavia. In J. Lonnqvist & T. Sahi (Eds.) *Depression: Preventative and risk factors* (vol. 89 supplement 377, pp. 50–58). Munksgaard.

Prior, P. M. (1999). *Gender and mental health.* MacMillan.

Raguram, R., Raghu, T. M., Vounatsou, P., & Weiss, M. G. (2004). Schizophrenia and the cultural epidemiology of stigma in Bangalore, India. *Journal of Nervous and Mental Disease, 192*, 734–744.

Roszak, T. (1999). *The gendered atom-reflections on the sexual psychology of science* (pp. 154–155). Conary Press.

Schomerus, G., Schwahn, C., Holzinger, A., Corrigan, P. W., Grabe, H. J., Carta, M. G., et al. (2012). Evolution of public attitudes about mental illness: A systematic review and meta-analysis. *Acta Psychiatrica Scandinavica, 125*, 440–452.

Seeman, M. V. (1983). Schizophrenic men and women require different treatment programs. *Journal of Psychiatric Treatment and Evaluation, 5*, 143–148.

Shankar, R., Kamath, S., & Joseph, A. A. (1995). Gender differences in disability: A comparison of married patients with schizophrenia. *Schizophrenia Research, 16*, 17–23.

Srivastava, N., & Anand, M. (2020). Understanding gender and mental health. In M. Anand (Ed.) *Gender and mental health: Combining theory and practice* (pp 3–18). Springer Nature.

Stoppard, J. M. (2000). *Understanding depression: Feminist social constructionist approaches.* Routledge.

Sweeny, A., & Taylor, B. L. (2022). In P. Beresford (Ed.), *The rutledge international handbook of mad studies.* Taylor and Francis.

Thara, R., & Joseph, A. A. (1995). Gender differences in symptoms and course of schizophrenia. *Indian Journal of Psychiatry, 37*(3), 124–128.

Thara, R., & Srinivasan, T. N. (2000). How stigmatising is schizophrenia in India? *International Journal of Social Psychiatry, 46*(2), 135–141.

Thara, R., Kamath, S., & Kumar, S. (2003). Women with schizophrenia and broken marriages: Doubly disadvantaged? Part II: Family perspective. *International Journal of Social Psychiatry, 49*, 233–240.

Vindhya, U. (2001). Mental health care: A review of gender differences. *International Journal of Diabetes in Developing Countries, 21*, 86-95. Retrieved from https://rssdi.in/newwebsite/journal/2001_april-june/article4.pdf

Wilhelm, K.A. (2014). Gender and mental health. *Australian & New Zealand Journal of Psychiatry, 48*(7), 603-605. https://doi.org/10.1177/0004867414538678

Wilkinson, R. G., & Pickett, R. (2009). *The spirit level: Why more equal societies almost always do better*. Penguin.

Woody, C. A., Ferrari, A. J., Siskind, D. J., Whiteford, H. A., & Harris, M. G. (2017). A systematic review and meta-regression of the prevalence and incidence of perinatal depression. *Journal of Affective Disorders, 219*, 86–92. https://doi.org/10.1016/j.jad.2017.05.003

World Health Organization. (2013). *Gender and women's mental health: Gender disparities and mental health: The facts*. Author. Retrieved from https://www.who.int/mental_health/prevention/genderwomen/en/.

World Health Organization. (2022). *World mental health report: Transforming mental health for all*. Retrieved from https://www.who.int/publications-detail-redirect/9789240049338

Zanca, F., et al. (2022). Gender. In D. Bhugra, D. Moussaoui & T. J. Craig (Eds.) *Oxford textbook of social psychiatry* (pp.207–218). OUP.

Zuchoswki, I. (2014). Gender-based violence and mental health. In Abraham P. Francis (Ed.), *Social work in mental health: Areas of practice, challenges and way forward* (pp. 97-117). New Delhi: Sage publications.

Chapter 5
Biopsychosocial Approach to Mental Health

Ananya Mahapatra and Prerna Sharma

Abstract The biopsychosocial model emphasizes the unified and interactive roles of biological, psychological, and social factors in understanding illness origins and effects on individual recovery and health. This framework emerged mainly as a counter to the narrow focus of the medical model on illness, which prioritizes biological aspects and individual pathology in illness causation while neglecting the intricate interactions and mutual influences of psychological and external socio-cultural elements with internal biological factors. The current chapter outlines the theoretical underpinnings of the Biopsychosocial Model and its conceptual evolution in mental health. It further discusses the role of the biopsychosocial framework in conceptualizing mental disorders and formulating practical strategies that can be implemented in clinical assessment, patient care, service delivery, research, and policymaking. It also highlights the advantages of the biopsychosocial approach in integrating humanistic perspectives in service delivery, thereby fostering therapeutic relationships that consider the lived experience of patients and acknowledge their role in the treatment process. Furthermore, the chapter also covers the limitations of the Biopsychosocial Model in its current form and its implications in mental health care and research.

Keywords Biopsychosocial · Mental health · Mental disorders

Introduction

In 1977, George Engel proposed a novel theoretical perspective for conceptualizing health and illness called the Biopsychosocial Model as a counterpoint and solution to the reductionist and "overly biological" approach of the Biomedical Model of disease. Since then, the Biopsychosocial Model has expanded in its scope to

A. Mahapatra (✉)
Dr. Baba Saheb Ambedkar Hospital and Medical College, New Delhi, India
e-mail: nnyaa09@gmail.com

P. Sharma
Center for Excellence in Mental Health, IHBAS, New Delhi, India

M. Anand (ed.), *Mental Health Care Resource Book*,
https://doi.org/10.1007/978-981-97-1203-8_5

become an epistemological paradigm, an integrative philosophy of clinical care, and a guiding framework for medical training and service delivery. The Biopsychosocial Model, in its conception of health and disease, included the biological and objectively measurable physiological parameters internal to patients and a myriad of relevant domains related to their psychological state and social circumstances. For the first time, this model expanded the purview of the medical framework to include the patient's subjective experiences, their socio-cultural setting, and the nature and quality of patient-clinician interaction as relevant factors in determining clinical diagnosis, health outcomes, and in planning clinical care. From an epistemological point of view, the Biopsychosocial Model propounded that physical or mental illness cannot be reduced purely to aberrations of individual pathology at a fundamental biological level. They must be conceived holistically as the outcome of a complex interaction of multiple levels of an organism, including societal, socio-cultural, psychological, physiological, and molecular. In the last few decades, the Biopsychosocial Model has played a primary role in effecting a radical change in the medical framework to make it more inclusive and humanistic and to foster participatory clinician-patient relationships. However, the importance of this model lies in the fact that it espouses the same not just from philosophical or moral grounds but rather from a practical standpoint in its claim that these factors integrate and interact in complex ways to affect health outcomes directly. Since its inception, the Biopsychosocial Model has found widespread applications in conceptualizing numerous medical as well as mental disorders. Given the complex nature of suffering in mental disorders, the Biopsychosocial Model has been critical in conceptualizing psychiatric illness. Engel, on the other hand, claimed that the biopsychosocial model was a "blueprint for research, a framework for teaching, and a design for action in the real world of health care." However, despite its staggering contribution in highlighting the varied dimensions of suffering in informing scientific clinical method, many researchers have also critiqued it for lacking "*scientific coherence*," promoting eclecticism, and have deemed it ineffectual in offering solutions or practical applications to the conceptual problems in psychiatric diagnosis, as well as clinical research (Benning, 2015). So much so that it has been called the "*conceptual status quo of contemporary psychiatry*" (Ghaemi, 2009).

This chapter will describe in detail the evolution and concepts of the Biopsychosocial Model and its applications in the field of mental health.

History and Evolution of the Biopsychosocial Framework

Cartesian mind–body dualism proponents emphasized viewing the mind and body as entirely separate entities: one is non-physical (the mind) and the other physical (the body). Cartesian Dualism proposed a causal interaction between these two substances meaning that the actions of the mind can have physical consequences in the body (manifest as actions), and the actions of the body can have non-physical consequences in the mind (manifest as perceptions).

In the 1930s, endocrinologist Hans Seley proposed the General Adaptation syndrome to highlight the role of psychological and stress-related factors in dysregulating physiological systems leading to adverse consequences on health (Papadimitriou, 2017). As the foundational ideas of psychosomatic medicine began to take root, researchers such as Flanders Dunbar and Franz Alexander espoused the role of personality factors and psychological conflict in the causation of certain specific bodily disorders.

Ironically, the term biopsychosocial is claimed to have been coined for the first time by Roy Grinker in the 1950s (a neurologist who trained in psychoanalysis under Sigmund Freud) to emphasize the role of biological factors in the causation of mental symptoms that were otherwise ignored by *"psychoanalytic orthodoxy"* (Ghaemi, 2009).

In the late 1970s, George Engel, drawing from the principles of the General Systems Theory (Engel, 1977), emphasized that given the complexity of the processes of health and illness, medical disorders cannot be reduced primarily to physiological or bodily parameters and that "all three levels, biological, psychological, and social, must be considered in every health care task" (Engel, 1977). The General Systems Theory, was initially outlined as a new paradigm for scientific inquiry, based on the premise that complex systems share organizing principles that can be modeled and subjected to an investigation drawing from this theory, the Biopsychosocial Model seeks to explain "illness" or "disease" in an individual as an entity that is derived from an individual who is part of a more extensive system comprising of "sub-personal levels" (i.e., nervous system, organs, tissues, cells, etc.) and "supra-personal levels" (factors related to their psychosocial context) (Asokan, 2009). According to this model, the determinants of physical as well as mental health disorders are the result of an interplay between biological, psychological, and social factors—with no factor having a "monopoly" on the explanation and/or cure (Babalola et al., 2017).

While Engel proposed the Biopsychosocial Model as a *"new model for medicine,"* because of the inherent complexity and multi-factorial nature of mental disorders, it became one of the mainstream ideologies in the conceptualization of psychiatric disorders since the 1980s. The Biopsychosocial Model perhaps emerged as a bridge of reconciliation between the decline of psychoanalysis and the advent of psychopharmacology and the DSM-III which aimed to operationalize psychiatric symptoms (Shorter, 2005).

Limitations of the Biomedical Model of Illness

The need for a new medical illness model arose primarily because of the restrictive and reductionist approach of the biomedical model for conceptualizing health and illness. The biomedical model devised as an explanation for the concept of "disease" is a scientific model under which it is guided by a shared set of assumptions and rules of conduct derived from the scientific method and has been the dominant model for clinical inquiry and research. The Biomedical model posits that the disease process can be fully explained by aberrations or deviations from the norm of bodily/somatic parameters (i.e., physiological, molecular, genetic, etc.), independent of social behavior or circumstances. Furthermore, it also seeks to explain mental or behavioral aberrations as a product of disorder biological function at a neurochemical or neurophysiological level. The biomedical model is thus influenced by the philosophical concept of reductionism, which asserts that complex occurrences stem from a singular fundamental principle, and mind–body dualism. This belief distinguishes the mental from the physical (Engel, 2012). In its efforts to take an exclusively scientific and analytical approach to the disease process, the biomedical model tended to become restrictive and narrow in its focus. It is by nature dehumanizing not only by excluding subjective patient experiences from consideration but also because it is dismissive of the notion that the subjective experiences of the patient were amenable for scientific exploration as determinants of health outcomes.

Engel critiqued this restrictive viewpoint of "disease" for its failure to include the varied social and culturally derived belief systems, which cannot be explained by the scientific model but are nevertheless essential when considering a person-centered approach to health care tasks. Another major issue with the biomedical model of illness is that because of its reductionist orientation and excessive focus on objective measurable biological parameters, any factor which could not be objectively verified or explained based on bodily processes was devalued or excluded from consideration. This led to further dehumanization of the process of scientific inquiry and reduced the human subject to a sum of its isolated organs and molecular functioning. This also furthered the implicit assumption that biological factors are more "real" than the factors related to the patient's subjective existence and are, therefore, more worthy of scientific observation and consideration.

The cold and impersonal biomedical orientation towards illness also leads to clinical service delivery practices which tend to overlook the human aspect of suffering. The biomedical model also neglects the role of empathy in clinician-patient interaction and is deemed to be disempowering for patients.

Engel in his seminal work (Engel, 1977), challenging the limitations of the biomedical model, pointed out that it had become a "cultural imperative" and achieved the status of dogma in Western medicine's conceptualization of disease: "*In science, a model is revised or abandoned when it fails to account adequately for all the data. A dogma, on the other hand, requires that discrepant data be forced to fit the model or be excluded. Biomedical dogma requires that all diseases, including "mental" diseases, be conceptualized in terms of the derangement of underlying physical mechanisms. This permits only two alternatives whereby behavior and disease can be reconciled: the reductionist, which says that all behavioral phenomena of disease must be conceptualized in terms of physicochemical principles; and the exclusionist, which says that whatever is not capable of being so explained must be excluded from the category of disease.*" The fundamental limitations of the Biomedical Model are listed in Table 5.1.

Table 5.1 Limitations of the biomedical model for mental illness

1. The biomedical model's reductionist perspective, which views all behavioral symptoms as stemming from biological malfunctions, fails to account for all aspects of a disorder adequately
2. This model leads to a dehumanized approach in medicine, concentrating solely on the disease and neglecting the unique characteristics of each patient
3. The model's principle of categorically excluding certain conditions from being classified as diseases is indefensible
4. By attributing mental disorders to brain structure anomalies, neurotransmitter imbalances, or genetic defects, the biomedical model has been unable to pinpoint any consistent biomarkers for specific psychiatric conditions
5. Major psychiatric classification systems like the DSM or ICD do not include biological testing for identifying, diagnosing, or categorizing psychiatric disorders, and there are no valid, reliable biological tests for diagnosing psychiatric illnesses
6. The uniform treatment methodology of the biomedical model contrasts sharply with a patient-centered approach in mental health care

Need for a Biopsychosocial Framework for Mental Health

Although initially proposed as a "new model" for all medical illnesses, the Biopsychosocial Model has been deemed especially crucial in conceptualizing psychiatric disorders. Since the mid-nineteenth century, the crisis of elucidating the nature and validity of psychiatric illnesses has led to the development of two radically divergent schools of thought. First, the Szazian "exclusionary" viewpoint considers mental illnesses to have an exclusively social origin, deems the concept of mental illness as a "myth," and calls for its exclusion from the jurisdiction of medicine. Second is the reductionist biomedical approach, which, in its efforts to legitimize the position of psychiatry as a discipline of medicine, seeks to explain all behavioral phenomena as a function of the neural and physiochemical processes (Engel, 1977). This called for the need for a new paradigm to take into account the various dimensions of mental and behavioral disorders—biological, psychological, social, and behavioral. A linear cause-effect model cannot explain the complexity of causation and clinical manifestation of psychiatric disorders. There are multiple interacting causes and contributing factors in varying dimensions—biological, social, cultural, and psychological—that determine the final clinical manifestation, course, and outcome of a psychiatric disorder. A Biopsychosocial approach to a psychiatric illness attempts to take into account these levels of interaction while formulating a psychiatric diagnosis and intervention. Figure 5.1 illustrates how biological, psychological, and social factors interact at multiple levels to determine mental health. It is important to note that a complex web of interaction exists amongst the various factors included in the different dimensions, and within the developmental trajectory of an individual's life, new factors are continually included that interact and affect the complex system of interactions between the existing factors.

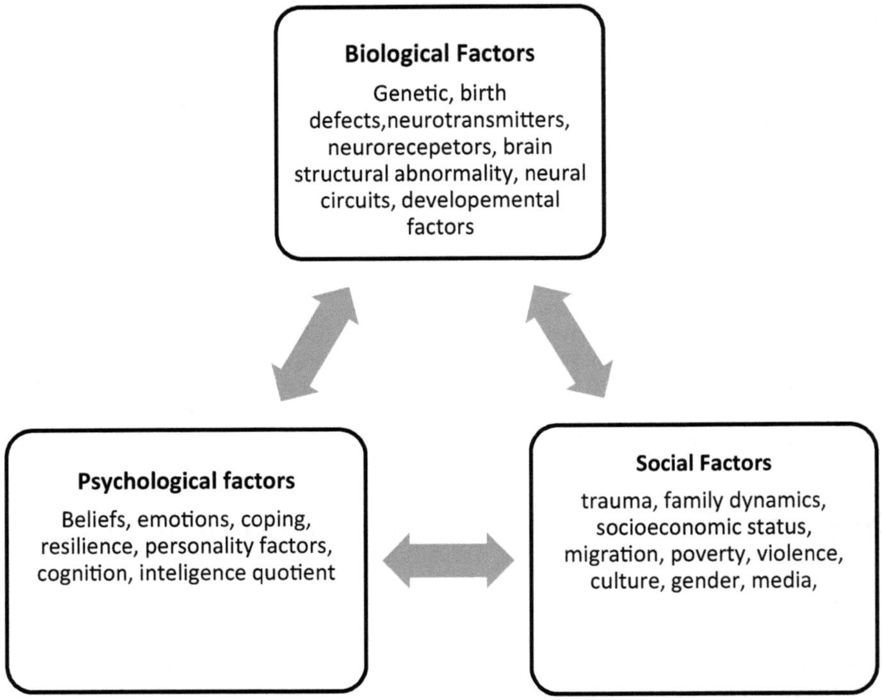

Fig. 5.1 The biopsychosocial model of mental health

Example of a Biopsychosocial Approach to a Mental Health Disorder

To further illustrate the Biopsychosocial Approach in conceptualizing a mental health disorder, let us consider the example of Schizophrenia. Schizophrenia is a severe mental illness that can progress to a chronic debilitating course. It is primarily a psychotic disorder that may present with positive symptoms (hallucinations, delusions), negative symptoms (anhedonia, asociality, alogia), disorganization, and cognitive deficits (executive dysfunction, social cognition deficits, etc.) leading to impaired social and occupational functioning. The biopsychosocial model can be utilized to understand the etiology of this disorder in a multi-factorial model, from the biomedical, psychological, and social aspects of health (Ader & Brown, 2004). The Biopsychosocial Model can also be an essential framework for understanding the types of management strategies that can be devised, keeping in mind the relationship between the biological and psychosocial mechanisms of schizophrenia.

Etiology of Schizophrenia from a Biopsychosocial Perspective

The Biopsychosocial Model posits that the etiology, course, and outcome of schizophrenia are related to not only factors associated with biological vulnerability (genetics, structural and functional brain defects, etc.) but also a complex interacting set of social and psychological factors such as stress related to poverty, migration, complex familial and cultural factors, etc. A multitude of interacting etiological factors has been identified to play a role in the causation and perpetuation of Schizophrenia. Although the exact role of these diverse sets of factors remains to be elucidated, research highlights that their interaction has a significant role in the manifestation and trajectories of the outcome of the disorder, which cuts across nations and cultures.

Biological Factors

The initial family studies reported that the incidence of schizophrenia was higher in relatives of patients with schizophrenia compared to the general population, thus highlighting a potential genetic component in its causation (Henriksen et al., 2017). Twin studies conducted after that documented that the concordance rate (i.e., both twins who have schizophrenia) was elevated in monozygotic (MZ) twins as compared to dizygotic (DZ) twins (Kendler, 1983). A meta-analysis of twin studies conducted by Sullivan et al. estimated the role of genetic liability to schizophrenia at 81%, whereas shared environmental influences were estimated to be 11% (Sullivan et al., 2003). Some of the candidate genes implicated by Genome-Wide Association Studies (GWAS) in the etiology of schizophrenia are DISC1, DTNBP1, NRG1, and COMT, but their potential pathogenetic involvement remains debated (Farrell et al., 2015).

A wide range of brain abnormalities has also been implicated in the etiology of schizophrenia. Brain structural abnormalities found in post-mortem studies as well as by structural neuroimaging such as computed tomography (CT) and magnetic resonance imaging (MRI) included enlarged lateral and third ventricles; loss of total grey matter, frontal, and temporal lobe volume; and a reduction in total brain size (Goldstein et al., 1999). The neurodevelopmental hypothesis of schizophrenia postulates that several brain abnormalities are present at the onset of illness and, to a certain extent, in first-degree relatives and, therefore, cannot be attributed to the progressive neurodegeneration caused by the disease. These factors are possibly trait markers of the illness, which are heritable, known as endophenotypes. However, most such findings are nonspecific and overlap with findings in other psychiatric disorders, such as bipolar disorder and major depression. Functional imaging studies using positron emission tomography (PET), which measures regional cerebral blood flow, have observed decreased metabolism in the frontal cortex, also called "hypofrontality," and left hemisphere dysfunction (Hill et al., 2004).

Abnormalities in levels of neurotransmitters in schizophrenia have primarily focused on the dopamine system. It has been hypothesized that the potency of an antipsychotic medication correlates with the amount of D_2 receptor blockade, which is a type of dopamine receptor abundantly found in the brain regions implicated in schizophrenia (Meltzer & Stahl, 1976). Secondly, drugs such as amphetamines, which increase dopaminergic activity, are known to precipitate symptoms of psychosis that are similar to paranoid schizophrenia (Featherstone et al., 2007). The dopamine hypothesis postulates that schizophrenia symptoms, such as hallucinations and delusions, are associated with hyperactivity of the mesolimbic dopaminergic system. Other neurotransmitters such as serotonin (5-hydroxytryptamine [5-HT]) and norepinephrine have also been implicated in the pathophysiology of schizophrenia (Carlsson et al., 1999). Recently, the role of the excitatory neurotransmitter glutamate in the pathophysiology of schizophrenia is gaining focus because several of the recently identified schizophrenia susceptibility genes target glutamatergic transmission (Coyle, 2006). Agonists of metabotropic glutamate receptors (mGluRs) are currently being investigated as potential therapeutic targets for schizophrenia.

Psychosocial Factors

The role of psychosocial factors in the etiology and course of schizophrenia has been a subject of scientific inquiry for just over 100 years. According to Kraepelin, schizophrenia was a "biological" disease process that inevitably ended in enduring cognitive deficits or "dementia" (Minkowski, 1987). Nonetheless, by the mid-twentieth century, it was being demonstrated that the course and outcome of schizophrenia were heterogeneous. Its clinical manifestations and behavioral abnormalities did not evolve uniformly negatively. Instead, it was found that they were subject to considerable influence from the socio-occupational and living conditions under which the patients lived and were cared for this observation that the patient's social and familial environment can mediate the course of severe mental illnesses, particularly schizophrenia, was a significant motivating factor for the worldwide reforms in the care of the mentally ill that took place in the second half of the twentieth century.

Trauma and social adversities in different forms, either during childhood or adulthood, have been extensively investigated as potential risk factors for schizophrenia. A meta-analysis by Varese et al. reported strong evidence that childhood adversity (defined as sexual abuse, physical abuse, emotional/psychological abuse, neglect, parental death, and bullying) was associated with an increased risk for psychosis in adulthood (Varese et al., 2012). Several research studies have also reported a significant association between childhood trauma and schizophrenic symptoms, with childhood trauma being associated with the most severe forms of positive symptomatology in adulthood, particularly hallucinations and affective symptoms (Matheson et al., 2013). Another meta-analysis study exploring the relationship between life events and psychosis has reported a threefold increased odds of life events in the period before psychosis onset, with the time under consideration ranging between 3 months and 3.6 years (Beards et al., 2013). Living in an urban environment has also been implicated in an increased risk of developing schizophrenia, in numerous studies. Numerous factors have been hypothesized for this phenomenon, such as greater exposure to prenatal influenza, income inequality, and social fragmentation, but none of them has been conclusive (Kirkbride et al., 2014).

Persons having schizophrenia are more likely to be single or unemployed, live in rented accommodation, in overcrowded conditions, and in poverty (Stilo et al., 2017). Previous research has also reported that migrant groups are at increased risk of schizophrenia and other psychotic disorders, which tend to persist into the second and third generations, implicating the role of acculturative stress and other psychosocial adversities related to the migration process (Bourque et al., 2011).

Using the Biopsychosocial Model for the Management of Schizophrenia

The understanding that the patient's psychosocial environment can have a significant effect on the course of severe mental illnesses, particularly schizophrenia, was a significant motivating factor for the worldwide reforms in the care of the mentally ill that took place in the second half of the twentieth century. The optimal therapeutic outcomes for people living with Schizophrenia are achieved only when pharmacological interventions (antipsychotic medications) are integrated with psychosocial intervention. This ensures the formulation of a treatment plan catering to a patient's individual needs, in keeping with his family, social, and cultural background and circumstances. However, while pharmacological interventions are widely implemented and researched, there is still a dearth of application of psychosocial interventions in an intensive manner, especially in low-middle-income countries with inadequate training and resources.

Despite the substantial burden of illness in schizophrenia, there has been a discrepancy between the beneficial effects of increased use of antipsychotic medications and achieving limited recovery or remission (Keating et al., 2017). Because the focus of the most common antipsychotic medications is on dopamine, which is associated with positive symptoms, there is an unmet need for patients with negative and cognitive symptoms who benefit from intense psychosocial and behavioral interventions. The Schizophrenia Patient Outcomes Research Team (PORT) project has played a significant role in the development and dissemination of evidence-based psychosocial treatments for schizophrenia (Kreyenbuhl et al., 2010). The methods and outcomes of the updated process in 2009 made recommendations for 16 psychopharmacologic and 8 psychosocial treatments for schizophrenia. Table 5.2 shows the psychosocial treatment recommendations for schizophrenia as per updated PORT Guidelines in the year 2009.

Table 5.2 Psychosocial treatment recommendations for schizophrenia as per updated PORT Guidelines (2009)

Assertive community treatment: Involves a comprehensive team including a medication provider, shared responsibility for patients among team members, direct provision of services by the team, frequent patient interaction, low staff-to-patient ratios, and community-based patient outreach
Supported employment: Features custom job creation, swift employment searches, continuous job support, and the integration of job and mental health services
Skills training: Concentrates on interpersonal abilities, utilizing methods like behavior-oriented instruction, demonstration, practice, constructive feedback, and positive encouragement
Cognitive behavior therapy: Central to this method are joint problem or symptom identification and crafting specific cognitive and behavioral approaches to manage these issues
Token economy interventions: Fundamental components include positive reinforcement contingent on defined behaviors, tailored treatment plans, and avoidance of punitive measures
Family-based interventions: Effective strategies encompass educating about the illness, crisis management, emotional support, and teaching coping strategies for illness symptoms and related challenges
Psychosocial interventions for alcohol and substance use disorder: Focus on motivational improvement and behavioral techniques aimed at treatment engagement, skill development for coping, relapse prevention, and integrating these approaches with mental health care
Psychosocial interventions for weight management: Comprising nutritional advice, managing caloric intake and portion sizes; behavioral self-management through motivation enhancement, goal setting, regular weight checks, daily monitoring of food intake and activity, and adjustments in diet and exercise routines

Applications of the Biopsychosocial Model in Clinical Practice

The most significant contribution of the Biopsychosocial Model in clinical practice has been to expand the horizons of the clinician's gaze. It was a call to change the restrictive biomedical way of understanding patients and their illnesses and to expand the domain of medical knowledge to address the diverse needs of each patient. This transformed how illness, suffering, and healing had been traditionally viewed, and incorporated the role of social, cultural, and psychological factors to provide a more holistic picture.

This has further led to develop patient-centered, relationship-centered, and client-centered approaches to an illness, which propose that reaching an accurate biomedical diagnosis is only part of the clinician's task. It is also of paramount importance that clinicians and health workers interpret illness and health from an intersubjective perspective by allowing the patients space and opportunity to articulate their concerns and expectations. These approaches help to mold the client–clinician relationship into a democratic and egalitarian relationship in which the clinician is mindful of the patient's needs as well as identity.

*Biopsychosocial-oriented clinical practice advocates a holistic and empathetic approach, which in psychiatric practice is essential to uphold the autonomy and dignity of the patient and validate their subjective lived experiences (*Alvarez et al.,

2012). It is also invaluable for clinical problem-solving as it helps incorporate multiple factors and considerations while formulating a patient management strategy.

Applications of the Biopsychosocial Model in Research

The stress–diathesis model for psychiatric disorders suggests that an interaction between biologically driven (genetic) predisposition with external (environmental) factors produces an individual's phenotype (manifestation of clinical illness) (Russo et al., 1995). However, the biopsychosocial approach in research studies explores how these individual factors interact to produce the disease. One of the mechanisms implicated has been the activation of the hypothalamic–pituitary–adrenal (HPA) axis, which occurs in response to environmental stress and has been implicated in the pathway from chronic stress. Chronic stress, such as childhood maltreatment, has been implicated in the etiopathogenesis of various psychiatric disorders, including psychosis. An altered HPA stress response and HPA axis hyperactivity have also been hypothesized to mediate the relationship between stress and symptoms of psychosis in schizophrenia (Barker et al., 2015).

Another major research breakthrough in understanding the link between genetic factors and environmental factors in causing psychiatric disorders has been epigenetics. Epigenetics posits that external environmental factors can influence changes at the DNA level (e.g., methylation), which are heritable and can lead to long-lasting phenotypic changes (Jablonka & Lamb, 2002). Thus, epigenetic processes may represent the interface between environmental and genetic risk factors for various psychiatric disorders. For example, in schizophrenia, they have been implicated as mediating the effects of childhood maltreatment in the development of psychosis (Read et al., 2009).

Limitations of the Biopsychosocial Model

While the Biopsychosocial Model was originally created as an alternative to biological reductionism, Borrell-Carrió and colleagues in 2004 argued against the model, stating that Engel's theoretical dedication to interactive dualism doesn't inherently encourage clinicians to be introspective and aware of their emotional demeanor, nor does it address issues like trustworthiness, authenticity, empathy, and inquisitiveness (Borrell-Carrió et al., 2004). According to them, the basic tenets of the Biopsychosocial Model in its current form present no guarantee that the clinician will cultivate the above. This is primarily due to the lack of a sound theoretical background related to the Biopsychosocial Model's content and its functioning. Since, to date, there is a lack of consensus on how these separate factors interact and result in the expression of the disease, the model provides no safeguards against either the dominance or the under-representation of any of the three domains of bio, psycho, or social.

The critiques of this model believe that this inevitably leads to undisciplined eclecticism (Benning, 2015). This has been further elucidated by Ghaemi, who wrote that the biopsychosocial Model, "*gives mental health professionals permission to do everything but no specific guidance to do anything*" (Ghaemi, 2011).

From a fundamental epistemological perspective, researchers have contended that the Biopsychosocial Model fails to conform to the criteria for a model (Mc Lafren, 1998). Whereas theories may be abstract, a stringent set of criteria, which are methodologically robust, are required in the case of models, to make them practically applicable. The Biopsychosocial Model has been critiqued for its difficulty in conceptualizing objective and measurable outcomes for the interacting factors, making it difficult to study its applications.

Because of these limitations, it is lately being recognized that *"while the biopsychosocial approach has its uses and had an important historical role, as an advance over both the biological and psychoanalytic dogmatisms. But it was only a temporary advance, not a final solution to our conceptual problem"* (Ghaemi, 2011).

Recently, researchers have moved beyond the multifactorial linear model to consider complexity theory as a more relevant model to conceptualize causality, dualism, and participation in care. Complexity theory shows how, in open systems, it is often impossible to know all the contributors to and influences on particular health outcomes (Borrell-Carrió et al., 2004). Describing how systems tend to self-organize provides guideposts to inform the clinician's actions. It also buffers the tendency to impose unrealistic expectations that one can know and control all of these contributors and influences.

Conclusion

Psychiatric disorders are not the result of a linear cause-and-effect medical model but are the result of a complex circular model of multiple causes and effects. The Biopsychosocial Model systematically explains the complex interplay of three major dimensions (biological, psychological, and social) in the etiology, course, and outcome of psychiatric disorders. This provided a holistic approach to the conceptualization of psychiatric illnesses. To understand and respond adequately to patients' suffering—and to give them a sense of being understood—clinicians must attend simultaneously to the biological, psychological, and social dimensions of illness.

However, even though the Biopsychosocial Model provides a holistic philosophy for clinical care, the model has been criticized for its lack of coherence and epistemological validity. In conclusion, the value of the Biopsychosocial Model has not been in the discovery of new scientific laws, as the term "new paradigm" would suggest, but rather in guiding the application of medical knowledge to the patients' individual needs.

References

Ader, R., & Brown, T. (2004). The biopsychosocial model: Interdisciplinarity in science and medicine. *Journal of Undergraduate Research, 3*, 6–9.

Alvarez, A. S., Pagani, M., & Meucci, P. (2012). The clinical application of the biopsychosocial model in mental health: A research critique. *American Journal of Physical Medicine & Rehabilitation, 91*(13), S173–S180.

Asokan, T. V. (2009). Towards an ideal paradigm. *Indian Journal of Psychological Medicine, 31*(2), 58–61.

Babalola, E., Noel, P., & White, R. (2017). The biopsychosocial approach and global mental health: Synergies and opportunities. *Indian Journal of Social Psychiatry, 33*(4), 291.

Barker, V., Gumley, A., Schwannauer, M., & Lawrie, S. M. (2015). An integrated biopsychosocial model of childhood maltreatment and psychosis. *The British Journal of Psychiatry, 206*(3), 177–180.

Beards, S., Gayer-Anderson, C., Borges, S., Dewey, M. E., Fisher, H. L., & Morgan, C. (2013). Life events and psychosis: A review and meta-analysis. *Schizophrenia Bulletin, 39*(4), 740–747.

Benning, T. B. (2015). Limitations of the biopsychosocial model in psychiatry. *Advances in Medical Education and Practice, 6*, 347.

Borrell-Carrió, F., Suchman, A. L., & Epstein, R. M. (2004). The biopsychosocial model 25 years later: Principles, practice, and scientific inquiry. *The Annals of Family Medicine, 2*(6), 576–582.

Bourque, F., van der Ven, E., & Malla, A. (2011). A meta-analysis of the risk for psychotic disorders among first-and second-generation immigrants. *Psychological Medicine, 41*(5), 897–910.

Carlsson, A., Waters, N., & Carlsson, M. L. (1999). Neurotransmitter interactions in schizophrenia—therapeutic implications. *Biological Psychiatry, 46*(10), 1388–1395.

Coyle, J. T. (2006). Glutamate and schizophrenia: Beyond the dopamine hypothesis. *Cellular and Molecular Neurobiology, 26*(4), 363–382.

Engel, G. L. (1977). The need for a new medical model: A challenge for biomedicine. *Science, 196*(4286), 129–136.

Engel, G. L. (2012). The need for a new medical model: A challenge for biomedicine. *Psychodynamic Psychiatry, 40*(3), 377.

Farrell, M. S., Werge, T., Sklar, P., Owen, M. J., Ophoff, R. A., O'Donovan, M. C., & Sullivan, P. F. (2015). Evaluating historical candidate genes for schizophrenia. *Molecular Psychiatry, 20*(5), 555–562.

Featherstone, R. E., Kapur, S., & Fletcher, P. J. (2007). The amphetamine-induced sensitized state as a model of schizophrenia. *Progress in Neuro-Psychopharmacology and Biological Psychiatry, 31*(8), 1556–1571.

Ghaemi, S. N. (2009). The rise and fall of the biopsychosocial model. *The British Journal of Psychiatry, 195*(1), 3–4.

Ghaemi, S. N. (2011). The biopsychosocial model in psychiatry: A critique. *American Journal of Psychiatry, 121*, 451–457.

Goldstein, J. M., Goodman, J. M., Seidman, L. J., Kennedy, D. N., Makris, N., Lee, H., & Tsuang, M. T. (1999). Cortical abnormalities in schizophrenia identified by structural magnetic resonance imaging. *Archives of General Psychiatry, 56*(6), 537–547.

Henriksen, M. G., Nordgaard, J., & Jansson, L. B. (2017). Genetics of schizophrenia: Overview of methods, findings and limitations. *Frontiers in Human Neuroscience, 11*, 322.

Hill, K., Mann, L., Laws, K. R., Stephenson, C. M. E., Nimmo-Smith, I., & McKenna, P. J. (2004). Hypofrontality in schizophrenia: A meta-analysis of functional imaging studies. *Acta Psychiatrica Scandinavica, 110*(4), 243–256.

Jablonka, E., & Lamb, M. J. (2002). The changing concept of epigenetics. *Annals of the New York Academy of Sciences, 981*(1), 82–96.

Keating, D., McWilliams, S., Schneider, I., Hynes, C., Cousins, G., Strawbridge, J., & Clarke, M. (2017). Pharmacological guidelines for schizophrenia: A systematic review and comparison of recommendations for the first episode. *British Medical Journal Open, 7*(1), e013881.

Kendler, K. S. (1983). Overview: a current perspective on twin studies of schizophrenia. *The American Journal of Psychiatry*.

Kirkbride, J. B., Jones, P. B., Ullrich, S., & Coid, J. W. (2014). Social deprivation, inequality, and the neighborhood-level incidence of psychotic syndromes in East London. *Schizophrenia Bulletin, 40*(1), 169–180.

Kreyenbuhl, J., Buchanan, R. W., Dickerson, F. B., & Dixon, L. B. (2010). The schizophrenia patient outcomes research team (PORT): Updated treatment recommendations 2009. *Schizophrenia Bulletin, 36*(1), 94–103.

Matheson, S. L., Shepherd, A. M., Pinchbeck, R. M., Laurens, K. R., & Carr, V. J. (2013). Childhood adversity in schizophrenia: A systematic meta-analysis. *Psychological Medicine, 43*(2), 225–238.

McLaren, N. (1998). A critical review of the biopsychosocial model. *Australian & New Zealand Journal of Psychiatry, 32*(1), 86–92.

Meltzer, H. Y., & Stahl, S. M. (1976). The dopamine hypothesis of schizophrenia: A review. *Schizophrenia Bulletin, 2*(1), 19.

Minkowski, E. (1987). The essential disorder underlying schizophrenia and schizophrenic thought. *The clinical roots of the schizophrenic concept*, 188–212.

Papadimitriou, G. (2017). The "Biopsychosocial Model": 40 years of application in Psychiatry. *Psychiatriki., 28*(2), 107–110.

Read, J., Bentall, R. P., & Fosse, R. (2009). Time to abandon the bio-bio-bio model of psychosis: Exploring the epigenetic and psychological mechanisms by which adverse life events lead to psychotic symptoms. *Epidemiology and Psychiatric Sciences, 18*(4), 299–310.

Russo, J., Vitaliano, P. P., Brewer, D. D., Katon, W., & Becker, J. (1995). Psychiatric disorders in spouse caregivers of care recipients with Alzheimer's disease and matched controls: A diathesis-stress model of psychopathology. *Journal of Abnormal Psychology, 104*(1), 197.

Shorter, E. (2005). The history of the biopsychosocial approach in medicine: before and after Engel. *Biopsychosocial medicine: An integrated approach to understanding illness*, 1–19.

Stilo, S. A., Gayer-Anderson, C., Beards, S., Hubbard, K., Onyejiaka, A., Keraite, A., et al. (2017). Further evidence of a cumulative effect of social disadvantage on risk of psychosis. *Psychological Medicine, 47*(5), 913–924.

Sullivan, P. F., Kendler, K. S., & Neale, M. C. (2003). Schizophrenia as a complex trait: Evidence from a meta-analysis of twin studies. *Archives of General Psychiatry, 60*(12), 1187–1192.

Varese, F., Smeets, F., Drukker, M., Lieverse, R., Lataster, T., Viechtbauer, W., & Bentall, R. P. (2012). Childhood adversities increase the risk of psychosis: A meta-analysis of patient-control, prospective-and cross-sectional cohort studies. *Schizophrenia Bulletin, 38*(4), 661–671.

Chapter 6
Community Mental Health: Evolution, Current Status, and Future Perspectives

K. R. Anish and P. Ginu George

Abstract Community mental health refers to the provision of mental health services in the community. Epidemiological studies across the globe indicate the presence of major mental health disorders such as major depression, schizophrenia, and bipolar affective disorder in all populations. Community mental health services are pivotal in addressing the established treatment gap in mental health care. The chapter unravels the past, present, and future of community mental health globally and in India. This chapter covers six broad aspects namely the concept of community mental health and the need for community mental health services; the evolution of community mental services; policies and programs linked to community mental health care; community mental health practice models, and; human resources for the community mental health. The chapter also focuses on future perspectives on community mental health.

Keywords Community mental health · Mental health care · National mental health programme · Mental health policy

Introduction

The WHO's Comprehensive Mental Health Action Plan for 2013–2030 acknowledges the importance of mental health in achieving health for all people. One of the objectives of this plan is to deliver comprehensive, responsive, integrated, and social care services in community-based settings. Though effective prevention and treatment options exist, there is still a wide disparity between those who can access care and those who do not. According to the World Health Organization's (2022) report, coverage of effective treatments remains relatively low. Therefore, there is

K. R. Anish (✉)
Department of Social Work, Rajagiri College of Social Sciences (Autonomous), Kalamassery, Cochin, India
e-mail: anish@rajagiri.edu

P. Ginu George
Rajagiri College of Social Sciences (Autonomous), Kalamassery, Cochin, India

M. Anand (ed.), *Mental Health Care Resource Book*,
https://doi.org/10.1007/978-981-97-1203-8_6

a great need to promote community mental health services to ensure everyone's mental health needs are met, especially those of the underprivileged. Community mental health provides a platform for the person in problem to utilize the available mental health services to restore their functioning and heal naturally in their preferred environment. "Community mental health care programs" indicate that the community's mental health needs and well-being are met within the community with the aid of local resources and the primary healthcare system. It includes "promotion of well-being, addressing stigma, psychosocial support, rehabilitation of those in need, prevention of harm from alcohol and drug abuse, treatment of the ill, using the primary health care system and the secondary health care system". The spectrum of interventions in community mental health ranges from mental health promotion to the rehabilitation of persons with severe mental disorders.

The mental health needs of the community are diverse and include the mental health of women, children and adolescents, refugees, survivors of disasters, persons attempting suicide, public mental health education, and promotion of mental health (Srinivasa Murthy et al., 1978; Chandrasekar et al., 1981; Parthasarathy et al., 1981; Chatterji et al., 2003; Srinivasa Murthy et al., 2005; Thara et al., 2008; Theerthalli et al., 2009).

Community mental health consists of the principles and techniques required to enhance the mental health of the people in the community by: (a) focusing on the strengths and ambitions of those who experience mental illnesses; (b) fostering a broad network of supports and services; and meeting needs in ways that are acceptable and accessible, (c) focusing services that are both evidence-based and recovery-oriented (d) emphasizing resources with sufficient capacity (Thornicroft et al., 2012). Community mental health programs ensure a continuum of care for the entire population or community. Services are systematically planned by considering the peculiarities of the population, specifying unmet needs, and identifying the population's high-risk needs. Community mental health also focuses on environmental causes of human distress than psychological distress (Bloom, 1977). The ideology behind community mental health is to ensure that everyone has fair access to services in their community in the "least restricted environment" (Thornicroft et al., 2012).

The World Mental Health Report (2022) reiterates the need for transformation of mental health care by reorganizing mental health services. The Mental health report document states:

> *"Community-based mental health care comprises a network of interconnected services that include: mental health services integrated into general health care; community mental health services; and services that deliver mental health care in non-health settings and support access to key social services. Social and informal support delivered by community providers (e.g., community workers, peers) complement formal services and help ensure enabling environments for people with mental health conditions. Overall, there is no single model for organizing community-based mental health services that apply to all country contexts. Yet every country, no matter its resource constraints, can take steps to restructure and scale up mental health care for impact."*

Thornicroft et al. (2012) allude that community mental health should include the following elements in low- and middle-income countries:

a. A concentration on population and public health requirements.
b. Case discovery and detection in the neighborhood.
c. Services available nearby (i.e., accessible in less than half a day).
d. Community involvement and decision-making in the design and delivery of systems for mental healthcare.
e. Individuals and families can empower themselves and use services.
f. Peer help and/or reciprocal assistance among service users.
g. Initial care is provided by community workers or primary care providers.
h. Stepped care choices for hospital beds or specialist staff referral, as needed.
i. Support and backup supervision from specialized mental health services.

WHO advocates creating comprehensive, responsive, integrated, and social care programs provided through local community platforms. Choosing the best combination of services, training non-specialist health workers to provide essential mental health care, promoting a recovery-oriented model of care, scaling up low-intensity psychological interventions, utilizing digital health to innovate, and integrating mental health into universal health coverage (UHC) and primary health care are some of the priority actions. A comprehensive range of interventions, including public awareness, early detection, treatment of acute illness, family education, long-term care, rehabilitation, reintegration, and protection of the human rights of the ill, are required to organize mental health services. Another crucial factor is the patient's unwillingness or unawareness to seek care on his own in particular clinical diseases or settings. These aspects must be considered when developing primary, secondary, and tertiary mental health services (Murthy, 2014).

The Evolution of Community Mental Health Services

Community mental health followed a series of stages in its development. It broadly includes the following aspects:

(a) The treatment of individual health issues in the neighborhood.
(b) The pooling of resources for mental healthcare.
(c) The concentration on community-level interventions.
(d) The promotion of positive mental health.

The origin of community mental health can be divided into three periods:

a. Isolation and safeguarding others: The construction of huge asylums that were situated distant from the populations they treated.
b. Deinstitutionalization and Service provision: An increase in mental health services offered in the community and therefore nearer to the clientele they served or deinstitutionalization.
c. Reforms in mental health services: The reform of mental health services according to an evidence-based approach, balancing and integrating community and hospital services elements (Thornicroft et al., 2012, 2016)

The community mental health movement began in the 1950s in the western world as a reaction to the institutionalization of psychiatric patients, which was discovered to have significant adverse effects. Patients who stay in psychiatric hospitals long-term lose their social skills, their social bonds erode, and they struggle to fit in and avoid stigma. The Civil Rights Act of 1964 passed in the USA and the consequent social changes led to the conviction that racial and ethnic minorities and other underprivileged groups' rights needed to be protected. The mental healthcare landscape for people of color changed significantly after the Civil Rights Act and the Community Mental Health Center Act of 1963.

A paradigm shift in mental health care occurred during the second half of the twentieth century, mainly as a result of three independent factors:

(a) A significant advancement in psychopharmacology led to the discovery of new classes of medications, especially neuroleptics and antidepressants, in addition to new psychosocial interventions.
(b) Under the sponsorship of the newly created United Nations, the human rights movement has become a truly global phenomenon.
(c) The development of new forms of psychosocial interventions.

These technological and societal developments helped shift the focus from the care provided in big institutions of confinement to more accessible and universal care in the community (WHO, 2001).

Features of Community Mental Health Services

In 1988, Echlin identified two models of community mental health services. The first is a base or building for a multidisciplinary team servicing a designated catchment area in the community. Others consider a central base to be a hindrance to the delivery of services and employment. Additionally, Dick (1985) notes two models as methods for treating psychiatric morbidity. First, there is a service that serves as a "funnel," giving local resources the majority of the work (e.g., primary health care, social services) and only maintains what cannot be managed by other means. The second is a specialized service that offers certain forms of therapy; however, if the available abilities do not meet the client's demands, the client cannot be assisted. Instead of being customer-need-led, it is service driven. Sayce (1987) listed three strategies, the first serves as the entry point for the majority of the locality's mental health referrals to a devolved psychiatric service; the second is a sessional model offering counseling and/or group work, and the third is a community development model with an emphasis on mental health. All these models shared common characteristics such as accessibility, focus on psychosocial intervention, multidisciplinary approach, comprehensiveness, and connections inside the community. The clients should have direct access to the service rather than requiring an intermediary referral by professionals. It should place more emphasis on psychosocial intervention strategies than medical (biophysical) ones. This entails placing more of an emphasis on social and familial aspects and making a wider variety of therapies and interventions available that would not be possible. Thirdly, emphasis is placed on multidisciplinary teamwork. For some, this entails increased equality between the different professions rather than medical leadership. It undoubtedly underscores the need for improved communication and coordination among mental health professionals. Fourthly, comprehensiveness is frequently emphasized. This is related to multidisciplinary teams that offer a range of talents. Therefore, it could be more accurate to refer to CMHCs as a component of an all-encompassing service (Sayce, 1989). Finally, connections inside the community are frequently valued. This may entail connections with other organizations, including "out posting" to general practitioners.

Community Mental Health in India

In the initial period, mental hospitals or asylums were the only places that could treat persons with mental illnesses. Later, the community psychiatry movement started to rehabilitate patients who underwent prolonged hospitalization. It also aims to protect the fundamental human rights of persons with mental illness and prevent institutionalization's ill effects. In India, many people with various mental problems are cared for in the community due to the power of the joint family, marriage, the close-knit community, increased tolerance of deviant conduct in the larger community, and faith-based coping and healing (Chavan et al., 2012). The primary driving force behind the community mental health movement was the need to "reach the untreated" due to the inadequate state of mental health care in India (Thara et al., 2008).

Dr. Vidya Sagar initiated family involvement in the treatment and rehabilitation of patients in the 1950s at Amritsar Mental Hospital. Later, the Mental Health Centre at Christian Medical College, Vellore, and the All-India Institute of Mental Health, now known as NIMHANS, Bengaluru, followed this model. During the 1970s and 1980s, attempts were made to understand the requirements of families with a mentally ill person. The focus of the following phase was to maximize the utilization of the current general healthcare infrastructure by integrating mental health services with general healthcare services. This happened concurrently with the growth and expansion of the general hospital psychiatry units.

In 1975, the WHO and the Post Graduate Institute of Medical Education and Research (PGIMER), Chandigarh, launched the Raipur Rani project, a model for rural mental treatment (Wig et al., 1981). In Raipur Rani block of Ambala district, Haryana, the project utilized the already-existing basic healthcare infrastructure to teach staff to recognize and treat individuals with mental illness. In 1976, the government opened a Community Mental Health Unit (CMHU) of the National Institute of Mental Health and Neuro Sciences (NIMHANS) in a rural Karnataka village called Sakalawara. The Sakalawara project focused on detecting and managing priority mental and neurological disorders like psychosis and epilepsy in a rural catchment by training general health practitioners. Initially, a triweekly primary healthcare clinic in Sakalawara provided mental health services before expanding to a daily clinic.

A community clinic in Thiruporur was founded in 1989 by the Schizophrenia Research Foundation (SCARF), an NGO in Chennai, and it was operational until 1999. During this time, numerous initiatives were started, including self-employment programs, referral systems, citizen groups, and staff training for primary health centers (Thara et al., 2008). Various programs and policies linked to community mental health services are listed below.

National Mental Health Programme (NMHP)

Numerous community mental health outreach programs were launched around the nation. The National Mental Health Programme (NMHP) of India, which was introduced in 1982, and the District Mental Health Programme (DMHP), which was introduced gradually starting in 1996, were the two most significant developments (Chadda et al., 2015). The National Mental Health Programme launched in 1982 mainly focused on decentralizing mental health services. The objective of NMHP was to guarantee the availability and accessibility of minimal mental healthcare for all in the near future, particularly to the most vulnerable and underprivileged sections of the population. It also aims to encourage the application of mental health knowledge in general healthcare and social development, promote community participation in the development of mental health services, and stimulate efforts toward self-help in the community.

District Mental Health Programme (DMHP)

Based on prior experiences in Bellary District, Karnataka State, DMHP was introduced in 1996 with four districts. DMHP envisioned a community-based strategy to solve the issue of mental health concerns in the community and accessibility to mental health care. It included training for mental health workers, providing services for the early diagnosis and treatment of mental diseases in the community, gathering data, gaining experience at the community level for future planning, raising awareness about mental health problems, and decreasing the stigma associated with them. The DMHP programme enhanced community awareness of mental illnesses and improved the satisfaction of clients with services. DMHP consists of the following components:

(a) Service provision: Outpatient and inpatient mental health services are provided, and there is a 10-bed inpatient facility.

(b) The outreach component includes satellite clinics run by the DMHP team at CHCs/PHCs, targeted interventions, life skills instruction and counseling in schools, college counseling services, workplace stress management programs, and services for suicide prevention.
(c) Health workers at district and sub-district levels are sensitized about mental health concerns through focused training.
(d) Awareness-raising events to disseminate information on mental disorders and associated stigma with the assistance of Panchayati Raj Institutions, faith healers, teachers, leaders, etc.
(e) Community involvement through connections with NGOs working in the field of mental health, family and caregiver groups, and self-help groups (Balagopal & Kapanee, 2019).

United Nations Conventions on the Rights of Persons with Disabilities (UNCRPD)

The UN General Assembly approved the United Nations Conventions on the Rights of Persons with Disabilities (UNCRPD) in December 2006. The goal was to advance respect for people with disabilities' innate dignity and to ensure that all people with disabilities may fully and equally enjoy all human rights and fundamental freedoms.

The National Mental Health Policy of India (2014)

During this decade, India has seen the establishment of a National Mental Health Policy and the passing of the Mental Healthcare Act. In order to protect people's right to live in the community, both the policy and the law acknowledged the rights to social and mental healthcare with a focus on community-based services. This strategy represents a change from legislation passed three decades ago, emphasizing issues relating to the institutional treatment of persons with mental illness.

The National Mental Health Policy of India (2014) outlines the government's guiding principles, goals, and focus areas for improving the population's mental health. The policy emphasizes everyone's access to mental health services while urging respect for the rights of people who struggle with mental illness (Balagopal & Kapanee, 2019).

The 2014 National Mental Health Policy of India outlines the following goals:

a. To provide mental healthcare accessible to everyone.
b. To enhance the utilization of comprehensive mental healthcare services and access to them, including vulnerable populations like the homeless and those residing in distant places and socioeconomically disadvantaged.
c. To lessen the prevalence and effects of mental health problem risk factors.
d. To lessen the likelihood and incidence of attempted and completed suicide.

e. To protect the rights of people with mental health issues and ensure well-being.
f. To lessen the stigma attached to mental health issues.
g. To increase the availability and fair distribution of human resources in the mental health sector.
h. To raise the amount of money spent on mental health care.
i. To determine the social, biological, and psychological factors influencing mental health and dispense proper remedies.

In the National Mental Health Policy 2014, mental health has been described holistically as a condition of well-being rather than only the absence of mental disorders. It emphasizes the concept that mental health, rather than being categorical, lies on a continuum and is characterized by its focus on "mental health problems," which range from the existence of psychosocial discomfort to mental illness and mental disability. It also recommends multifaceted strategies in mental healthcare. The importance of integrated care has been emphasized in light of the demand for a primary healthcare strategy that makes mental health services widely available and easily accessible.

Mental Health Care Act, 2017

The Mental Healthcare Act (MHA) 2017, which attempts to align Indian laws with the Convention on the Rights of Persons with Disabilities, which India adopted in 2007, is a significant advancement for mental healthcare in India (The Gazette of India)0.2017). The primary emphasis is on the rights of people with mental illnesses and the right to mental healthcare in non-custodial settings agreeable to the client. The Act also recognizes the ability of individuals with mental illness to choose their course of treatment, provided they have the ability to comprehend treatment-related facts, comprehend choice consequences, and effectively express decisions. The Act also ensures that every person has the legal right to utilize mental health services provided by or supported by the relevant government, including access to mental healthcare and treatment. The provision of geographically accessible mental health care is the focus of this initiative. The Act envisages accessible, reasonably priced, and high-quality mental healthcare services available in the community.

The formulation and implementation of mental health care in the community in India is complicated due to low budgetary spending, a lack of human resources, and varying levels of social and economic development among states, despite the recent governmental emphasis given to mental health.

Challenges for Mental Healthcare in India

Murthy (2014) identified the following challenges in the provision of mental healthcare services in India.

Large "Unmet Need": There is a significant gap in meeting the demand for mental healthcare within the community.
Poor Understanding: There is a lack of awareness and understanding in the general population regarding psychological distress, with many not recognizing it as a condition that requires medical intervention.
Limited Acceptance: The general population shows limited acceptance of modern medical care for mental disorders, suggesting a stigma or reluctance to seek help for such issues.
Availability Challenges: Mental health services, including both professionals and facilities, are limited within public health services, creating barriers to access.
Underutilization: Even when mental health services are available, there is poor utilization by individuals suffering from mental illnesses and their families, indicating potential issues with accessibility or willingness to seek help.
Recovery and Reintegration Challenges: There are problems in the recovery and reintegration of individuals with mental illnesses back into society, suggesting a need for comprehensive support systems.
Lack of Institutionalized Mechanisms: There is a lack of organized mechanisms for the delivery of mental healthcare, highlighting the need for structured and institutionalized approaches to address mental health issues effectively.

Role of the Voluntary Sector

The contribution of voluntary organizations to the creation of small-scale, locally appropriate, community-based psychiatric care facilities like daycare facilities, vocational training facilities, sheltered workplaces, halfway houses, and long-term care facilities is another significant development in Indian community psychiatry. Currently, community-based mental health services are provided in various primary care settings, including district hospitals, GHPUs, community psychiatry programs, and office-based practices. In the private sector, numerous private general hospitals and psychiatric nursing homes are also available (Chadda et al., 2015). Faith-based organizations also facilitated community-based care for homeless mentally ill persons (Anish, 2013).

Community Mental Health Practice Models in India

1. Satellite Clinics and Care and Support Programme of Antara

In 1997, Antara began operating its Mobile Mental Health Clinics, also known as Satellite Clinics, to offer psychiatric treatments to those who lived in rural locations. The Community Mental Health Unit's Care and Support Programme (CSP) was established in 2008 as a result of Antara's observation that clients from socioeconomically disadvantaged backgrounds had a high rate of dropout, relapse, and hospitalization, which necessitated the development of community-based services. (Balagopal & Kapanee, 2019).

2. Rural Mental Health Programme of the Banyan

The Banyan was established in 1993 in Chennai to offer complete treatment to homeless women who had mental illnesses. Following the 2004 tsunami, Relief and rehabilitation efforts in response to the plight of the Kovalam villagers led to the creation of something more tangible—a community mental health center program. The Rural Mental Health Program has formed formal and informal coalitions with various community stakeholders, including the Dargah, local self-government institutions (panchayat), members of self-help groups, government employees of anti-poverty programs, and patients and caregivers themselves. (Balagopal & Kapanee, 2019).

3. Mental Health Programme of Mental Health Action Trust

A community mental health initiative called Mental Health Action Trust (MHAT), run by volunteers, offers free bio-psychosocial mental healthcare to the most vulnerable among the impoverished and homeless people with mental illnesses are supported by a network in collaboration with the Institute of Palliative Medicine (IPM), Kozhikode of palliative care facilities in a few of Kerala's northern districts. The initiative was started in response to a request from the neighborhood. Community-based clinics offer free medical care, nutritional assistance, and financial support for providing clients with transportation options, livelihood opportunities, financial assistance, counseling, and connecting clients with social organizations and government agencies. Schoolchildren, door-to-door campaigns, business owners, and other local community members provide all of the funding for the community program (Balagopal & Kapanee, 2019).

Human Resources for Community Mental Health

The voluntary sector plays a vital role in community mental health. Individuals from the local community who are not trained in mental health or health care can offer a range of services. Lay volunteers, community workers, employees of advocacy groups, organizers of self-help/user groups, humanitarian relief workers, traditional health workers, and other professionals, including teachers and police officers, are a few examples of those who work at this level of service provision. Despite having little to no formal training in mental health care, many informal community-care providers are the primary providers of mental health services in many developing nations. They are usually accessible and generally well-accepted in local communities. They can help integrate people with mental disorders into the community and thus play an important supportive role in formal mental health services (Murthy, 2014).

Recent Trends in Community Mental Health Care

The availability of a wider variety of treatments is one of the most significant improvements that has happened. Most second-generation antipsychotics and antidepressants are widely accessible and affordable in India. This has made it possible for experts to make full use of them. One of the only developing nations with the widespread use of these medications is likely India. The expanding significance of families in the nation's mental healthcare system is the other significant change. Another change over the past 20 years is the accessibility of a wide range of medical and non-medical care options. Notably, India greatly benefits from the expanding involvement of Non-Governmental Organizations (NGOs), which offer suicide prevention, disaster care, and school health programs, where non-specialists and volunteers play a crucial role (Murthy, 2014).

Significance of Community Mental Health in the Post-Pandemic Period

The COVID-19 pandemic has substantially and widely impacted social structures, the economy, and healthcare systems. People's mental health has been significantly affected due to these health, social, and economic effects. Many people have expressed psychological distress and signs of post-traumatic stress disorder, anxiety, or despair (WHO, 2022). Kathirvel (2020) also pointed out that the long-term impacts of the pandemic, the restrictive measures like social isolation and quarantine, and the socio-economic effects all point to an increase in the frequency of common mental health disorders during the post-pandemic period. Mental health services have been severely disrupted while mental health needs have increased. Early in the pandemic, when personnel and infrastructure were frequently redeployed to COVID-19 relief, this was particularly true. Social restrictions at the time also made it difficult for people to receive care. And in many instances, lack of information and disinformation about the virus fueled people's anxieties and worries, preventing them from seeking medical care.

The most important steps in solving the issue are improving access to mental health services, including telepsychiatry, early diagnosis, treatment, psychosocial support, screening, and support for specific groups, such as frontline HCP, when necessary, putting in place long-term strategies to lessen the effects of the economic downturn on mental health, and addressing stigma during the pandemic (Kathirvel, 2020). Community-based programs frequently adapted more quickly and devised creative ways to offer psychosocial support through digital technology and unofficial assistance. One of the recommendations of WHO to countries is to ensure that mental health and psychosocial assistance are widely accessible, especially by expanding access to self-help and fostering neighborhood projects. Community-based mental health programs are vital to understanding the felt needs of the population and designing appropriate interventions to cope with pandemic-related mental.

Implications for Future Practice

Thornicroft et al. (2012) proposed key recommendations to enhance community mental health services in the future. First, they emphasize measuring the treatment coverage of individuals with mental illness and setting specific goals for improvement over defined time frames. Acknowledging the reduced life expectancy of those with mental health issues, healthcare systems are urged to develop and test strategies addressing this health disparity.

To combat stigma, evidence-based interventions should be consistently implemented at both the population and community levels. Mental health professionals should ensure accessible and acceptable care, balancing services between hospitals and communities. The authors advocate for prudent investment in proven treatments while avoiding ineffective or harmful ones, regardless of economic conditions.

Enhancing shared decision-making between healthcare professionals and service consumers is crucial. Interdisciplinary teamwork and leveraging diverse professional competencies are vital for comprehensive and effective community care. Additionally, promoting recovery-focused programs and increasing mental health care delivery, especially integrated care for long-term conditions, are recommended. Lastly, aligning mental health services with global Sustainable Development Goals and integrating evidence-based practices into broader initiatives can contribute to widespread improvements in mental health.

Conclusion

Community mental health emphasizes the shift of care from institutions to the community. It aims to reduce the treatment gap as most vulnerable groups still do not receive mental health services. Community mental health services successfully address the mental health needs of the general public. This chapter has provided a comprehensive exploration of community mental health, tracing its evolution, assessing its current status, and offering insightful perspectives for the future. The historical journey has illuminated the transformative shifts from institutionalization towards community-based care, emphasizing the significance of understanding societal, cultural, and systemic factors in shaping mental health practices. The current status analysis underscores both achievements and persistent challenges and the future perspectives outlined in this chapter set a forward-looking agenda. The emphasis on interdisciplinary collaboration, shared decision-making, and strategic investment in proven treatments reflects a commitment to enhancing the quality and accessibility of mental health care.

As we move forward, it is clear that the evolution of community mental health is an ongoing process, requiring continuous adaptation to societal changes, technological advancements, and a deeper understanding of the complexities surrounding mental well-being. This chapter serves as both a reflection on the journey so far and a roadmap for the evolving landscape of community mental health, urging stakeholders to collectively strive for a more inclusive, compassionate, and effective mental health ecosystem.

References

Anish, K. R., (2013). An evaluation of psychosocial rehabilitation facilities for homeless mentally ill in India. *Artha–Journal of Social Sciences, 12*(2).

Balagopal, G., & Kapanee, A. R. M. (2019). Mental healthcare services in the community: Where does India stand? In G. Balagopal & A. R. M. Kapanee (Eds.), *Mental health care services in community settings: Discussions on NGO approaches in India* (pp. 1–37). Springer. https://doi.org/10.1007/978-981-13-9101-9_1.

Bloom, B. L. (1977). *Community mental health: A general introduction*. Brooks/Cole.

Chadda, R., Patra, B., & Gupta, N. (2015). Recent developments in community mental health: Relevance and relationship with the mental health care bill. *Indian Journal of Social Psychiatry, 31*, 153. https://doi.org/10.4103/0971-9962.173296

Chandrashekar, C. R., Isaac, M. K., Kapur, R. L., & Sarathy, R. P. (1981). Management of priority mental disorders in the community. *Indian Journal of Psychiatry, 23*(2), 174–178.

Chatterji, S., Patel, V., Chatterji, A., & Weiss, A. H. (2003). Evaluation of a community-based rehabilitation model for chronic schizophrenia in rural India. *The British Journal of Psychiatry,* 57–62.

Chavan, B. S. (2012). Community Mental Health in India. New Delhi: Jaypee Brothers Medical.

Dick, P., Cameron, L., Cohen, D., Barlow, M., & Ince, A. (1985). Day and full time psychiatric treatment: a controlled comparison. *The British Journal of Psychiatry: The Journal of Mental Science, 147*, 246–249. https://doi.org/10.1192/bjp.147.3.246

Kathirvel, N. (2020). Post COVID-19 pandemic mental health challenges. *Asian Journal of Psychiatry, 53*, 102430. https://doi.org/10.1016/j.ajp.2020.102430

Murthy, R. S. (2014). Mental health initiatives in India (1947–2010). In A. Francis (ed.), *Social work in mental health: Contexts and theories for practice* (pp. 28–61). SAGE Publications India Pvt Ltd. https://doi.org/10.4135/9789351507864.n3

Parthasarathy, R., Chandrashekar, C. R., Isaac, M. K., & Prema, T. P. (1981). A profile of the follow up of the rural mentally ill. *Indian Journal of Psychiatry, 23*(2), 139–141.

Srinivasa Murthy, R., Kala, R., & Wig, N. N. (1978). Mentally ill in a rural community: Some initial experiences in case identification and management. *Indian Journal of Psychiatry, 20*(2), 143.

Srinivasa Murthy, R., Kishore Kumar, K. V., Chisholm, D., Thomas, T., Sekar, K., & Chandrashekari, C. R. (2005). Community outreach for untreated schizophrenia in rural India: A follow-up study of symptoms, disability, family burden and costs. *Psychological Medicine, 35*(3), 341–351. https://doi.org/10.1017/s0033291704003551

Thara, R., Padmavati, R., Aynkran, J. R., & John, S. (2008). Community mental health in India: A rethink. *International Journal of Mental Health Systems, 2*, 11. https://doi.org/10.1186/1752-4458-2-11

Theerthalli, J., Venkatesh, B. K., Kishorekumar, K. V., Arunachala, U., Venkatasubramanian, G., Subbakrishna, D. K., & Gangadhar, B. N. (2009). Prospective comparison of course of disability in antipsychotic-treated and untreated schizophrenia patients. *Acta Psychiatrica Scandinavica, 119*(3). https://doi.org/10.1111/j.1600-0447.2008.01299.x

Thornicroft, G., Deb, T., & Henderson, C. (2016). Community mental health care worldwide: Current status and further developments. *World Psychiatry: Official Journal of the World Psychiatric Association (WPA), 15*(3), 276–286. https://doi.org/10.1002/wps.20349

Thronicroft, G., Atalay, A., Robert, D. E., Hiroto, I., & Jair, M. (2012). *Community mental health: Putting policy into practice globally*. John Wiley & Sons.

WHO (2001). The World Health Report: 2001: Mental health: new understanding, new hope. Geneva: World Health Organization.

WHO (2022). World mental health report: transforming mental health for all. Geneva: World Health Organization.

Wig, N. N., Murthy, R. S., & Harding, T. W. (1981). A model for rural psychiatric services-raipur rani experience. *Indian Journal of Psychiatry, 23*(4), 275–290.

World Mental Health Report. (2022). Retrieved November 2, 2022, from https://www.who.int/teams/mental-health-and-substance-use/world-mental-health-report.

Chapter 7
Contextualizing Law and Policy Framework on Mental Health

Saumya Uma

Abstract The right to a standard of living adequate for health and well-being has been proclaimed as a human right by the Universal Declaration of Human Rights. As a logical corollary, mental health is an essential, inter-linked, and indivisible component of the human right to health. All persons are entitled to receive timely, quality, affordable mental health care and to be treated with dignity and respect, without any form of discrimination. However, this chapter argues that the human right to mental health comprises of much more than access to quality health care. Mental health as a human right is not merely the absence of mental illnesses but a complete state of well-being that addresses underlying determinants of health as well. This chapter discusses the components of mental health as a human right and the related international standards; it presents and critiques the current law and policy framework pertaining to mental health in India; and identifies the gaps in the same which ought to be addressed in the near future.

Keywords Mental health · Law · Policy · Programs

Introduction

Mental health issues are often touted as "first world problems," implying that in developing countries, where physical survival and the achievement of basic needs of food, water, shelter, and livelihood are an ordeal, mental health is a luxury to have and ought to be a low priority of state policy. Despite disparities in challenges faced by ordinary people in developed and developing countries, the fact remains that the absence of mental health and well-being is anything but selective; in fact, it may be exacerbated in developing countries due to poor socio-economic and political factors.

The World Health Organization (2019) evaluated financial loss in India in terms of loss in productivity, due to mental health conditions, in the time period 2012–2030,

S. Uma (✉)
Professor of Law, Jindal Global Law School, O.P.Jindal Global University, Sonipat, India
e-mail: saumya@jgu.edu.in

M. Anand (ed.), *Mental Health Care Resource Book*,
https://doi.org/10.1007/978-981-97-1203-8_7

at 1.03 trillion dollars. Other surveys estimate a loss of $14 billion a year in India due to mental health issues (The Hindu, 2022). A study conducted by Assocham in 2017 unveiled that 42.5% of employees in the Indian private sector are distressed with general anxiety disorder or depression, as compared to government employees. This is due to longer working hours and exploitative conditions at work, leading to fatigue, stress, and frustration (Joshi, 2018). Scholars have documented the prevalence of mental illnesses and a state-wise burden of the same in India (Sagar et al., 2020). The cyclical link between mental ill-health and poverty has been traced, documented, and analyzed in various reports (Narasimhan et al., 2019). It is evident from these and other such findings of research that addressing mental health issues through law and policy is an urgent need for India.

The right to a standard of living adequate for health and well-being has been proclaimed as a human right by the Universal Declaration of Human Rights. As a logical corollary, mental health is an essential, inter-linked, and indivisible component of the human right to health. All persons are entitled to receive timely, quality, affordable mental health care and to be treated with dignity and respect, without any form of discrimination. However, the human right to mental health comprises of much more than access to quality health care. Mental health as a human right is not merely the absence of mental illnesses but a complete state of well-being, that addresses underlying determinants of health as well.

Mental health law provides normative standards of behavior and treatment, which enable individuals and communities with mental illnesses to assert their human rights. Mental health policy draws upon the legislative framework to attain its objectives and operationalize the same. It is the convergence of law and policy on mental health that contributes to the accessibility of mental health care and augment the quality of the health services provided. Mental health care includes medical (psychiatric) as well as social/community-based care.

Against this backdrop, the chapter is largely divided into three parts: in the first part, it discusses the components of mental health as a human right and the ensuing international standards. In the second part, it provides an overview of the present law and policy framework pertaining to mental health in India. In the third part, it critiques the national law and policy framework vis-à-vis established international human rights standards and identifies gaps in law and policy that ought to be addressed through advocacy, practice-based skills, and field-based actions.

A. Mental health as a human right

The Universal Declaration of Human Rights (UDHR) was adopted by the United Nations (UN) General Assembly on 10 December 1948. Article 25 of the UDHR reads as follows:

> *Everyone has the right to a standard of living adequate for the health and well-being of himself and of his family, including food, clothing, housing and medical care and necessary social services, and the right to security in the event of unemployment, sickness, disability, widowhood, old age or other lack of livelihood in circumstances beyond his control.*

Although Article 25 does not explicitly mention mental health, it is complimented by a definition of health given in the Preamble to the ***Constitution of World Health***

Organization (WHO) 1946, which states that health is "a state of complete physical, mental and social well-being and not merely the absence of disease or infirmity.". Additionally, Article 12(1) of the ***International Covenant on Economic, Social and Cultural Rights*** (to which India is a state party and thereby bound by its provisions) elaborated on Article 25 of the UDHR and stated that "the States Parties to the present Covenant recognize the right of everyone to the enjoyment of the highest attainable standard of physical *and mental health*" (emphasis added). However, it is a fact that many international conventions containing provisions on the human right to health predominantly focus on aspects of equal access to public health, medical care, food and nutrition, clean drinking water, hygiene and environmental sanitation with only fleeting references to mental health.[1] This indicates that even within international jurisprudential standards on human right to health, the focus on mental health is a relatively recent phenomenon, given its intangible and imperceptible nature.

Right to mental health is intrinsically inter-linked, indivisible from and inter-dependent on the right to physical health as well as other human rights. For instance, the existence of violence, armed conflict and mass crimes have adverse ramifications on mental health, clearly demonstrating the links between prevalence of peace and mental well-being (Murthy & Lakshminarayana, 2006). Other studies have noted the absence of mental health and well-being among asylum seekers, refugees, and immigrants (Steel et al., 1999). Recent studies by the WHO have indicated that the COVID-19 pandemic, the lockdown and quarantine have negatively impacted not only the physical well-being but also led to mental health issues such as anxiety, depression, panic, obsessive behaviors, paranoia, and post-traumatic stress disorders (World Health Organization, 2022). At the same time, mental health warrants a specific focus, both in international and domestic legal standards.

A significant international human rights standard on mental health consists of the ***Principles for the Protection of Persons with Mental Illness and the Improvement of Mental Health Care,*** adopted by the United Nations General Assembly in 1991 (The United Nations General Assembly, 1991). It consists of various entitlements of persons with mental illnesses, such as the right:

- to receive the best mental health care available;
- to be treated with humanity and respect;
- to be free of discrimination on the grounds of mental illness;
- to equal right to medical and social care as others;
- to live, work, and receive treatment in the community, as far as possible; and
- to mental health care that is based on internationally accepted ethical standards.

The principles also contain fundamental freedoms of persons with mental illness such as.

- from misuse of mental health skills and knowledge;
- from administration of medication for the convenience of others or as a punishment;
- from administration of treatment without informed consent, for voluntary patients, subject to some exceptions; and

- from physical restraint or involuntary seclusion except in accordance with official guidelines.

Additionally, the principles place certain obligations on states including for appropriate structuring and resourcing of mental health facilities, and for the establishment of an impartial review body which, in consultation with mental health practitioners, review the cases of involuntary patients with mental illnesses.

In 1996, drawing upon the 1991 UN Principles discussed above, and largely inspired from a comparative analysis of mental health laws in 45 selected countries conducted by the WHO, it outlined 10 basic principles of mental health care. ***WHO's Principles of Mental Health Care 1996*** are as follows (World Health Organisation, 1996):

1. All persons should benefit from the best possible measures to promote mental well-being and prevent mental disorders;
2. All persons in need should have access to basic mental health care;
3. Mental health assessments should be performed in accordance with internationally accepted medical principles and instruments;
4. All persons with mental disorders should be provided with health care which is the least restrictive possible;
5. Consent is needed before any type of interference with a person can occur;
6. If a patient experiences difficulty appreciating the implications of a decision, although not unable to decide, the patient shall benefit from the assistance of an appropriate third party of his or her choice;
7. There should be a review procedure for any decision made by official, surrogate, or representative decision-makers and health care providers;
8. For decisions affecting integrity or liberty, with a long-lasting impact, there should be automatic periodical review mechanisms;
9. All decision-makers acting in official or surrogate capacity should be qualified to do so; and
10. All decisions should be made in keeping with the body of law in force in the jurisdiction involved and not on any other basis, or an arbitrary basis.

The WHO principles aim at ensuring the protection and advancement of human rights of persons with mental illnesses, in a universal manner, cutting across diversity in geopolitical contexts, cultures or legal traditions. Needless to say, it was expected that these principles will form the foundation for domestic legislations, policies and practices. However, similar to the words of Eleanor Roosevelt—the chairperson of the Drafting Committee of UDHR—who predicted that the challenge was not in drafting the Declaration but in living it, the challenge with UN Principles of 1991 and WHO Principles of 1996 was the challenge of implementation and incorporation within domestic legal systems (Gardner, 1998).

In order to facilitate this process, in 2005, WHO published a ***Mental Health Policy, Plan, and Program*** as a part of a resource book to enable countries to formulate, implement, review the adequacy and comprehensiveness of existing legislations on mental health domestically and make amendments to the same (if required) in accordance with international standards (World Health Organisation, 2005). The resource book also contains a check list to assist countries with this process (World Health Organisation, 2005). The incorporation of international standards may be undertaken through general anti-discrimination legislations, specific legislations on mental health, related policies, regulations, rules, programs, and interventions or a combination of these strategies. The WHO principles and resource book are useful as a yardstick to assess and critique the domestic legal framework on mental health.

The global efforts towards achieving mental well-being of all in a holistic manner received a shot in the arm with the ***UN Convention on the Rights of Persons with Disabilities (UNCRPD) 2007,*** passed by the UN General Assembly in December 2006. This Convention contains extensive provisions aimed at protecting and promoting the human rights of persons with mental disabilities as well, in addition to those with mental illnesses. While the Convention does not define "disability," it contains an inclusive (non-exhaustive) definition of "persons with disabilities," which is:

> *Persons with disabilities include those who have long-term physical, mental, intellectual or sensory impairments which in interaction with various barriers may hinder their full and effective participation in society on an equal basis with others.* (Article 1)

The UN Committee on the Rights of Persons with Disabilities (UNCRPD) (2015) has stated that persons with a "mental illness" (referred to as having a "psychosocial disability") are included within the purview of the Convention. Though mental illness is not always associated with mental disability, the coverage of UNCRPD covers both, and hence a hair-splitting distinction between the two is not necessary. The UNCRPD is instrumental in ensuring an elimination of legislations, policies, programs, and interventions that discriminate against persons with mental illnesses and disabilities. Significantly, it allows involuntary treatment to persons with mental illnesses only in exceptional circumstances—when a person's decision-making capability (DMC) for a specific treatment decision is impaired.

In 2013, WHO released a ***Mental Health Action Plan for 2013–2020.*** The Plan further developed upon and provided clarity to its Mental Health Policy, Plan and Program of 2005. While the 2005 document aimed at presenting evidence-based guidance for the development and implementation of mental health policy, plans, and programs at the national level, the Plan for 2013–2020 aimed at concrete outcomes. It promoted mental well-being (in addition to treating persons with mental illness), working at a preventive level on mental illnesses, providing care, enhancing recovery and promoting human rights of affected persons, and reducing the mortality, morbidity, and disability for those persons who live with mental illnesses.

B. **Policy and programmatic responses in India**

Indian official responses to the issue of mental health consist of both hard law (statutes specifically on mental health and those that refer to specific aspects of mental health) as well as soft law (such as policies and programs) dealing with the same. These categories are not watertight compartments but complementary in nature in order to make the human right to mental health a reality in India.

The Indian government launched the ***National Mental Health Programme (NMHP) in 1982***. This was triggered by the high incidence of mental illness in the country, and the absolute lack of infrastructure to address the same. In 1996, in an effort to decentralize the program and to increase the outreach of mental health care facilities to the community level, a ***District Mental Health Programme (DMHP)*** was added. The three main focus areas or components of NMHP 1982 are: (a) treatment of the mentally ill; (b) rehabilitation; and (c) prevention and promotion of positive mental health (Government of India, 2021). Although the strategies envisaged by the NMHP 1982 were lofty—such as eradicating stigmatization of mentally ill persons, and integration of mental health with primary health care services, much of the planned interventions remained on paper. In 2003, the Programme was re-strategized after considerable introspection and focused on modernization of state mental hospitals and upgradation of psychiatric wings of medical colleges/general hospitals.

National Mental Health Plan-365 in 2013 was a plan formulated by the Indian government to describe, clarify, and outline the roles and responsibilities of each stakeholder for action pertaining to mental health. The major stakeholders whose work has been outlined in the Plan are the persons with mental illness, central government, state governments and governments of union territories, municipalities, Panchayati raj (local governance) institutions, non-governmental organizations, health care personnel and institutions, medical colleges, research institutions, educational institutions including schools and colleges, private sector including corporate entities as well as media personnel. The Plan is an important attempt at assigning tasks and responsibilities, and fixing responsibility, as well as to facilitate a well-coordinated response to the issue of mental health.

The National Mental Health Plan was followed by the ***National Mental Health Policy (NMHP) 2014*** which is of special significance (Union Ministry of Health and Family Welfare, 2014). The Policy was formulated after India became a signatory to the World Health Assembly 2012, which stated that "there is need of a comprehensive, coordinated response from the health and social sectors at the community level to address the issue of burden of the mental illness" (World Health Organisation, 2012). The Policy aims at informing, clarifying, strengthening, and prioritizing the government's roles and responsibilities vis-à-vis mental health. It provides a clear plan for mental health interventions, based on an integrated, participatory and rights-based approach, aimed at providing quality mental healthcare facilities. It is ambitious and path-breaking in some ways, with far-reaching consequences, particularly in emphasis on rights-based treatment, non-institutional care and community-based rehabilitation. The objectives of the Policy, as set out in para 3.2, are as follows:

1. To provide universal access to MH care;
2. To increase access to and utilization of comprehensive MH services by PWMI (including prevention services, treatment and care, and support services);
3. To increase access to MH services for vulnerable groups;
4. To reduce the prevalence and impact of risk factors associated with MH problems;

5. To reduce the risk and incidence of suicide and attempted suicide;
6. To ensure respect for rights and protection from harm of PWMI;
7. To reduce the stigma associated with MH problems;
8. To enhance availability and equitable distribution of skilled human resources for MH;
9. To progressively enhance financial allocation and improve utilization for MH promotion and care; and
10. To identify and address the bio-psycho-social determinants of MH problems and to provide appropriate interventions.

The cross-cutting issues highlighted in the Policy (in para 4) are both interesting and informative. They include the following: stigma, right-based approach, vulnerable populations, adequate funding, support for families, inter-sectoral coordination, institutional care, promotion of mental health, and research. Acknowledging the stigma surrounding mental illnesses is the first step to addressing them, so the Policy has taken a first step in recognizing that stigma is a barrier to seeking professional help. It calls upon government, opinion makers, media personnel and community leaders to deal sensitively, compassionately and responsibly with persons with mental illnesses instead of stigmatizing them. The Policy's emphasis on vulnerable populations—such as the poor, the homeless, those inside custodial institutions, orphaned persons with mental illnesses, children of mentally ill persons, elderly caregivers, internally displaced persons, persons affected by disasters and emergencies, and other marginalized persons, stems from its apt use of an intersectional lens to address the issue of mental health. As a logical corollary of the Policy's shift from institutional care to community care, it emphasizes on support for families for the emotional and social costs involved with the role of a caregiver. In short, the Policy contains lofty ideas and principles that are founded upon human rights standards and ground realities.

In April 2020, after the breakout of the COVID-19 pandemic, the Union Ministry of Health and Family Welfare published a document titled ***Mental Health in the times of Covid-19 Pandemic: Guidance for General Medical and Specialised Mental Care Settings*** (National Institute of Mental Health & Neurosciences, 2020). The Department of Psychiatry at National Institute of Mental Health and Neurosciences (NIMHANS) was instrumental for developing the set of guidelines due to the emerging challenges on impact of COVID-19 on mental health. The Guidance document covers various mental health concerns of laypersons, as well as those with mental illness. Additionally, it addresses the safety concerns of psychiatrists and other mental health care providers. The document acknowledges that mental health concerns may keep changing in different phases of the pandemic, yet the guidelines are relevant as a form of guidance. In Part A of the document, focused on community and general medical settings, the issues it addresses include the following:

- Mental health assessment of COVID-19 patients in health care and community settings;
- Mental health issues related to home quarantine;
- Mental health issues related to quarantine or isolation in hospitals;
- COVID-19 and mental health issues among children and adolescents;

- COVID-19 and mental health among older adults;
- Addressing mental health issues among pregnant and post-partum women during COVID-19;
- Challenges faced by persons with disabilities during the pandemic;
- Psychological issues of frontline health workers;
- Social stigma and COVID-19;
- Domestic violence and COVID-19;
- Management of alcohol and tobacco use during the pandemic;
- Risk assessment and management of aggression and suicidal tendencies in the context of the pandemic;
- Yoga and COVID-19;
- Use of digital platforms for COVID-19 and beyond.

In Part B of the document, which focuses on specialist mental health services, the issues addressed include the following:

- Protective measures in psychiatric hospitals;
- Recalibrating district mental health programs during COVID-19 pandemic;
- Severe mental illnesses and COVID-19;
- Rapid tranquilization;
- Electroconvulsive therapy for patients with severe mental illnesses during the COVID-19 pandemic;
- Mental health rehabilitation in times of COVID-19 pandemic;
- COVID-19 and the recommended standards of personal hygiene and sanitation.

This document aims at providing clear guidance to medical professionals and front-line health personnel in addressing issues pertaining to mental health—both among others and among themselves—in the context of the COVID -19 pandemic.

C. **Legal framework in India**

The Indian legal framework closely follows the policy responses and are interconnected and complementary in nature. The latest legislation governing mental healthcare in India is the ***Mental Healthcare Act (MHA) 2017***. The UN Principles of 1991 and WHO's Principles of 1996, as well as the latter frameworks formulated by WHO (discussed above) influenced and informed domestic law, and came to be incorporated into the domestic legal framework through MHA 2017.

The Preamble to the MHA 2017 states as follows:

> "*An Act to provide for mental healthcare and services for persons with mental illness and to protect, promote and fulfil the rights of such persons during delivery of mental healthcare and services and for matters connected therewith or incidental thereto.*"

The emphasis on protection, promotion, and fulfillment of rights of persons with mental illnesses foregrounds the paradigm shift that MHA 2017 makes from its predecessor—MHA 1987—which did not have a rights-based approach to treatment of persons with mental illnesses, and which prioritized institutionalization over community care.

The definition of mental illness is stated in Sect. 7.2(s) of the MHA 2017 as "a substantial disorder of thinking, mood, perception, orientation or memory that grossly impairs judgment, behaviour, capacity to recognise reality or ability to meet the ordinary demands of life, mental conditions associated with the abuse of alcohol and drugs, but does not include mental retardation which is a condition of arrested or incomplete development of mind of a person, specially characterised by sub normality of intelligence." The definition is broader, more elaborate and inclusive in comparison with MHA 1987.

The MHA 2017 is divided into 16 chapters, out of which Chapters II and V are crucial in understanding mental health from a rights-based perspective, and Chapter VI is crucial in understanding state responsibility towards persons with mental illnesses. Chapter II contains provisions pertaining to how mental health should be determined, and deals with the capacity to make decisions related to mental health care and treatment. Chapter V lists and elaborates on various rights of persons with mental illnesses. Chapter VI provides various directions and guidance to the government in executing and implementing the legislation, while also emphasizing on preventive programs on mental health.

The rights of persons with mental illnesses, stated in Sects. 18–28, include the following:

- Right to access mental healthcare (S. 18).
- Right to community living (S. 19).
- Right to protection from cruel, inhuman, and degrading treatment (S. 20).
- Right to equality and non-discrimination (S. 21).
- Right to information (S. 22).
- Right to confidentiality (S. 23).
- Restriction on release of information in respect of mental illness (S.24).
- Right to access medical records (S. 25).
- Right to personal contacts and communication (S. 26).
- Right to legal aid (S. 27).
- Right to make complaints about deficiencies in provision of services (S. 28).

An understanding of rights of persons with mental illnesses would be incomplete if it was not juxtaposed with duties of the government, which include promotion of mental health and preventive programs (S. 29), awareness raising on mental health and illnesses and reduction of stigma associated with the same (S. 30), human resource development and training (S. 31) and coordination with appropriate government (S. 32). The government is also duty-bound to establish and maintain Central Mental Health Authority (detailed in Chapter VII) and State Mental Health Authority (detailed in Chapter VIII) at the central and state levels respectively, as oversight mechanisms over the work of mental health professionals and establishments. Significantly, MHA 2017 decriminalized suicide and prohibited barbaric treatments such as chaining, compulsory tonsuring, the use of electroconvulsive therapy (ECT) among adults without muscle relaxants and anesthesia, and prohibited the use of ECT altogether on minors. Significantly, the 2017 Act also provides for "advance directive" through which a person with mental illness has a right to give a directive in advance as to how they want to be treated and who their nominated representative should be (Ss. 5–13).

Given the history of international legal standards on human right to health, and the slow recognition of mental health as a vital aspect, it is significant that the MHA 2017 affirms the integration of mental health services into general healthcare services at the primary, secondary and tertiary levels and in all government-run health programs (S. 18(5)(a) of Mental Health Act, 2017). This is a step in the right direction towards ensuring that mental health is treated on par with physical health and well-being. The government is also obliged to provide mental health services at "affordable cost, of good quality, available in sufficient quantity, accessible geographically, without discrimination on the basis of gender, sex, sexual orientation, religion, culture, caste, social or political beliefs, class, disability or any other basis and provided in a manner that is acceptable to persons with mental illness and their families and care-givers" (S. 18(2) of Mental Health Act, 2017).

MHA 2017 also intersects with other legislations such as ***The Protection of Human Rights Act, 1993; The National Trust Act, 1999; Protection of Women from Domestic Violence Act (PWDVA), 2005; Protection of Children from Sexual Offences Act (POCSO), 2012***, and such other legislations. Although it is a standalone legislation focusing on mental health care, it is imperative that it is read in conjunction with ***The Rights of Persons with Disabilities (RPD) Act 2016***, particularly in reference to persons with mental disabilities. Both MHA 2017 and RPD 2016 were enacted subsequent to India's ratification of the UN Convention on Rights of Persons with Disabilities in 2006. Further, PWDVA defines 'domestic violence' as encompassing "verbal and emotional abuse" for which civil remedies are provided to any woman in a domestic relationship with the respondent (Protection of Women from Domestic Violence Act, 2005). The mental health ramifications of substantive and procedural law given in POCSO have been discussed elsewhere (DH News Service, 2017).

D. **Critically examining the national legal and policy framework**

Both the MHA 2017 and the NMHP 2014 are positive attempts at conforming to international standards on mental health, containing important paradigm shifts in official recognition of and responses to mental health issues. The legal instruments create a progressive framework of rights of persons with mental illnesses, responsibilities of state and central governments in protecting, respecting, and fulfilling their rights as well as in proactively working at the preventive level on mental health. While these are important milestones, there is a gap that exists between the provisions on paper and their implementation at the ground level.

Critique of the National Mental Health Policy 2014

The fulcrum of the Policy relied on an integrated care model, by which primary health centers will provide mental health services through general practitioners. However, in reality, there has been little focus on training and capacity building of general practitioners (Gupta & Sagar, 2014). Additionally, the policy emphasizes on aspects of justice for vulnerable groups including juveniles, children in conflict with the law (CCL) and homeless children. However, this would be possible only through the coordinated effort of various stakeholders such as lawyers, NGO actors, educators and media personnel, who will need to be on the same page including on mental illness and the commission of legal offences as a consequence. The differing approaches of the stakeholders to such offences (punitive, deterrent, retributive and rehabilitative) weaken the possibilities of a coordinated response, and reduce the possibilities of improving the lives of CCL with mental illnesses. The ground-level implementation of the Policy has been found to be abysmally low, due to poor mental health resources, lack of participation of community leaders and civil society actors (Gupta & Sagar, 2014). Moreover, the Policy, in its shift towards community-based care model, vouched to support families of persons with mental illness and support such caregivers and their families through social welfare schemes. However, research finds that this too has not been achieved to a satisfactory extent due to factors such as stigma and discrimination, cumbersome procedures for obtaining disability certificates and lack of awareness about social welfare schemes among care givers (Rao et al., 2016).

A major concern raised is about the allocation of funds for the implementation of NMHP in the national budget. In the Union budget for 2022–2023, it has been observed that a key share of the funds is assigned for the centrally funded institutes of Mental Health, while the National Mental Health Programme (NMHP) has received only 6% of the total funds assigned for mental health (India Mental Health Observatory, 2022). Further, funds allocated for the District Mental Health Programme increase over a 5-year period; however, the Union budget for 2022–2023 continues to provide districts with funds meant for year 1 of implementation (or less) and not the amount they are entitled to in subsequent years (Indian Mental Health Observatory, 2022).

Critique of the Mental Healthcare Act 2017

As in the case of the NMHP 2014 discussed above, in the case of MHA 2017 too, there are many roadblocks to a proper and effective implementation at the ground level. For instance, it ambitiously focuses on affordable, accessible, quality mental health services to all, with a focus on services at the district and sub-district levels. However, given the poor and inadequate medical infrastructure at the local levels, adding on mental health services to the physical health services provided hitherto seems to impose an unfair financial and logistical burden on state governments, unless it is offset by funds from the central government (Mishra & Galhotra, 2018). In fact, though the central and state governments have shared responsibilities in relation to the implementation of the Act, there is no provision envisaging a sharing of funds between them.

Strangely, the definition of "mental health professional" given in the Act is limited to clinical psychiatrists and specialists containing a postgraduate degree in Ayurveda, Homeopathy, Siddha, and Unani, but does not include psychotherapists and psychoanalysts. This may have been an inadvertent exclusion on the part of the legislators, but one that can have negative repercussions.

Concerns have also been raised about provisions related to the advanced directive. Given the low level of awareness, educational background, social and cultural background of persons with mental illness, it is difficult to gauge as to how many will make informed and rational decisions (Rao, 2018). Moreover, since the advanced directive maybe revoked, canceled, or modified by the person concerned endlessly, this may impair the treatment to be administered (Rao, 2018). On another note, it is imperative that a gender perspective is infused into the implementation of the Act and the Policy, as women and girls, as well as members of the LGBTQIA + community with mental illness are more vulnerable in the patriarchal society that exists in India.

Conclusion

International human rights standards related to mental health provide a foundational framework for the formulation and implementation of legislations, policies, programs, schemes, and strategic interventions at the national level. Both the Mental Healthcare Act 2017 and National Mental Health Policy 2014 are important and recent milestones in Indian official responses to mental health issues. The government's issuance of guidelines in the context of the COVID-19 pandemic is a positive step. While the lacuna between the letter of the law/policy and its implementation at the ground level needs to be addressed on a war footing, we cannot deny the significance of the normative framework, which enables each one of us to assert our entitlements and freedoms vis-à-vis mental health.

Notes

1. See for instance Article 5 of the International Convention on the Elimination of All Forms of Racial Discrimination, ICERD (1965); Article 12 of the Convention on the Elimination of All Forms of Discrimination against Women, CEDAW (1979); Article 24 of the Convention on the Rights of the Child, CRC (1989); Articles 28, 43 and 45 of the International Convention on the Protection of the Rights of All Migrant Workers and Members of Their Families, ICMW (1990); and Article 25 of the Convention on the Rights of Persons with Disabilities, CRPD (2006).

References

DH News Service. (2017, January 12). The Pocso Act and child mental health. *Deccan Herald*. Retrieved September 15, 2022, from https://www.deccanherald.com/content/591189/pocso-act-child-mental-health.html.

Gardner, R. N. (1998, December 10). Eleanor Roosevelt's legacy: Human rights, *New York Times*.

Government of India. (2021). National health policy. Retrieved September 14, 2021, from https://www.nhp.gov.in/national-mental-health-programme_pg.

Gupta, S., & Sagar, R. (2014). National mental health policy, India. Where have we reached? *Indian Journal of Psychological Medicine, 44*(5), 510–515.
The Hindu. (2022, September 8). Mental health issues cost Indian firms $14 billion a year, says Deloitte. Retrieved from https://www.thehindu.com/business/Industry/mental-health-issues-cost-indian-firms-14-bn-a-year-says-deloitte/article65866768.ece
India Mental Health Observatory. (2022). *Budget for mental health: Analysis of union budget 2022–23.* Budget Brief. Retrieved from https://cmhlp.org/wp-content/uploads/2022/02/IMHO-Union-Budget-for-Mental-Health-2022-23.pdf.
Joshi, P. A. (2018, October 10). *World mental health day: Nearly half of India Inc employees suffer from depression.* The Economic Times. Retrieved September 2022, from https://economictimes.indiatimes.com/magazines/panache/world-mental-health-day-nearly-half-of-india-inc-employees-suffer-from-depression/articleshow/66119215.cms?utm_source=contentofinterest&utm_medium=text&utm_campaign=cppst.
Mishra, A., & Galhotra, A. (2018). Mental healthcare act: Need to wait and watch. *International Journal of Applied and Basic Medical Research, 8*(2), 67–70.
Murthy, R. S., & Lakshminarayana, R. (2006). Mental health consequences of war: A brief review of research findings. *World Psychiatry, 5*(1), 26–30.
Narasimhan, L., et al. (2019). Responsive mental health systems to address the poverty, homelessness and mental illness nexus: The Banyan experience from India. *International Journal of Mental Health Systems, 13*, 54.
National Institute of Mental Health and Neurosciences. (2020). Mental health in the times of COVID-19 pandemic. In *Guidance for general medical and specialised mental health care settings*. Retrieved from https://www.mohfw.gov.in/pdf/COVID19Final2020ForOnline9July2020.pdf.
Rao, S. S. (2018). The mental health care act 2017: A critical review. *Telangana Journal of Psychiatry, 4*(2), 55–56.
Rao, G. P., Ramya, V. S., & Bada, M. S. (2016). The rights of persons with disability bill, 2014: How "enabling" is it for persons with mental illness? *Indian Journal of Psychiatry, 58*, 121.
Sagar R., et al (2020). The burden of mental disorders across the states of India: the global burden of disease study 1990–2017. *The Lancet Psychiatry*, *7*(2), 148–161. https://doi.org/10.1016/s2215-0366(19)30475-4.
Steel, Z., Silove, D., Bird, K., et al. (1999). Pathways from War trauma to posttraumatic stress symptoms among tamil asylum seekers, refugees and immigrants. *Journal of Traumatic Stress, 12*, 421–435.
The United Nations Committee on the Rights of Persons with disability. (2015). *Guidelines on article 14 of the convention on the rights of persons with disabilities. Office of the High Comissioner of Human Rights.*
The United Nations General Assembly. (1991). Resolution 46/119 of 17 December 1991. Retrieved from https://www.ohchr.org/en/instruments-mechanisms/instruments/principles-protection-persons-mental-illness-and-improvement.
Union Ministry of Health and Family Welfare, Government of India. (2014). Retrieved from http://nhm.gov.in/images/pdf/National_Health_Mental_Policy.pdf.
World Health Organisation. (2019). Mental Health. Retrieved from https://www.who.int/india/health-topics/mentalhealth#:~:text=WHO%20estimates%20that%20the%20burden,estimated%20at%20USD%201.03%20trillion.
World Health Organization. (1996). WHO/MNH/MND/96.9. Retrieved September 5, 2022, from https://bioethics.gr/api/files/download/2123/mental_healthcare_law_who.pdf?attachment=false.
World Health Organization. (2005). Mental health policy, plans and programmes, Updated version. Retrieved from https://apps.who.int/iris/handle/10665/42948.
World Health Organization. (2012). Sixty-fifth world health assembly: The global burden of mental disorders and the need for a comprehensive, coordinated response from health and social sectors

at the country level. Retrieved from https://apps.who.int/gb/ebwha/pdf_files/WHA65/A65_R4-en.pdf.
World Health Organization. (2022). The impact of Covid 19 on mental health cannot be made light of. Retrieved June 16, 2022, from www.who.int.

Saumya Uma acknowledges the research assistance of Ms. Adithi Rajesh—a student at Jindal Global Law School. The opinions expressed in this article are the author's own.

Part II
Practice Skills in Mental Health

Chapter 8
Skill Sets and Novel Approaches for Rehabilitation of Persons with Mental Disorders

Smita N. Deshpande, Mary E. Hawk, and Vishwajit L. Nimgaonkar

Abstract Mental illnesses account for a substantial portion of global disease burden: they are a top contributor to years lived with disability, and fifth largest contributor to disability-adjusted life years (Charlson, Ferrari et al., 2018). Current best treatment practices include medications, which are largely palliative, but not curative. Indian government initiatives including the pathbreaking Rights of Persons with Disability Act, 2016 (RPWD Act) (Ministry of Social Justice and Empowerment India, 2016) are hampered by societal lack of knowledge of rights, prejudice against persons with mental illness (PMI) and stigma due to mental illness preventing optimal utilization. While stigma is a more overarching term indicating knowledge attitudes and behaviour towards people with mental illness, prejudice indicates the negative attitude of the public towards those with mental illnesses. Social changes in India, such as shrinking families, ageing parents and consequent lack of family support lead to further marginalization of PMI. Meeting the needs of PMI should go beyond clinical treatment of the individual. Novel models and innovative approaches are required to integrate PMI into society and create conditions whereby the benefits of existing treatment and policies can be fully realized. The socio-ecological model is a framework for understanding the needs of PMI, and critically, to pinpoint approaches to maximize care. We discuss novel approaches to support PMI that operate at the individual, community, and policy level of the socio-ecological model. Proximal approaches, which involve treating the individual experiencing mental illness directly, include palliative care and cognitive remediation. Housing first is a supportive model of care that operates at the community level, while policy-based interventions are distal, and

---

S. N. Deshpande (✉)
Department of Psychiatry, St John's Medical College Hospital, St John's National Academy of Health Sciences, Bengaluru, India
e-mail: smitadeshp@gmail.com

M. E. Hawk
Chair of Behavioral and Community Health Sciences, University of Pittsburgh School of Public Health, Pittsburgh, USA

V. L. Nimgaonkar
Psychiatry and Human Genetics, University of Pittsburgh, Pittsburgh, USA

M. Anand (ed.), *Mental Health Care Resource Book*,
https://doi.org/10.1007/978-981-97-1203-8_8

therefore likely to have the broadest impact. We discuss the current base of evidence for each of these models; they need to be evaluated in Indian settings.

Keywords Person with mental illness · Rehabilitation · Integration · Remediation · Palliation · Community · Policy

Introduction

Nearly one billion people worldwide experience mental disorders/illnesses including severe ones such as schizophrenia or bipolar disorder, and common ones such as anxiety and depression. Experiences of mental illness have been exacerbated by the COVID-19 pandemic, which increased rates of anxiety and depression by 25% in the first year (World Health Organization, 2021a, b). In India, suicide rates rose markedly during the pandemic years (Scroll.in September 2 2022). It should be recognized and emphasized that mental health is an essential part of health overall, as it helps us attain resilience and achieve our full potential. In addition, full community participation is an essential component of mental health (World Health Organization, 2021a, b).

Mental illnesses comprise an entire group listed under "Mental and Behavioural Disorders" in the International Classification of Diseases-11 (ICD-11) (World Health Organization, 2022a, b). Mental illnesses such as depression, bipolar affective disorder, schizophrenia, anxiety disorders, dementia, substance use disorders (the most common of which include tobacco and alcohol use), intellectual disabilities, and mental illnesses with onset in childhood and adolescence, including autism are disabling and cause high burden (World Health Organization, 2021a, b).

Psychosocial Disability

Complicating the occurrence of mental illnesses is *psychosocial disability,* which refers to hurdles experienced by PMI that prevent full realization of their potential and full participation in society. These barriers may be social, physical, or legal. The Indian Rights of Persons with Disability Act, 2016 (RPWD Act) (Empowerment and India December 27 2016) aims to reduce the impact of psychosocial disabilities by asserting that all people with disabilities are entitled to dignity and respect. However, the protections afforded by the RPWD act to PMI are limited due to myths, stigma, discrimination, and exclusion that prevail in our society against mental illnesses.

Treatment Gap

A complicating factor related to psychosocial disability is the treatment gap. Simply put, the treatment gap is the difference in the numbers of people with a particular condition who need treatment but do not get it (Kale, 2002). The treatment gap for mental illnesses is huge in India- above 85% for certain conditions—extending to 91.8% even for socially accepted but unhealthy practices such as tobacco use (Gururaj, Varghese et al., 2016; Singh, 2018). India's National Mental Health Programme (NMHP) aims to close this gap by bringing mental health treatment to the community (Director General of Health Services., 1982). The WHO has formulated a model list of essential medicines (World Health Organization, 2021a, b), which include medicines for psychosis, bipolar disorder, anxiety disorders, depression, and obsessive–compulsive disorder. Even these essential psychotropic medicines are not available in the free government supply at the community level all the time, in all places. In addition, successful treatment of mental illnesses requires both medications and psychosocial interventions (World Health Organization, 2021a, b), and many criticize the NMHP as overly focused on pharmacotherapy to the exclusion of psychosocial interventions (Jain & Jadhav, 2009), which remain less widely available despite their potential impact (World Health Organization, 2021a, b).

A Socio-Ecological Model of Mental Health

Mental illnesses are multifactorial: a number of discrete, disparate factors can contribute to their onset and course. Many of these factors have reciprocal and interactive effects (Harrison, Cowen et al., 2019). These factors range from prenatal exposures (maternal infection or poor nutrition) to individual experiences such as childhood abuse or trauma. These factors can immediately precede illness onset (precipitative) and their outcome can be influenced by individual-familial-social supportive or pejorative relationships. In terms of scientific aetiology, they can thus be biological-psychological-social-environmental in origin. The socio-ecological model provides a framework for understanding factors that contribute to mental illness as a series of concentric circles (Evans, Barer et al., 1994; Kousoulis & Goldie, 2021). Initially proposed by Bronfenbrenner as a systems theory of child development (Bronfenbrenner July 13–17 1975), this model describes various levels, which interact dyadically and multiply to influence human development. This model is being increasingly used to describe mental health issues and influence public health policy (Kausoulis & Goldie, 2021). The subfactors within this model are not mutually exclusive.

Individual factors include variables that are both enabling and disabling such as biological or genetic factors, and psychological vulnerability or coping skills. Factors at the interpersonal level of the model include social relationships, such as supports from family, friends, as well as experiences rooted in the family, such as substance use and parenting skills or nurturing of children. Community-based factors contributing to mental health and mental illness include those occurring in schools, workplaces, and even faith-based groups, or in any community setting where interpersonal interactions occur. It should also be noted that disadvantaged neighbourhoods, violence, and discrimination can also occur at the community level and contribute to suboptimal mental health. At the most distal level of the model are policy and societal factors, such as government investments, environmental forces, and cultural issues such as oppression, racism, and other forms of marginalization (Guy-Evans November, 2020).

Since these policy and social factors are far reaching, investing in interventions that operate at the individual and group levels can have the greatest impact but may also be the most challenging to achieve. It is also important to consider reciprocity across levels, which means that factors on any given level can affect factors at more proximal or distal levels. For example, parenting relationships and skills (which operate at the interpersonal level) produce effects on specific members of a family (the individual level). However, family characteristics can also influence "up" in the model, contributing to the healthy or unhealthy functioning of communities. The main takeaways from the socio-ecological model are that factors influencing mental health do not occur in vacuums, and that mapping specific enabling and obstructive factors across all levels of the model will help not only to build on individual assets and strengths but also direct public health policy.

Individual-Level Models of Care

Cognitive remediation using yoga and meditation

Major mental illnesses such as schizophrenia, bipolar disorder, and major depression extract a huge human toll. Schizophrenia alone contributes 13.4 million disability-adjusted life years globally (Charlson, Ferrari et al., 2018). Medications for these illnesses are only partially effective against deficits in cognitive and community functioning. In addition, medications may themselves cause harmful side effects such as metabolic syndrome, which leads to obesity, other non-communicable metabolic diseases, physical inertia, morbidity and mortality (Cloutier, Greene et al., 2018; Goff & Hill, 2011; Newcomer & Haupt, 2006; Gautam & Meena, 2011).

We explored yoga as a cognitive enhancement tool for serious mental disorders over the last 10 years. Yoga is a culturally ingrained and highly popular practice in India, which comprises a set of spiritual and physical practices that have evolved over the past 5,000 years in India (Aranya, 1983). Yoga includes practices of self-restraint, routines, postures and physical exercises, as well as regulated mindful breathing to achieve focus and self-improvement. Positive cognitive effects of yoga have been reported in healthy persons in perceptual accuracy, processing speed, memory scores, and some other functions (Vani, Nagarathna et al., 1997; Subramanya & Telles, 2009a, b, c; Chattha, Raghuram et al., 2008). In a comprehensive review of randomized controlled trials, yoga training significantly improved cognitive functioning among older adults, improving gross memory functioning and executive functions (Hoy, Östh et al., 2021).

Yoga was associated with beneficial effects on those with depression, for sleep disorders and as an augmentation therapy in a systematic review (Balasubramaniam, Telles et al., 2012). Yoga practice has several benefits—improved quality of life (Visceglia & Lewis, 2011; Broderick, Knowles et al., 2015). In addition, some research has documented improvements in neurocognitive functions and clinical symptoms among persons with schizophrenia or stabilized psychosis (Duraiswamy, Thirthalli et al., 2007; Varambally, Gangadhar et al., 2012; Manjunath, Varambally et al., 2013; Ikai-Tani, Tani et al., 2020; Vogel, van der Gaag et al., 2019) and in community social functioning for persons with schizophrenia (Varambally, Vidyendaran et al., 2013; Behere, Arasappa et al., 2011).

Overall, the literature quoted above supports yoga as an augmentation treatment for improvement in symptom severity, various cognitive functions and social functioning for persons with schizophrenia. However, it must be noted that the beneficial effects of yoga cited in the literature to date describe relativity short-term studies. Longitudinal research is needed to fully understand the potential effects of yoga on mental illness.

Our group has been conducting studies on the effect of a 21-day formalized yoga protocol on cognitive functions in people with schizophrenia (Bhatia, Agarwal et al., 2012; Deshpande, Bhatia et al., 2016; Bhatia, Mazumdar et al., 2016; Bhatia, Gujral et al., 2021). We developed a manualized protocol in consultation with experts at the Central Council of Research in Yoga and Naturopathy (AYUSH), Government of India, Delhi and used it for all our studies (Deshpande & Pandey, 2021). In our initial pilot study, we found significant beneficial effects of yoga for cognitive functions in four groups—schizophrenia, bipolar disorders, major depression, and even stable cardiovascular disorders with differing patterns of cognitive changes in each diagnostic group, with small to medium effect sizes (Bhatia, Agarwal et al., 2012). In our second study, speed of attention on a computer-based cognitive task improved among schizophrenia patients after 21 days of yoga practice (Bhatia, Mazumdar et al., 2017). In our third trial, we added a simple meditation component to the yoga training (Bhatia, Kumari et al., 2022) and found changes in the positive direction.

In addition to these positive clinical outcomes, yoga appears to be a feasible approach to caring for PMI. Our findings demonstrate that persons with schizophrenia could perform meditation adequately, and that the practice is acceptable to all groups of people including younger persons with schizophrenia, and enhanced specific cognitive functions in all those who undertook it regularly in our studies (Bhatia, Gujral et al., 2021).

Given these findings, yoga practice can be incorporated into the treatment of PMI to improve both physical and mental health parameters. Since yoga is culturally acceptable and encouraged by society, it can be incorporated easily.

Palliative Care for Severely Disabling Mental Illnesses

Unlike palliative care for those with terminal illnesses, in its application to the treatment of PMI, palliative care does NOT indicate life-threatening or end-of-life scenarios, but rather care for certain severe, chronic, disabling and sometimes life-threatening mental illnesses such as treatment refractory schizophrenia, chronic mood disorders, or severe personality disorder. In many such patients, comorbidity with other mental and physical disorders (e.g., substance use disorder or diabetes) is common. Previous research demonstrates that palliative care approaches to treating mental illness may increase patient centredness and improve quality of life by prioritizing mutually agreed upon goals of treatment (Strand, Sjöstrand et al., 2020). In this sense, most treatments of mental disorders are palliative rather than curative.

In such scenarios, therapeutic nihilism and lack of a "permanent cure" may culminate in the patient being left to their own devices. If instead a palliative approach is adopted, then even with existing limited treatments, quality of life may improve for both patient and caregivers.

The WHO describes the following aims of palliative care: improving quality of life, early identification, impeccable assessment and treatment of pain and other problems including physical, psychosocial, and spiritual (World Health Organization, 2022a, b). Adapting this description for serious mental illnesses, the goal could be symptom control and participation in activities of daily living rather than a permanent 'cure' or a return to 'normal or regular' life.

In effect, this is what many mental health professionals may be actually practising for their treatment-resistant cases. A case management or assertive community-based treatment model—uniquely the domain of social workers—will need to be developed for such cases. Apart from medications in reasonable doses, psychosocial, or psychotherapeutic interventions and environmental manipulations could result in a much better outcome (Vita & Barlati, 2018).

Community-Level Approaches to Care

Homelessness and mental disorders: housing and supported living services

The closing of large-scale mental health institutions where the mentally ill were incarcerated for life gave rise to the problem of the homeless mentally ill all over the world. In India, families had "admitted" their mentally ill family members in "mental hospitals" and forgotten all about them. When hospitals closed down and the long-term inmates were sent home, many ended up on the street because families could not accept them back. Apart from the mentally ill becoming homeless, homelessness itself may lead to mental health conditions such as depression, suicidal thoughts, trauma, and drug abuse (Padgett, 2020).

World over, between 20 and 25% of a nation's homeless may be suffering from mental illness (Moorkath, Vranda et al., 2018). About 400,000 "wandering mentally ill" are estimated to exist in India, the largest group being the severely mentally ill—15% by some estimates (Singh, Shah et al. 2016). In one study, only half of the homeless mentally ill could be rehabilitated with their families after admission and improvement in a national institute (Gowda, Gopika et al., 2017). With family size diminishing and family support dwindling, this issue is bound to increase. Vulnerable populations such as women (Moorkath, Vranda et al., 2018) or those at extremes of age—children and the elderly—will likely be the most vulnerable to ending up on the street. With the passage of the rights-based Mental Health Care Act 2017 (MHCA, 2017; The Mental Health Care Act 2017), India has to address this problem after considering various models.

How has India tackled the issue of housing for the homeless mentally ill? Halfway homes were mentioned in the MHCA 2017. Several are in operation across India, most managed by NGOs or family organizations. The dearth of Indian publications on the subject testifies to the scarcity of this service. Some programs have been successful (the Banyan for abandoned women is a shining example) (Rao, 2004). The Richmond Fellowship (Kalyanasundaram, Hemchand et al., 2022), Anjali in Kolkata, SCARF (Schizophrenia Research Foundation) in Chennai are others. In addition, several psychiatrists work in this area—Dr Bharat Vatvani from Mumbai won the Magsaysay Award for his selfless and individual work to rehabilitate the wandering mentally ill through his organization the Shraddha Rehabilitation Foundation (https://thelogicalindian.com/exclusive/bharat-vatwani/). Ashadeep works in Guwahati, while Anvita works in Varanasi. These are laudable initiatives but need to be scaled up for the vast number of people who need such services, and then tested for effectiveness via large-scale studies. To implement such programmes all over the country, the Government needs to roll out a pan-India large-scale program. The mentally ill, after treatment and subsidence of their symptoms need some type of supported housing which can provide safe shelter and if possible regular food and medication supervision. Here, we consider the "Housing First" model, which is working in Europe and North America.

The "Housing First" model

The Housing First model as its name suggests, prioritizes providing permanent housing to homeless people, which in turn improves security and quality of life. Housing is provided without any preconditions and without prior "graduation" from other programs. In the case of PMI or those with substance use disorders, this program does not insist on treatment adherence or "perfect" health or social behaviour as a precondition to housing. This is an important distinction, since these expectations can be difficult to achieve for those who are homeless.

Housing First began in New York and is now operating in multiple sites across North America. As noted above, this model does not require adherence to treatment/abstinence from drugs as a pre-condition to obtaining supported housing. It is applied to many different groups—mentally ill, drug users, homeless youths, and even indigent families (Padgett, 2020). Another program called Critical Time Intervention (CTI) facilitates housing needs before discharge from mental health institution (Herman, Conover et al., 2011) and is also effective.

A review found Housing First to improve housing stability, lessen the need for emergency health care, and fewer and shorter hospitalizations (Baxter, Tweed et al., 2019). Another review reported that several different programs with differing approaches, as well as case management services may continue to help reduce homelessness and its consequences (Munthe-Kaas, Berg et al., 2016). Adding psychiatrist and team-based services enhanced supportive care housing (Barker, Lee-Evoy et al., 2022).

Policy-Level Approaches to Care

Rights-based care for the mentally ill: nothing for us without us:

In India, both the Rights of Persons with Disability Act (2016) (Ministry of Social Justice and Empowerment 2016) and the Mental Health Care Act 2017 (Ministry of Health & Family Welfare, 2017) are rights-based laws following from the United Nations Convention on the Rights of Persons with Disabilities (United Nations, 2006). Despite the enactment of these policies, stigma and discrimination against persons with mental illnesses continue not only in India but all over the world (Health, 2021).

For these policies to be effective, structural approaches must be implemented. There is an urgent need to integrate mental healthcare at all levels of general health care and incorporating mental healthcare in all public health programmes and policies. "Mental hygiene" training should begin in school with hygiene and drug abuse issues. Using a "life course" approach, the focus should be to inculcate healthy mental practices for all. Treatment for mental disorders should be integrated into all levels of public healthcare. Non-discriminatory health insurance should be made available for mental health conditions as well.

The rights granted under the RPWD act itself are said to "underemphasize" rights of persons with mental disability. Reservations in jobs for the mentally ill are inadequate compared to their prevalence. Moreover, the procedure for certification of mental disability is cumbersome and difficult (Balakrishnan, Kulkarni et al., 2019). The disability assessment tool for mental disability in India (Indian Disability Evaluation and Assessment Scale—the IDEAS) (Grover, Shah et al., 2014) needs research and refinement to improve its coverage of all mental illnesses (Math, Gowda et al., 2019). These authors list several challenges associated with certifying disability for various other disorders including neurodevelopmental disorders (Math, Gowda et al., 2019).

While the RPWD Act is a step in the right direction, the prevalent ignorance and stigma against mental illness influenced the relative lack of emphasis on their disability rights.

Conclusion

SMI is a "wicked" public health issue—a term used to describe a problem that is complex, not easily solved, and a significant and persistent threat worldwide. Given factors contributing to mental illness occur across all levels of the socio-ecological model, approaches to treat SMI must also be enacted across multiple levels. We propose several approaches and provide examples. In developing future interventions, we should consider other approaches of care not traditionally applied to the issue of mental illness, such as housing first. Overall, when considering treatment approaches, attention must be given to those likely to have the broadest impact, often meaning those at the policy or societal levels. Despite the fact that these can be furthest reaching, they can also be the most difficult to implement. If effective, innovative, and sustainable interventions are to succeed, commitment is needed across stakeholders. These stakeholders must not be limited to families who have too often been left to care for those with mental illness but must include clinical providers, researchers, community leaders, and the government.

References

Aranya, S. H. (1983). *Yoga Philosophy of Patanjali*. State University of New York Press.

Balakrishnan, A., et al. (2019). The rights of persons with disabilities act 2016: Mental health implications. *Indian Journal of Psychological Medicine, 41*(2), 119–125.

Balasubramaniam, M., et al. (2012). Yoga on our minds: A systematic review of yoga for neuropsychiatric disorders. *Frontiers of Psychiatry, 3*, 117.

Barker, L. C., et al. (2022). Delivering collaborative mental health care within supportive housing: Implementation evaluation of a community-hospital partnership. *BMC Psychiatry, 22*(1), 36.

Baxter, A. J., et al. (2019). Effects of housing first approaches on health and well-being of adults who are homeless or at risk of homelessness: Systematic review and meta-analysis of randomised controlled trials. *Journal of Epidemioliy and Community Health, 73*(5), 379–387.

Behere, R. V., et al. (2011). Effect of yoga therapy on facial emotion recognition deficits, symptoms and functioning in patients with schizophrenia. *Acta Psychiatrica Scandinavica, 123*(2), 147–153.

Bhatia, T., et al. (2016). *Cognitive remediation with yoga for patients with schizophrenia*. World Congress of Psychiatric Genetics, Israel.

Bhatia, T., et al. (2022). Feasibility, acceptability and evaluation of meditation to augment yoga practice among persons diagnosed with schizophrenia. Acta Neuropsychiatr, pp. 1–14.

Bhatia, T., et al. (2012). Adjunctive cognitive remediation for schizophrenia using yoga: An open, non-randomized trial. *Acta Neuropsychiatrica, 24*(2), 91–100.

Bhatia, T., et al. (2017). A randomised controlled trial of adjunctive yoga and adjunctive physical exercise training for cognitive dysfunction in schizophrenia. *Acta Neuropsychiatry, 29*(2), 102–114.

Bhatia, T., et al. (2021). Adjunctive yoga training for persons with schizophrenia: Who benefits? *Acta Neuropsychiatrica, 33*(3), 113–120.

Broderick, J., et al. (2015). Yoga versus standard care for schizophrenia. *Cochrane Database of Systematic Reviews* 10.

Bronfenbrenner, U. (1975, July 13–17). The ecology of human development in retrospect and prospect. Conference on Ecological Factors in Human Development held by the International

Society for the Study of Behavioral Development (Guildford, England, July 13–17, 1975). Guildford, England.
Charlson, F. J., et al. (2018). Global epidemiology and burden of schizophrenia: findings from the global burden of disease study 2016. *Schizophrenia Bulletin, 44*(6), 1195–1203.
Chattha, R., et al. (2008). Treating the climacteric symptoms in Indian women with an integrated approach to yoga therapy: A randomized control study. *Menopause, 15*(5), 862–870.
Cloutier, M., et al. (2018). The economic burden of bipolar I disorder in the United States in 2015. *Journal Affect Disorders, 226*, 45–51.
Deshpande, S. N., & Pandey, S. N. (2021). *Yoga Protocol for Major Mental Disorders and Stable Cardiovascular Disorders.* Delhi, Central Council for Research in Yoga and Naturopathy, Government of India.
Deshpande, S. N., et al. (2016). Cognitive remediation in schizophrenia-the view from India. *Asian Journal of Psychiatry, 22*, 124–128.
Director General of Health Services. (1982). National Mental Health Programme for India. M. o. H. a. F. Welfare. New Delhi, MoHFW.
Duraiswamy, G., et al. (2007). Yoga therapy as an add-on treatment in the management of patients with schizophrenia–a randomized controlled trial. *Acta Psychiatrica Scandinavica, 116*(3), 226–232.
Empowerment, M. O. S. J. A., & G. O. India. (2016, December 27). Rights of Persons with Disability Act; Act No. 49 of 2016. RPWD Act 2016. New Delhi India, Government of India.
Evans, R. G., et al. (1994). *Why are some people healthy and others not?* Routledge.
Gautam, S., & Meena, P. S. (2011). Drug-emergent metabolic syndrome in patients with schizophrenia receiving atypical (second-generation) antipsychotics. *Indian Journal of Psychiatry, 53*(2), 128–133.
Goff, D. C., & Hill, M. (2011). The treatment of cognitive impairment in schizophrenia. *Pharmacology Biochemistry & Behavior, 99*(2), 245–253.
Gowda, G. S., et al. (2017). Clinical outcome and rehabilitation of homeless mentally ill patients admitted in mental health institute of South India: "Know the Unknown" project. *Asian Journal of Psychiatry, 30*, 49–53.
Grover, S., et al. (2014). Internal consistency & validity of Indian disability evaluation and assessment scale (IDEAS) in patients with schizophrenia. *Indian Journal of Medical Research, 140*(5), 637–643.
Gururaj, G., et al. (2016). *National Mental Health Survey of India,* 2015–16.
Guy-Evans, O. (2020, November 09). *Bronfenbrenner's ecological systems theory.* Retrieved September 4, 2022, from www.simplypsychology.org/Bronfenbrenner.html.
Harrison, P., et al. (2019). *Shorter Oxford textbook of Psychiatry* (7th ed.). Oxford University Press India.
Health, O. W. (2021). *Comprehensive mental health action plan 2013–2030.* World Health Organization.
Herman, D. B., et al. (2011). Randomized trial of critical time intervention to prevent homelessness after hospital discharge. *Psychiatric Services, 62*(7), 713–719.
Hoy, S., et al. (2021). Effects of yoga-based interventions on cognitive function in healthy older adults: A systematic review of randomized controlled trials. *Complementary Therapy Medicine, 58*, 102690.
Ikai-Tani, S., et al. (2020). Quality of life changes in response to yoga therapy in patients with schizophrenia: Reanalysis of Three randomized controlled trials. *Asian Journal of Psychiatry, 54*, 102250.
Jain, S., & Jadhav, S. (2009). Pills that swallow policy: Clinical ethnography of a community mental health program in northern India. *Transcultural Psychiatry, 46*(1), 60–85.
Kale, R. (2002). Global campaign against epilepsy: The treatment gap. *Epilepsia, 43*(Suppl 6), 31–33.

Kalyanasundaram, S., et al. (2022). Psychiatric rehabilitation during COVID-19 pandemic: Richmond fellowship society (I), Bangalore branch experience. *Journal of Psychosocial Rehabilitation and Mental Health, 9*(1), 117–122.
Kousoulis, A. A., & Goldie, I. (2021). A visualization of a socio-ecological model for urban public mental health approaches. *Frontiers in Public Health, 9*, 654011.
Manjunath, R. B., et al. (2013). Efficacy of yoga as an add-on treatment for in-patients with functional psychotic disorder. *Indian Journ, 5*(Suppl 3), S374-378.
Math, S. B., et al. (2019). The rights of persons with disability act, 2016: Challenges and opportunities. *Indian J Psychiatry, 61*(Suppl 4), S809–S815.
Ministry of Social Justice and Empowerment and G. o. India. (2016). Rights of persons with disability Act; Act No. 49 of 2016. RPWD Act 2016. Ministry of Social Justice and Empowerment and G. o. India. New Delhi India, Government of India.
Ministry of Social Justice and Empowerment. (2016). Rights of Persons with Disability Act; Act No. 49 of 2016. RPWD Act 2016. Ministry of Social Justice and Empowerment and G. o. India. New Delhi India, Government of India.
Ministry of Health and Family Welfare. (2017). The mental health care act no. 10 of 2017. No 10 of 2017. G. o. India. Delhi, Government of India. 10 of 2017.
Moorkath, F., et al. (2018). Lives without roots: Institutionalized homeless women with chronic mental illness. *Indian Journal of Psychological Medicine, 40*(5), 476–481.
Munthe-Kaas, H., et al. (2016). *Effectiveness of Interventions to Reduce Homelessness: A Systematic Review.*
Newcomer, J. W., & Haupt, D. W. (2006). The metabolic effects of antipsychotic medications. *Canidian Journal of Psychiatry, 51*(8), 480–491.
Padgett, D. K. (2020). Homelessness, housing instability and mental health: Making the connections. *Bjpsych Bulletin, 44*(5), 197–201.
Rao, P. N. (2004). Rehabilitation of the wandering seriously mentally ill (WSMI) women-The Banyan experience. *Social Work Health Care, 39*(1–2), 49–65.
Scroll.in. (2022, September 2). Deaths by suicide highest ever in India in 2021, domestic problems biggest reason, shows NCRB data. Scroll.in. India, Scroll.
Singh, G., et al. (2016). The clinical presentation and outcome of the institutionalized wandering mentally ill in India. *Journal of Clinical and Diagnostic Research, 10*(10), VC13-VC16.
Singh, O. P. (2018). District mental health program - Need to look into strategies in the era of mental health care Act, 2017 and moving beyond Bellary model. *Indian Journal of Psychiatry, 60*(2), 163–164.
Strand, M., et al. (2020). A palliative care approach in psychiatry: Clinical implications. *BMC Medical Ethics, 21*(1), 29.
Subramanya, P., & Telles, S. (2009a). Changes in midlatency auditory evoked potentials following two yoga-based relaxation techniques. *Clinical EEG and Neuroscience, 40*(3), 190–195.
Subramanya, P., & Telles, S. (2009b). Effect of two yoga-based relaxation techniques on memory scores and state anxiety. *Biopsychosocial Medicine, 3*, 8.
Subramanya, P., & Telles, S. (2009c). Performance on psychomotor tasks following two yoga-based relaxation techniques. *Perceptual and Motor Skills, 109*(2), 563–576.
United Nations. (2006). *Convention on the rights of persons with disabilities*. United Nations.
Vani, P. R., et al. (1997). Progressive increase in critical flicker fusion frequency following yoga training. *Indian Journal Physiology and Pharmacology, 41*(1), 71–74.
Varambally, S., et al. (2012). Therapeutic efficacy of add-on yogasana intervention in stabilized outpatient schizophrenia: Randomized controlled comparison with exercise and waitlist. *Indian Journal of Psychiatry, 54*(3), 227–232.
Varambally, S., et al. (2013). Yoga-based intervention for caregivers of outpatients with psychosis: A randomized controlled pilot study. *Asian Journal of Psychiatry, 6*(2), 141–145.
Visceglia, E., & Lewis, S. (2011). Yoga therapy as an adjunctive treatment for schizophrenia: A randomized, controlled pilot study. *Journal of Alternative and Complementary Medicine, 17*(7), 601–607.

Vita, A., & Barlati, S. (2018). Recovery from schizophrenia: Is it possible? *Current Opinion in Psychiatry, 31*(3), 246–255.
Vogel, J. S., et al. (2019). The effect of mind-body and aerobic exercise on negative symptoms in schizophrenia: A meta-analysis. *Psychiatry Research, 279*, 295–305.
World Health Organization. (2021a). *Comprehensive mental health action plan 2013–2030*. World Health Organization.
World Health Organization. (2021b). *World Health Organization Model List of Essential Medicines – 22nd List, 2021*. World Health Organization.
World Health Organization. (2022a). *Health Topics- Palliative Care*. World Health Organization.
World Health Organization. (2022b). *ICD 11 for mortality and morbidity statistics (version 02/ 2022)*. World Health Organization.

Chapter 9
Therapeutic Alliance in Psychotherapy: Clinical Significance and Skills Training

M. Manjula and Reshma Antony

Abstract Therapeutic alliance is relevant across diverse therapies and has a long history in psychotherapy. Theoretical definitions of the alliance have three common components across the therapy approaches including the collaborative nature of the relationship, the affective bond between client and therapist, and the client's and therapist's ability to mutually agree on treatment goals and tasks. Therapeutic alliance scales have the patient's/ client's version, the therapist's version as well as the independent rater versions. The moderating effect of the therapeutic alliance is dependent on the kind of the assessment instrument used. Higher level of therapeutic alliance has been associated with better outcomes across the brief psychotherapies and the relationship between the outcome and alliance was modest. The current chapter covers the concept of therapeutic relationship and its various dimensions, the general principles and role of the therapist. It also covers the desirable personal attributes of the therapist such as being flexible, honest, respectful, trustworthy, confident, warm, interested, genuine and open that contribute positively to the alliance. The chapter also focuses on the methods of training to improve the therapeutic alliance building skills of the therapist.

Keywords Therapeutic alliance · Client and therapist perceptions · Assessment of therapeutic alliance · Outcome and therapeutic alliance · Therapeutic alliance building skills

Understanding Therapeutic Relationship

The therapeutic alliance or the working alliance refers to 'the collaborative relationship between therapist and client where the two establish a bond and agree on the goals of therapy and tasks to be undertaken to achieve them' (Tryon, 2011). The deliberate establishment of a therapeutic relationship is an indispensable skill as it is the vehicle and context in which therapeutic change takes place. Though therapeutic

M. Manjula (✉) · R. Antony
Department of Clinical Psychology, NIMHANS, Bengaluru, India
e-mail: drmanjula71@gmail.com

M. Anand (ed.), *Mental Health Care Resource Book*,
https://doi.org/10.1007/978-981-97-1203-8_9

alliance was talked about in psychoanalytic approach, it became one of the common factors across the therapies (Martin et al., 2000). Therapeutic alliance is indeed the base and the soul of psychotherapy which can be understood as the "treatment by psychological means, of problems of an emotional nature in which a trained person deliberately establishes a professional relationship with the patient/ client with the object of removing, modifying or retarding existing symptoms, mediating disturbed patterns of behaviour and promoting positive personality growth and development" (Wolberg, 1967). There are various theoretical perspectives that approach the therapeutic relationship differently, and the same is reflected in the therapy process starting from the very first contact of the client with the therapist. Few significant perspectives adopted in the therapeutic alliance are discussed as below:

The Existential Perspective

The Existential school of thought emphasizes the role of individual in his/her growth and maturation. A meaningful therapeutic contract is developed between the client and therapist, an arrangement in which both parties contribute and benefit. The therapist strives to establish an open and honest relationship with the client, maintaining transparency in all aspects of the therapy. This involves answering questions fully and attempting to demystify the process of therapy to enable a therapeutic relationship that is 'equal' (May & Yalom, 1989). The goal of therapeutic alliance in the existential context is to foster awareness in the client using the authentic relationship between therapist and client. The relationship with the therapist acts as the container of the clients' struggles and emotions, the acceptance of which enables them to make choices in alignment with their growth. Therefore, as per the existential perspective, the therapeutic relationship is characterized by mutual respect, individual uniqueness, authenticity, and the pursuit of meaning (Dattilio, Freeman & Blue, 1998).

The Psychodynamic Perspective

The Psychodynamic school of thought emphasizes the role of intrapsychic conflicts and early childhood experiences in the current pathologies. Three relational components are important in the study of the therapeutic alliance from a psychodynamic perspective viz. transference, countertransference and resistance. Transference refers to responding to the therapist in a way that is similar to the way one responded to another person (such as a parent) in childhood. Countertransference refers to the therapist's response to the client in a similar way he or she responded to another person in their life. The therapeutic alliance, therefore, is developed to elicit transference and countertransference distortions in the client and therapist. These are then interpreted by the therapist to allow for the resolution of conflicts. From the attachment perspective, the therapeutic relationship is seen as the developmental crucible that enables the client to explore and experience life while providing a 'secure base' for regulating himself (Wallin, 2007). The interactional affect regulation then allows the client to internalize the 'secure base' so that he can function better.

The Humanistic Perspective

The Humanistic school of thought redirects focus on the 'person' rather than on the 'problems' presented by the client. In the context of humanistic therapy, this person-centredness means that it is not the therapeutic techniques that are of prime importance, but the emphasis is on the therapeutic relationship. The therapist becomes the instrument of change by denouncing his/ her 'clinical' role and providing a space to the client for individual growth. This type of relationship then necessitates a change in the client's personality, as proposed by Carl Rogers (1961), 'If I can provide a certain type of relationship, the other person will discover within himself or herself the capacity to use that relationship for growth and change, and personal development will occur'. According to Rogers, integrity, genuineness, unconditional positive regard for the client, empathic understanding and effective communication of these with the client would enable a therapeutic relationship.

The Behaviourist Perspective

The Behavioural school of thought emphasizes the role of maladaptive behavioural patterns and faulty learning as the underlying cause of behavioural disturbances. The behavioural therapist conceptualizes the client's concerns behaviourally and attempts to develop a supportive relationship with him or her to facilitate change. The therapeutic relationship forms the foundation upon which the techniques and skills are learnt. It is not the primary instrument of change but one that ensures the necessary trust required to facilitate self-disclosure and to learn the skills that the client might find challenging. They take an active and directive stance, as opposed to one that is passive and attempting to elicit transference distortions.

The Cognitive-Behavioural Perspective

The Cognitive Behavioural perspective attempts to understand the client's dysfunctional assumptions and beliefs, and how they lead to maladjustment. Beck (1979) emphasizes the role of the therapeutic relationship in Cognitive Behavioural Therapy, starting from the very first interaction. The therapist develops trust and rapport with the client by communicating genuine interest in the client and a desire to help him/ her. One of the principles of CBT is 'collaborative empiricism', which refers to exploring the validity of the clients' thoughts together in the session using 'guided discovery'. Such collaboration requires a well-developed therapeutic alliance to be in place. Therefore, a considerable amount of time is spent on establishing the therapeutic alliance, which can then be used to effectively work with the clien's core beliefs X (Beck, 2011).

Therapeutic effects of the Therapeutic Alliance (TA) have been emphasized in all therapies. It is considered as one of the common factors across the therapies, and there is a growing consensus in the clinical psychology on the combined contribution of common and specific factors in the outcome of psychotherapy (Laska et al., 2014). Presented below are the transtheoretical observations by Bordin (1979) about the therapeutic (working) alliance across different perspectives:

a. All genres of psychotherapy have embedded therapeutic alliances and can be differentiated most meaningfully in terms of the kind of working alliance each requires
b. The effectiveness of therapy is a function in part, if not entirely, of the strength of the therapeutic alliance
c. Different approaches to psychotherapy are marked by the difference in the demands they make on the client and therapist
d. The strength of the therapeutic alliance is a function of the closeness of fit between the demands of the particular kind of alliance and the personal characteristics of the client and therapist.

Dimensions of the Therapeutic Relationship (Bordin, 1979)

1. The development of bond
2. The assignment of tasks
3. The agreement on goals

The Development of Bond

A therapeutic bond refers to the human relationship between the client and therapist. According to Carl Rogers, if the therapist treats the client like an object, he or she will tend to become an object. Bordin (1979) emphasizes the significant difference that trust, genuine concern and respect can bring about in the therapeutic relationship thereby elevating the quality of the relationship from one that is clinical and detached, to the one that is humane.

The Assignment of Tasks

The tasks dimension of the therapeutic relationship encompasses the therapist's skills and the client's perception of the therapist's ability to help (Johnson, 2002). It includes the activities undertaken by the therapist and client, and how effectively the therapist can link the assigned activities to the client's understanding of his or her difficulties. The tasks take different forms depending upon the orientation, giving reinforcements might be a therapist's task in Behaviour therapy, while interpreting might be the one in Psychoanalytic therapy. The therapeutic relationship gets enhanced by these concrete exchanges also.

The Agreement on Goals

This dimension focuses on agreeing upon a set of goals at the outset of therapy and the commitment towards these during therapy. The client's perception that the set goals are achievable also plays a role in the therapy. The specific goals set for a client depend also on the theoretical stance of the therapist, wherein a behavioural therapist may focus on specific goals such as developing coping strategies, while a psychoanalytic therapist may set broader goals such as reconstructing the client's personality.

Assessment of Therapeutic Alliance

There are a number of scales available to assess the therapeutic alliance. The scales are available in mainly three versions—observer rated, self-rated—client and therapist rated. Most frequently used measures in the research are California Psychotherapy Alliance scales (Gaston & Ring, 1992; Marmar et al., 1989), the Penn helping alliance scales (Alexander & Luborsky, 1987), the Therapeutic alliance scale (Hartley & Strupp, 1983) and Working alliance Inventory (Horvath, 1982). The literature indicates that therapist-based measures are most stable as compared to observer's rating of alliance (Horvath & Symonds, 1991). The core aspects of alliance across the measures seem to be the attachment and collaboration in the therapy process. The other factors which seem to play a role are therapist's and clients' positive or negative contributions to therapy are: shared goals for therapy, capacity to form relationship, acceptance of therapy tasks and active participation in therapy (Horvath & Luborsky, 1993).

General Principles of Therapeutic Alliance and Addressing Ruptures in Therapeutic Alliance

Safran and Muran (1998) list the following general principles which can facilitate therapeutic alliance:

(a) Facilitating therapeutic bond by conveying warmth, respect and genuine interest.
(b) Outline the therapeutic rationale the techniques and methods at the beginning of the therapy
(c) Establishing realistic goals and maintain the therapeutic focus
(d) Explain the purpose of the therapeutic tasks
(e) Maintain a balance between activity and receptivity—confrontation of the defensiveness has to be balanced with responsiveness to patients' emotions
(f) Identify and minimize enactment of vicious cycles
(g) Identification and addressing therapeutic ruptures early in the therapy—struggles over control, matching of therapist activity with the expectation of the patient, preparing patients for termination (addressing their fears and concerns).

A process outcome study carried out at Switzerland found that inability of the therapist to bond with the client by maintaining a distant alliance predicted alliance ruptures and alliance ruptures predicted premature termination (Tschuschke et al., 2021).

Client and Therapist Perspectives on Therapeutic Relationship

Client and therapists' experiences of therapeutic relationship can be different. A meta-analysis by Igra et al. (2020) examined the moderating role of client diagnosis and alliance instruments used in estimation of therapeutic alliance. They found that the client diagnosis (Schizophrenia Spectrum Disorders, Personality Disorders and Substance Use Disorders) did not have any moderating effect; however, the type of instrument had a moderating effect on the agreement of therapeutic alliance between client and therapist. A metanalytic review showed that therapeutic alliance played a moderating role in the perception of therapist empathy and genuineness (Nienhuis et al., 2018).

The therapist and patient negative ratings of the alliance at early treatment predicted drop out whereas positive rating of the patient in the first half of the treatment predicted subsequent improvement in the clinical condition (Spinhoven et al., 2007). Therapist rated alliance at session four could predict the outcome in the depression scores whereas the client rated alliance did not predict change in a study comparing internet-based interventions for depression (Vernmark, 2017).

Joyce and Piper (1998) examined the role of therapist and patient expectancies regarding the therapy sessions and its relation to therapeutic alliance and therapy outcome during short term dynamic psychotherapy. They found that the expectancy ratings were strongly related therapeutic alliance and moderately with therapy outcome. Expectancy along with the quality of object relations (capacity for mature relationships) predicted alliance or outcome. Patient rated alliance comes across as a consistent predicted of outcome (Joyce et al., 2007).

The Role of Therapist and Client Characteristics and Techniques in TA

There are various factors that affect the development of therapeutic alliance between the client and the therapist. These include the qualities of the client and therapist and therapist technical activity in the sessions (Moras & Strupp, 1982).

Therapist's attributes: Therapist's personal attributes are found to have an impact on the therapeutic alliance. A review by Ackerman and Hilsenroth (2001) identified therapist characteristics such as being rigid, uncertain, critical, distant, tense and distracted to contribute negatively. Additionally, therapist in session techniques such as over structuring or failure to structure the therapy, inappropriate self-disclosure, inappropriate use of silence, belittling, superficial interventions, unyielding transference interpretation to have negative impact on the TA. The same authors carried out a review to identify the therapist's personal attributes and in-session activities that positively influence TA. They found that personal attributes of being flexible, honest, respectful, trustworthy, warm, confident, interested and open contributed positively. Additionally, techniques such as exploration, reflection, and attending to patient's experiences contributed positively to the alliance (Ackerman & Hilsenroth, 2003). Therapist personality is also found to play an important role in the therapeutic alliance. In a study by Finlay (2018) using NEO-FFI indicated that higher agreeableness in the therapist was related to higher client reported therapeutic alliance. It was also noted in the research that therapist who achieve better outcomes score higher on interpersonal skills such as warmth and empathy (Anderson et al., 2009). More perceived social support and comfort with closeness led to stronger therapeutic alliance (Dunkle & Friedlander, 1996).

Some of the therapist skill related aspects that contributed to the therapeutic alliance were explicitly discussing the nonverbal communication of the client (Grace et al., 1995), interpreting his/ her core conflicts early in the treatment (Crits-Christoph et al., 1993), ability to repair the ruptures (Safran & McMain, 1990), greater training and experience (Mallinckrodt & Nelson, 1991).

Client's attributes: With respect to the client characteristics/ attributes and their relation to TA, both interpersonal and intrapersonal variables such as poor interpersonal/family relationships, hostile, dominant interpersonal problems, little hope in therapy, poor object relations, defensiveness, and lack of psychological mindedness are associated with poor therapeutic relationship (Connolly et al., 2016). However, there is no clarity on whether these factors influence alliance in the beginning of the therapy or throughout.

Positive expectations by the client about motivation for therapy at intake were associated with positive therapeutic alliance (Joyce & Piper, 1998; Marmar et al., 1989). Similarly, adult attachment styles in patients and therapeutic alliance are found to be related wherein greater attachment security was associated with stronger therapeutic alliance and greater attachment insecurity was associated with weaker therapeutic alliance in meta-analytic reviews (Diener & Monroe, 2011; Smith et al., 2010). However, it has to be kept in mind that the therapeutic alliance emerges from the mutual interaction between the therapist and the client, thus the interpersonal dynamics has to be paid attention to (Tschacher et al., 2015).

Therapeutic Alliance and Outcomes in Psychotherapy

Therapeutic relationship has been found to be related to the effectiveness of a therapy. The relationship between the therapeutic alliance and outcome has been very well established as stronger alliance has predicted positive outcomes (Fluckiger et al., 2018; O'Connor et al., 2019). A sound therapeutic relationship motivates the client to overcome his/her illness, cooperate in the therapy willingly and see the therapist as a person capable of helping (Fluckiger et al., 2012; Norcross & Wampold, 2011; Friedlander et al., 2011).

Metanalytical studies have shown that higher level of therapeutic alliance was associated with better outcomes across the therapies and the relationship between the outcome and alliance was modest (an average effect size of 0.22—0.26) (Horvath & Symonds, 1991; Horvath et al., 2011; Martin et al., 2000).). The effect of therapeutic alliance however was found to be larger than the effects of therapist adherence to treatment or therapist competence (Webb et al., 2010). Another review noted that the positive outcomes are irrespective of the therapeutic approaches and the kind of the measures used (Ardito & Rabillino, 2011). Agreement on the therapeutic goals at the beginning of the therapy is found to be related to the reduction of depressive symptoms at the end of therapy (Webb et al., 2011). Additionally using techniques which targets symptom reduction in the initial sessions strengthens working alliance (Bedi et al., 2005).

Therapeutic alliance may vary across the time points in therapy. Though the importance of therapeutic alliance in the initial sessions is proposed to influence the motivation to change, reduction in symptoms and experience of quality of life in clients, the findings have been inconsistent (Horvath & Marks, 1991). In the literature related to the patterns of the therapeutic alliances across the therapy suggests two major models: (a) A linear model characterized by progressive increase in the alliance rating, and (b) A high-low-high model—which is characterized by initial high alliance and middle low and finally high alliance. In the initial sessions clients will have hope and believe in improvement, however in the middle sessions they may realize that all the problems may not be addressed as expected thereby giving rise to low alliance. Once they start seeing the results and accept the outcomes, they will have high alliance. The literature is inconsistent with respect to high-low-high alliance (Stevens et al., 2007). A few studies have noted that a linear trend of alliance was found in more than half of the clients whereas local rupture-and-repair patterns were found in about half of the clients (Bordin, 1989; Stevens et al., 2007). However, there was no relationship between outcome and either of the patterns. The alliance is found to fluctuate across the sessions as well as within a session. Thus, it was opined that aggregate of the early few sessions would provide a better prediction of the outcomes (e.g., sessions 3–9) (Crits-Christoph et al., 2012). More than the trend, early detection of alliance ruptures (poor understanding and breakdown in communication etc.) and resolution of the same was found to be critical to successful therapy (Saffron & Muran, 2006; Parry et al., 2016).

Therapeutic alliance was similar across the face-to-face interventions, mixed/combined interventions and technology-based interventions. It was also noted that many therapists may be apprehensive of the technical glitches interfering with the therapeutic alliance. In the online therapies it has been noted that any technical issues can be dealt with back-up plans (Lopez et al., 2019; Wehmann et al., 2020). Therapeutic alliance was found to be equally strong across the range of diagnosis. The clients rated bond and presence equally strong as in-person therapies (Simpson & Reid, 2014). The clients who dropped out of therapy and their therapists rated the therapeutic alliance as more problematic as compared to those in the 'good' outcome group. However, there has been no significant difference between those with 'poor' outcome and 'good' outcome patients' group with respect to the rating of therapeutic alliance (Samstag et al., 1998).

Therapeutic alliance played an important role across psychotherapies (Cognitive Behavior Therapy and Interpersonal Therapy), Active and Placebo Pharmacotherapy in the outcomes of depression. A study found that the rating of patient contribution to the alliance was significantly related to the outcome whereas therapist's contribution was not linked to the outcome (Krupnick et al., 1996). However, in psychodynamic therapies, the accuracy of therapist's interpretations also contributed to maintaining good therapeutic relationship. This implies that what the therapist does or the intervention components adopted by the therapist also play a major role in maintaining therapeutic relationship (Crits-Christoph et al., 1993). It has been consistently noted in the literature that patient rated alliance predicted the outcomes compared to the therapist ratings (Joyce et al. (2007)). Additionally, patient's treatment preference played a major role on the therapeutic alliance (Iacoviello et al., 2007).

A metanalytical review on the relationship between therapeutic alliance and dropout in adults undergoing individual psychotherapy, a moderately strong relationship was found between the two. Higher education level in the clients had lower drop out, lengthier therapy had more dropouts and inpatient setting had lower drop out compared to therapy carried out at counseling and research centers (Sharf et al., 2010).

Strength of the early therapeutic alliance was associated with later drop out in personality disorders. While cluster A patients had difficulty in establishing therapeutic relationship, therapists evaluated alliance negatively in cluster B patients. Therapists' evaluation was lower compared to the client's evaluation most of the time (Lingiardi et al., 2005).

Significance of Training for Therapists in Addressing Ruptures in Therapeutic Alliance

Though therapeutic relationship is considered as one of the general core components of the psychotherapies, most training programs (counseling and psychotherapy) do not give importance to training in the relationship factors. Often therapists find it difficult to recognize and address the ruptures. This is applicable to both novice therapists as well as senior/experienced therapists. Some of the reasons for the same are the therapist giving personal reactions to the ruptures and avoid rifts in the alliance without addressing them, avoiding discomfort of addressing them by responding defensively.

Summers and Barber (2003) recommend various methods of skills training to improve the therapeutic alliance including early supervisory focus of therapeutic alliance; focus on the therapeutic formulation; attention to therapeutic ruptures; setting appropriate, realistic and negotiated goals; and identifying patient and therapist tasks in therapy.

Some of the principles outlined by Safran and McMain (1990) in resolving therapeutic ruptures entail attending to ruptures in alliance, awareness of one's own feelings, accepting responsibility, empathizing with the client's experience and maintaining the stance of observer.

The question as to whether training the therapists in enhancing their skills to foster therapeutic alliance would result in better alliance and outcome in therapy has been addressed recently and there are attempts to develop and test such interventions. One such therapy is given by Crits-Christoph et al. (1998) named as manual-based alliance-fostering therapy. The techniques used in this therapy are based on a number of existing psychotherapies such as client-centered therapy, motivational enhancement therapy, and cognitive behavior therapy and these techniques are organized around Bordin's (1979) conceptualization of therapeutic alliance i.e., tasks, goals and bond. The techniques for maximizing the agreement on goals included establishing explicit goals, and regular review of goals. For maximizing agreement on tasks, patients were socialized to therapy and the tasks were reviewed regularly for enhancing bond; motivation enhancement and monitoring the patient involvement to increase personal role and the collaborative environment was established through empathic stance of the therapist, use of the word we, and back and forth communication. In addition, therapists were trained in the components of core conflictual relationship theme. One study using training of therapists in alliance fostering therapy, it was found that from pre to post training there was moderate to large increases in the alliance. However, this study did not have a control group, thus it is difficult to conclude on the effectiveness of the intervention (Crits-Christoph et al., 2006).

Beitman's (1999) modular psychotherapy training emphasizes on training in therapeutic alliance in the beginning of the training. The therapists are trained to observe and rate their therapeutic alliance during their sessions and video interviews with respect to role of task, goal and bond. In another training by Grace (1990) for counselors there was emphasis on explicitly addressing the verbal and non-verbal behaviours of the clients which was associated with improved therapeutic relationship. Kurcias (2000) gave a step-by-step teaching of the therapeutic alliance skill in her trainees. According to her the initial focus of the supervision is to recognize the therapeutic alliance, formulation of patient and therapist, therapeutic relationship and handling ruptures.

Another study reported that training the students in conceptual and observational skills relating to therapeutic alliance resulted in significant improvement in knowledge of conceptualization and observational skills. However, this study did not assess its relation to the therapeutic outcomes (Carpenter et al., 2008). It is also reported that the clinician students who received personal therapy reported higher confidence, goal and task agreement and self-reported alliance as compared to those without personal therapy. It was also noted that the number of therapy sessions attended by their clients were two times more than those without (Gold & Hilsenroth, 2009). Summers and Barber (2003) recommend the following in training the therapists in therapeutic alliance: evaluation of the training programs in terms of when the task, goal and bond should be addressed educationally; collection of alliance ratings for competency assessment and program evaluation; rating of alliance across the therapy e.g. at sessions 2, 5, 10 and follow-up. Probably paying attention to consistent lower ratings by the clients and when there are large discrepancies between the client and therapist rating would help in training is their suggestion.

Though therapeutic alliance is considered as a core element of any psychotherapy most of the doctoral programs and clinical training programs do not include systematic, evidence based training into their programs. A survey conducted by Constantino et al. (2017) obtained data from the Directors of the counseling and clinical programs accredited to American Psychological Association found that the systematic training in TA was not happening in most of these programs.

Conclusion

Therapeutic alliance is identified as one of the pan theoretical common factors across the psychological therapies. The core aspect of the therapeutic alliance across the therapies and assessment tools seems to be the attachment between the therapist and client and the amount of collaboration between the two in the process of therapy. The other contributing factors include the personal characteristics of the therapist and the client based attributes, mutual agreement on goals of therapy, therapeutic techniques adopted, acceptance of the tasks and active participation. Additionally, identification of therapy ruptures and repairing them early in therapy play an important role in therapy outcomes. Both therapist and client rating of the therapeutic alliance predict the therapy outcomes. Therapeutic relationship significantly contributes to the therapy outcomes irrespective of the kind of the therapy used. The therapeutic relationship may vary across the time points in therapy; however, the strength of the initial therapeutic relationship seems to play an important role in the therapy outcomes. The training of the therapist in enhancing therapeutic skills is not a part of many training programs. It is an upcoming topic of interest in the therapy research and training.

References

Ackerman, S. J., & Hilsenroth, M. J. (2001). A review of therapist characteristics and techniques negatively impacting the therapeutic alliance. *Psychotherapy, 38*, 171–185.

Ackerman, S. J., & Hilsenroth, M. J. (2003). A review of therapist characteristics and techniques positively impacting the therapeutic alliance. *Clinical Psychology Review, 23*(1), 1–33.

Alexander, L. B., & Luborsky, L. (1986). The Penn helping alliance scales. In L. S. Greenberg & W. M. Pinsoff (Eds.), *The psychotherapeutic process: A research handbook* (pp. 325–366). Guilford Press.

Anderson, S., Tambling, R., Yorgason, J., & Rackham, E. (2018). The mediating role of the therapeutic alliance in understanding early discontinuance. *Psychotherapy Research, 29*, 1–12.

Ardito, R. B., & Rabellino, D. (2011). Therapeutic alliance and outcome of psychotherapy: Historical excursus, measurements, and prospects for research. *Frontiers in Psychology, 18*(2), 270.

Beck, J. S. (2011). *Cognitive Behavior Therapy, Second Edition: Basics and Beyond*. Guilford Publications.

Beck, A. T., Rush, A. J., Shaw, B. F., & Emery, G. (1979). *Cognitive therapy of depression*. Guilford Press.

Bedi, R., Davis, M., & Williams, M. (2005). Critical incidents in the formation of the therapeutic alliance from the client's perspective. *Psychotherapy Theory Research Practice Training., 42*, 311. https://doi.org/10.1037/0033-3204.42.3.311

Beitman, B. D., & Yue, D. (1999). *Learning psychotherapy: A time-efficient, research-based, and outcome-measured psychotherapy training program. W W Norton & Co.*

Bordin, E. S. (1979). The generalizability of the psychoanalytic concept of the working alliance. *Psychotherapy: Theory, Research & Practice, 16*(3), 252–260.

Carpenter, J., Escudero, V., & Rivett, M. (2008). Training family therapy students in conceptual and observation skills relating to the therapeutic alliance: An evaluation. *Journal of Family Therapy, 30*(4), 411–424.

Connolly J. P. (2016). *Principles of organization of psychic energy within psychoanalysis: A systems theory perspective*. thesis, Pretoria: University of South Africa. Unpublished doctoral thesis.

Constantino, M. J., Morrison, N. R., Coyne, A. E., & Howard, T. (2017). Exploring therapeutic alliance training in clinical and counseling psychology graduate programs. *Training and Education in Professional Psychology, 11*(4), 219–226.

Crits-Christoph, P., Connolly Gibbons, M. B., Crits-Christoph, K., Narducci, J., Schamberger, M., & Gallop, R. (2006). Can therapists be trained to improve their alliances? A pilot study of Alliance-Fostering Therapy. *Psychotherapy Research., 13*, 268–281.

Crits-Christoph, P., & Crits-Christoph, K. (1998). *Alliance-fostering therapy for major depressive disorder.* University of Pennsylvania; Unpublished manuscript.

Crits-Christoph, P., Gibbons, M. B., Hamilton, J., Ring-Kurtz, S., & Gallop, R. (2011). The dependability of alliance assessments: The alliance-outcome correlation is larger than you might think. *Journal of Consulting and Clinical Psychology, 79*(3), 267–278.

Crits-Christoph, P., Barber, J., & Kurcias, J. (1993). The accuracy of therapists interpretations and the development of the therapeutic alliance. *Psychotherapy Research, 3*(1), 25–35.

Dattilio, F., & Hanna, C. M. (2012). Collaboration in cognitive-behavioral therapy. *Journal of Clinical Psychology, 68*, 146–158.

Diener, M. J., & Monroe, J. M. (2011). The relationship between adult attachment style and therapeutic alliance in individual psychotherapy: A meta-analytic review. *Psychotherapy, 48*(3), 237–248.

Dunkle, J. H., & Friedlander, M. L. (1996). Contribution of therapist experience and personal characteristics to the working alliance. *Journal of Counseling Psychology, 43*(4), 456–460.

Finlay, Michael. (2018). The relationship between psychotherapist personality and therapeutic alliance. *Loma Linda University Electronic Theses, Dissertations & Projects.* 519.

Flückiger, C., Del Re, A. C., Wampold, B. E., Symonds, D., & Horvath, A. O. (2012). How central is the alliance in psychotherapy? A multilevel longitudinal meta-analysis. *Journal of Counselling Psychology, 59*(1), 10–17.

Flückiger, C., Del Re, A. C., Wampold, B. E., & Horvath, A. O. (2018). The alliance in adult psychotherapy: A meta-analytic synthesis. *Psychotherapy, 55*(4), 316–340.

Friedlander, Myrna, Escudero, Valentín, Heatherington, Laurie, & Diamond, Gary. (2011). The therapeutic alliance in couple and family therapy. Psychotherapy (Chicago, Ill.). 48, pp. 25–33.

Gaston, L., & Ring, J. M. (1992). Preliminary results on the inventory of therapeutic strategies. *Journal of Psychotherapy Practice and Research, 1*(2), 135–146.

Gold, S. H., & Hilsenroth, M. J. (2009). Effects of graduate clinicians' personal therapy on therapeutic alliance. *Clinical Psychology and Psychotherapy, 16*(3), 159–171.

Grace, M., Kivlighan, D. M., Jr., & Kunce, J. (1995). The effect of nonverbalskills training on counselor trainee nonverbal sensitivity and responsiveness and on session impact and working allianceratings. *Journal of Counselling and Development, 73*, 547–552.

Hartley, D. E. & Strupp, H. H. (1983). The therapeutic alliance: Its relationship to outcome in brief psycho-therapy. *Empirical studies in psychoanalytic theories*, 1–37.

Horvath, A. O., Del Re, A. C., Flückiger, C., & Symonds, D. (2011). Alliance in individual psychotherapy. *Psychotherapy (Chic), 48*(1), 9–16.

Horvath, A. O., & Luborsky, L. (1993). The role of the therapeutic alliance in psychotherapy. *Journal of Consulting and Clinical Psychology, 61*(4), 561–573.

Horvath, A. O. (1982). Working alliance inventory (Revised). *Instructional Psychology Research Group, 82* (1). Simon Fraser University, Burnaby, British Columbia, Canada.

Horvath, A. O., & Symonds, B. D. (1991). Relation between working alliance and outcome in psychotherapy: A meta-analysis. *Journal of Counseling Psychology, 38*, 139–149.

Horvath, A. O., & Marx, R. W. (1991). The development and decay of the Working Alliance during time-limited counselling. *Canadian Journal of Counselling, 24*, 240–259.

Iacoviello, B. M., McCarthy, K. S., Barrett, M. S., Rynn, M., Gallop, R., & Barber, J. P. (2007). Treatment preferences affect the therapeutic alliance: Implications for randomized controlled trials. *Journal of Consulting and Clinical Psychology, 75*(1), 194–198. https://doi.org/10.1037/0022-006X.75.1.194. PMID: 17295580.

Igra, L., Lavidor, M., Atzil-Slonim, D., Arnon-Ribenfeld, N., De Jong, S., & Hasson-Ohayon, I. (2020). A meta-analysis of client-therapist perspectives on the therapeutic alliance: Examining the moderating role of type of measurement and diagnosis. *European Psychiatry, 63*(1), E67. https://doi.org/10.1192/j.eurpsy.2020.67

Johnson, L. N., & Wright, D. W. (2002). Revisiting Bordin's theory on the therapeutic alliance: implications for family therapy. *Contemporary Family Therapy*, 13.

Joyce, A. S., & Piper, W. E. (1998). Expectancy, the therapeutic alliance, and treatment outcome in short-term individual psychotherapy. *Journal of Psychotherapy Practice & Research, 7*(3), 236–248.

Joyce, A. S., Piper, W. E., & Ogrodniczuk, J. S. (2007). Therapeutic alliance and cohesion variables as predictors of outcome in short-term group psychotherapy. *International Journal of Group Psychotherapy., 57*(3), 269–296.

Krupnick, J. L., Sotsky, S. M., Simmens, S., Moyer, J., Elkin, I., Watkins, J., & Pilkonis, P. A. (1996). The role of the therapeutic alliance in psychotherapy and pharmacotherapy outcome: Findings in the national institute of mental health treatment of depression collaborative research program. *Journal of Consulting and Clinical Psychology, 64*(3), 532–539.

Kurcias, J. (2000). Therapy trainees and developmental changes in the alliance. *Dissertation Abstracts International: Section B: the Sciences & Engineering, 60*(11-B), 5779, US: Univ. Microfilms International.

Laska, K. M., Gurman, A. S., & Wampold, B. E. (2014). Expanding the lens of evidence-based practice in psychotherapy: A common factors perspective. *Psychotherapy, 51*, 467.

Lingiardi, V., Filippucci, L., & Baiocco, R. (2005). Therapeutic alliance evaluation in personality disorders psychotherapy. *Psychotherapy Research, 15*(1–2), 45–53.

López-López, J. A., Davies, S. R., Caldwell, D. M., Churchill, R., Peters, T. J., Tallon, D., et al. (2019). The process and delivery of CBT for depression in adults: A systematic review and network meta-analysis. *Psychological Medicine, 49*(12), 1937–1947.

Mallinckrodt, B., & Nelson, M. L. (1991). Counselor training level and the formation of the psychotherapeutic working alliance. *Journal of Counseling Psychology, 38*, 133–138.

Marmar, C. R., Weiss, D. S., & Gaston, L. (1989). Toward the validation of the California therapeutic alliance rating system. *Psychological Assessment., 1*, 46–52.

Martin, D. J., Garske, J. P., & Davis, M. K. (2000). Relation of the therapeutic alliance with outcome and other variables: A meta-analytic review. *Journal of Consulting and Clinical Psychology, 68*(3), 438–450.

May, R., & Yalom, I. D. (1989). Existential psychotherapy. In R. J. Corsini & D. Wedding (Eds.), *Current psychotherapies* (pp. 363–402). F E Peacock Publishers.

Moras, K., & Strupp, H. H. (1982). Pretherapy interpersonal relations, patients' alliance, and outcome in brief therapy. *Archives of General Psychiatry, 39*(4), 405–409.

Nienhuis, J. B., Owen, J., Valentine, J. C., Winkeljohn, B. S., Halford, T. C., Parazak, S. E., Budge, S., & Hilsenroth, M. (2018). Therapeutic alliance, empathy, and genuineness in individual adult psychotherapy: A meta-analytic review. *Psychotherapy Research., 28*(4), 593–605.

Norcross, J. C., & Wampold, B. E. (2011). Evidence-based therapy relationships: Research conclusions and clinical practices. In J. C. Norcross (Ed.), *Psychotherapy relationships that work: Evidence-based responsiveness* (pp. 423–430). Oxford University Press.

O'Connor, K., Jr., Hill, C. E., & Gelso, C. J. (2019). Therapist-client agreement about their working alliance: Associations with attachment styles. *Journal of Counseling Psychology, 66*(1), 83–93. https://doi.org/10.1037/cou0000303

Parry, R., Pino, M., Faull, C., & Feathers, L. (2016). Acceptability and design of video-based research onhealthcare communication: Evidence and recommendations. *Patient Education and Counseling, 99*(8), 1271–1284. https://doi.org/10.1016/j.pec.2016.03.013

Rogers, C. R. (1961). *On becoming a person.* Houghton Mifflin.

Safran, J. D., Crocker, P., McMain, S., & Murray, P. (1990). Therapeutic alliance rupture as a therapy event for empirical investigation. *Psychotherapy: Theory, Research, Practice, Training, 27*(2), 154–165.

Safran, J. D., & Muran, J. C. (1998). The therapeutic alliance in brief psychotherapy: General principles. In J. D. Safran & J. C. Muran (Eds.), *The therapeutic alliance in brief psychotherapy* (pp. 217–229). American Psychological Association.

Safran, J. D., & Muran, J. C. (2006). Has the concept of the therapeutic alliance outlived its usefulness? *Psychotherapy (chicago, Ill.), 43*(3), 286–291.

Samstag, L. W., Batchelder, S. T., Muran, J. C., Safran, J. D., & Winston, A. (1998). Early identification of treatment failures in short-term psychotherapy. An assessment of therapeutic alliance and interpersonal behavior. *Journal of Psychotherapy Practice and Research, 7*(2):126–143.

Sharf, J., Primavera, L. H., & Diener, M. J. (2010). Dropout and therapeutic alliance: A meta-analysis of adult individual psychotherapy. *Psychotherapy (chicago, Ill.), 47*(4), 637–645.

Simpson, S. G., & Reid, C. L. (2014). Therapeutic alliance in videoconferencing psychotherapy: A review. *Australian Journal of Rural Health., 22*(6), 280–299.

Smith, A. E., Msetfi, R. M., & Golding, L. (2010). Client self-rated adult attachment patterns and the therapeutic alliance: A systematic review. *Clinical Psychological Review, 30*(3), 326–337.

Spinhoven, P., Giesen-Bloo, J., van Dyck, R., Kooiman, K., & Arntz, A. (2007). The therapeutic alliance in schema-focused therapy and transference-focused psychotherapy for borderline personality disorder. *Journal of Consulting and Clinical Psychology, 75*(1), 104–115.

Stevens, C. L., Muran, J. C., Safran, J. D., Gorman, B. S., & Winston, A. (2007). Levels and patterns of the therapeutic alliance in brief psychotherapy. *American Journal of Psychotherapy., 61*(2), 109–129.

Summers, R. F., & Barber, J. P. (2003). Therapeutic alliance as a measurable psychotherapy skill. *Academic Psychiatry., 27*(3), 160–165.

Tryon, G., & Winograd, G. (2011). Goal consensus and collaboration. *Psychotherapy* (Chicago, Ill.), *48*, 50–57.

Tschacher, W., Haken, H., & Kyselo, M. (2015). Alliance: A common factor of psychotherapy modeled by structural theory. *Frontiers in Psychology, 1*,. https://doi.org/10.3389/fpsyg.2015.00421

Tschuschke, V., Koemeda-Lutz, M., von Wyl, A., et al. (2022). The impact of Clients' and therapists' characteristics on therapeutic alliance and outcome. *Journal of Contemporary Psychotherapy, 52*, 145–154.

Vernmark, K. (2017). *Therapeutic Alliance and Different Treatment Formats When Delivering Internet-Based CBT for Depression.* https://doi.org/10.3384/diss.diva-142389

Wallin, D. J. (2007). *Attachment in psychotherapy*. Guilford Publications.

Webb, C. A., DeRubeis, R. J., Amsterdam, J. D., Shelton, R. C., Hollon, S. D., & Dimidjian, S. (2011). Two aspects of the therapeutic alliance: Differential relations with depressive symptom change. *Journal of Consulting and Clinical Psychology., 79*(3), 279–283.

Wehmann, E., Köhnen, M., Härter, M., & Liebherz, S. (2020). Therapeutic alliance in technology-based interventions for the treatment of depression: Systematic review. *Journal of Medical Internet Research, 11*; 22(6), e17195. https://doi.org/10.2196/17195.

Wolberg, L. R. (1967). *The Technique of Psychotherapy,* Vol. 2. United Kingdom: William Heinemann (Medical Books).

Chapter 10
Motivational Interviewing: Walking Towards Change

Prerna Srivastava and Kannappa V. Shetty

Abstract Motivational Interviewing (MI) is an evidence-based counseling and a collaborative approach. It targets clients' ambivalence and helps them bring about behavioral changes through negotiation. Miller observed that people tend to become defensive and show resistance when they are confronted directly about their shortcomings. The highlight of this technique is that the entire articulation about commitment to changes is made by the client himself rather than the therapist. The current chapter focuses on the MI as a 'skilful clinical method' and as a technique adopted by mental health professionals and entails its central principles and strategies including OARS (Open questions, Affirming, Reflecting and Summarizing), decisional balance sheet, change plan worksheet, etc. It reflects the usage of the technique in treatment of alcohol and related disorders and expansion of MI in the treatment of gambling disorder, eating disorder, risky sexual behaviour, diabetes, pain, and stress management. The chapter also feature the application of MI in various fields including healthcare, rehabilitation, dentistry, public health, education, and IT & BT sectors. The chapter also consists of several case illustrations for the use of MI in various mental disorders. Thus, motivational interviewing is an essential counselling technique that can be used independently or as an adjunct to various other interventions.

Keywords Motivational interviewing · Alcohol dependence · Substance dependence · Life style disorders · Mental health · Wellness · Rehabilitation

P. Srivastava
Clinical Psychologist, Mumbai, Maharashtra, India

K. V. Shetty (✉)
Assistant Professor, School of Social Work, Indira Gandhi National Open University, New Delhi, India
e-mail: vksettymsw@gmail.com

M. Anand (ed.), *Mental Health Care Resource Book*,
https://doi.org/10.1007/978-981-97-1203-8_10

Introduction

The origin of Motivational Interviewing (MI) lies in the observations made by Miler (1992) about the impact of therapist's style of delivering therapy made on the behavioral outcome of the substance used disorder clients. He noted that client centered therapy style accounted for significant variance in therapy outcome as well as in the relapse rate. Studies also found significant difference in substance use outcome depending on the therapist. Miller (1992) observed that people tend to become defensive and show resistance when they are confronted directly about their shortcomings. The highlight of this technique is that the entire articulation about commitment to changes is made by the client himself/ herself rather than the therapist (Rollnick, Miller, & Butler, 2008) defined Motivational Interviewing (MI) as '*a directive, patient-centred counselling style for eliciting behaviour change by helping patients to explore and resolve ambivalence.*' They enlisted collaboration, evocation, and autonomy as key components of MI. This was based on Beam's self-perception theory (Bem, 1972) which states that the attitude of people is derived from their observation of their own behaviour. Hence, hearing themselves talk about making a change might help re-evaluate and bring about changes in their behaviour. The motivational Interviewing also derives from the transtheoretical model of change (Prochoska & Velicer, 1997) which divides the readiness to change into five stages viz. Precontemplation, Contemplation, Determination, Action, and Maintenance.

Miller and Rollnick (2012) emphasized that MI is a '*skilful clinical method*' rather than a collection of techniques which can be easily acquired. Bien et al. (1993) enlisted 6 components that they observed to be present in most of the effective brief intervention. They used an acronym FRAMES – Feedback, Responsibility, Advice, Menu, Empathic style, and Self efficacy. This along with MI formed the 'Drinker's Check-up' programme and later was called Motivational enhancement Therapy.' The therapy was found to significantly change drinking behaviour (Miller & Rollnick, 2012).

The motivational interview was traditionally used in the treatment of alcohol and substance dependence. Studies have indicated that it is equivalent or superior to interventions like Cognitive Behaviour Therapy, Behaviour Therapy, and pharmacotherapy (Burke & Arkowitz, 2003). However, it has now evolved to be used in healthcare, rehabilitation, dentistry, public health, education sector, and social work. It has been used for gambling disorders (Yakovenko et al., 2015) as well as eating disorders (Weiss et al., 2013) and risky sexual behaviours (Bassett et al., 2022). It is used to improve treatment adherence (Palacio et al., 2016) as well as to enhance healthier lifestyle (Boom et al., 2022). MI has been used in stress management, diabetes and HIV management, and pain management (Hall et al., 2012) in addition to being used in organizations to help facilitate change amongst the staff (Arbuckle et al., 2020).

Although a significant number of trials have proved the efficacy of MI, there has been few contradictory findings as well. Few studies have shown no significant improvement in alcohol use, nicotine use, substance use and eating disorder. Further few studies have shown that efficacy varies across population (Miller & Rose, 2009).

Pillars of Motivational Interviewing

(1) Change talk

Miller and Rollnick (2012) gave the hypothesis of 'change talk' which helps clients verbalize thoughts about change. 'Sustain talk' is the talk which would help maintain the status quo. A major emphasis is on the client therapist relationship, focusing on the empathic understanding. Although change is a natural process, brief counseling plays a significant role in bringing about the change. It is highlighted that the role of the counselor/therapist as a determining factor in bringing about the change and enlisted three essential components of motivation, which are readiness, willingness, and ability to change. Miller and Rollnick (2012) gave 4 categories of change talk.

- Disadvantages of status quo
- Advantages of change
- Optimism for change
- Intention to change

(2) Ambivalence

Ambivalence is a normal experience and is experienced in various spheres of life including jobs and relationships. It is considered as a stage in the change process where an individual needs to resolve the conflict which might arise due to ambivalence in order to bring about a positive change in life. In case of addiction, the client may need help in resolving the ambivalence. The therapist must be cautious about the paradox responses which might hinder the positive change and even might push the client further into addiction. Too much persuasion from the family members is considered as a common cause of paradoxical response. Miller and Rollnick (2012) pointed out that often by giving a mere option to choose rather than persuading for a single option helps in avoiding the paradoxical response and resolving the ambivalence.

It may be added that a key feature of MET is that it considers motivation as interpersonal process rather than an internal process. Many therapeutic approaches assume that client is already motivated and gives less importance to the motivation process, however MET puts great importance on the motivation for change.

(3) Discrepancy

When the therapist argues with the client to bring about the change, it is more like 'wrestling'. However, MI is said to be like 'dancing' where there is a smooth movement between the therapist and the client. The therapist subtly leads the client toward change. Discrepancy is an important aspect in promoting motivation to change. It is the perceived difference between the current state and the desired state. It is advised in the MI technique to avoid asking questions which highlight righting reflexes like "why are you wanting to change," "why do you think that you are not addicted", etc. Such questions often evoke defensive statements.

Key Components of Motivational Interviewing

- Collaboration between the counselor/therapist and the client
- Evocation of client's motivation.
- Autonomy of the client in bringing about the change

Principles of Motivational Interviewing

- The therapist must express empathy through reflective listening.
- The therapist creates and amplifies discrepancy.
- Rolling with resistance, i.e., using the resistance to provide momentum to bring about the change, usually through active problem solving.
- Supporting client's self-efficacy i.e., his/her belief about ability to bring about the change.

Motivational Interviewing: The Process

Motivational interviewing is usually administered in three phases described as below:

(1) ***Phase 1*** – The first phase in MI focuses on Building motivation for change and employs various strategies (discussed below) in order to build the motivation of the client to enter the change process. Some of these strategies are OARS, reframing, etc.
(2) ***Phase 2*** – The second phase in MI focuses on strengthening client's commitment for change. This is the phase where active work towards bringing about the change is done. Decisional balance sheet is used to understand the pros and cons of both action and inaction. Change plan worksheet is used to sketch out a plan for change. Resistance is dealt with. Abstinence is focused on. Maintenance of commitment is aimed for.
(3) ***Phase 3***- The third phase in MI entails maintaining the change and is the follow through Phase. It aims at maintaining the acquired change through reviewing, renewing, and redoing.

Miller and Rollnick (2012) further enlisted five "early" methods which are to be used right from the beginning of the interviewing. These are.

(1) ***Open Questions***: MI focuses on open ended questions such as "Tell me more about Alcohol…what are the good things about having Alcohol?" Asking three questions in a row should be avoided. Close ended questions such as "Do you like drinking?" should be avoided.
(2) ***Affirming***: Affirmation is essential for rapport establishment. Statements such as "I really appreciate you opening up about it" "I am proud that you are trying", etc. can be used as affirmation.
(3) ***Reflective listening***: Reflective listening is also a form of affirmation. It is an essential component of motivational interviewing. It is an important skill to be acquired by a therapist. It is not merely summarizing or repeating client's statements. It is skillful way of directing the conversation towards a desired outcome. Presented below is an illustration of reflective listening by the therapist:

Client: I tend to drink too much; people often point it out

Therapist: So, people worry about you drinking too much

C: Yeah, it gets annoying sometimes. I know it is not the right thing to do. I do not need to be reminded about it.

T: Right! You are aware that drinking too much is not good for you

C: I am! I do not do it purposefully. I try but it just happens. People do not understand that. They think I enjoy drinking

T: You put in efforts to control your intake, but exercising control is a difficult thing. It must be very frustrating for you to go through the ordeal.

(4) ***Summarize***: Summarizing serves as a reinforcer and aids the change process. It should be done at regular intervals. It can be of collective type (presenting all the change statements said by the client), Linking (establishing a link between different statements, mostly in case of ambivalence; use of 'on one hand', 'and' instead of 'but' is advised) and Transitional (used at the end of the session and to highlight the transition between the stages of change). Presented below is an illustration of summarizing by the therapist:

Let me quickly go through what we have discussed so far. You were brought here by your wife because she along with other closed ones thinks that you might be drinking more than what is normal limit. This constant pestering annoys you. However, you are not happy with your drinking behavior and you constantly put efforts to limit your intake. But it is extremely difficult thing to do. The fact that you are here is commendable and I really appreciate your awareness and constant efforts. It shows that you really care about it and that you are serious about bringing about a change. We discussed about the problems that might have aroused due to excessive drinking. You rightly pointed out the symptoms as constant cravings, reduced concentration, forgetfulness, and a sense of being lost most of the time. You also very bravely pointed out that most of the time you choose drinking over your other activities, which concerns you dearly. On one hand you are concerned about these problems, and on the other hand you also feel tempted towards the positive feelings which alcohol provides. You feel relaxed and at peace. You do not want to lose that feeling. You are confused about your situation. Have I covered everything or is there anything which I missed?

The above four skills are together abbreviated as OARS (Open ended questions, Affirmation, Reflective Listening and Summarizing).

(5) ***Eliciting Change Talk***: The aforesaid four strategies are used by the therapist to elicit ambivalence. The fifth strategy is used to address that ambivalence by helping the client come up with the disadvantages of their current behavior, the advantages of change, and by eliciting optimism and intention to change. This can be done by asking questions, asking for elaborations, exploring goals and values of the client, looking into advantages and disadvantages of the behaviour (decisional balance), and looking back and in future.

Structure of the Therapy

The very first step in the therapy process is to identify which stage of change the client is in. The stages are divided into six categories:

(1) ***Precontemplation stage***: The client either is not aware of his/her problem behaviour or he/she does not find it serious enough to do anything about it. There are no thoughts about making a change.
(2) ***Contemplation stage***: In this stage the client is aware about his problem behaviour. However, an ambivalence exists regarding the positive side of indulging in problem behaviour. They are seriously considering making a change. It is very important to address ambivalence at this stage.
(3) ***Preparation stage***: This stage is also known as determination stage. In this stage the client is ready to make a change. He/ she is in planning phase on how to bring about a change. This stage too is marked with ambivalence. At this stage, the therapist is mostly supportive and helps the client in building the self-efficacy and in dealing with resistance.
(4) ***Action stage:*** This stage is achieved once the ambivalence is resolved. The client would make active efforts to change problem behaviour. The therapist's role at this stage is to help achieve the change and develop new coping strategies to deal with the change.
(5) ***Maintenance stage***: This stage appears when the desired change has been achieved. This is usually marked after 6 months of desired change. The goal of the therapy at this stage is to maintain the change through constant positive feedback and reviewing.
(6) ***Relapse:*** Maintenance of change such as being abstinent is a difficult process and clients often relapse. The therapist's role at this stage is to help the client look at it as a part of healing process, a mere roadblock and not as a complete failure of the process. The therapy must be reinitiated depending on client's current status. It usually takes a couple of attempts before a client can successfully quit a problem behaviour.

A 4-session Programme

The 4-Session programme as outlined by Miller (1992) comprises of a set of tests that are run during Pre-session 1 depending on the problem area. This might include MAST, AUDIT, DrInC questionnaire in case of alcohol dependence along with biochemical tests such as liver function test and neuropsychological assessments.

(1) ***Session 1-*** Majorly comprises of the first phase of the therapy. The session begins with discussing the problem area and rationale of the treatment. All the required information is provided to the client. The concept of "free choice" is communicated to the client wherein the client is informed that he has complete freedom to choose to bring about a change and only he alone can bring about the change. Stage of change is assessed. Motivational interviewing using strategies discussed above is used to build the motivation to change. A Personal Feedback Report is presented to the client to make him aware of his drinking status. It includes all the detailed report of his drinking habits along with his assessment scores. The session ends with a summary of the session along with a brief note on the follow-up session.

(2) ***Session 2-*** The second session is usually scheduled after a week or 14 days. It begins with a brief recapitulation of the previous session. The personal feedback form is discussed if it was not done in the previous session. If the commitment of change was not obtained in the first session, then this session focuses on that. If the commitment is obtained, then phase 2 of the therapy begins. If the commitment is not obtained by the end of this session, then the client is given time to work upon his thoughts and is asked to take it over in the third session.

(3) ***Session 3 and 4***: These sessions are arranged on 6th week and 12th week respectively. They are basically used for maintenance of the change process. If relapse happens, the motivation is renewed and the client is encouraged to continue his path towards abstinence. If the client successfully maintains abstinence, then the self-efficacy is reinforced. This marks phase 3 of the therapy process.

(4) ***Termination***: The entire therapy is reviewed and recapitalized. The client is given a summary of the process and is invited to add their perspective. Relapse prevention is done by asking the client to predict future hindrances and planning out ways to deal with them. Positive feedback is provided and self-efficacy is reinforced in order to maintain the change.

Identifying Resistance in Clients

- *Arguments* – The client would try to challenge and put the therapist's down by questioning his/her accuracy and integrity. He/she may also display hostile behavior.
- *Interruptio*n- The client may frequently interrupt the therapist in order to defend oneself.

- *Negation*- The client may negate one's problem by blaming others, disagreeing with the counselor, making excuses, etc.
- *Ignorance*- The client may ignore the therapist by being inattentive or being uncooperative towards the counselor.

Traps to Avoid During MI

Miller and Rollnick (2012) recommended few traps to avoid in the process of initiating MI:

- Avoid following closed question–answer pattern which would render the client passive. Even in case of open-ended question, the tendency to ask a follow up question after each response might produce similar effect. Hence, reflective listening is advised.
- The therapist/counselor must avoid taking sides during the interview process as it would lead to client to incline towards the opposite side of the ambivalence.
- The therapist must avoid projecting an 'expert' image. Rather the client should be the expert who knows his/her situation and resources the best.
- The therapist/counselor should avoid labeling at all costs e.g., usage of terms like 'Alcoholic' should be strictly avoided.
- The therapist must not press on talking about his/her perception of the problem in the initial stage. The client must be allowed to talk about what he/she thinks is the concern. For example, a client may first want to talk about his health issues or relationship issues and the counselor attempt to press on the abstinence/alcohol use problem might irk the client and lead to dropout.
- Blaming should be avoided by depicting non-judgmental attitude and reframing clients into a problem-solving approach.

Dealing with the Client's Resistance

- Resistance is never confronted directly in the MI process. Rather it is advised to roll with it. This means agreeing with the client using reflective statements like "alcohol gives you the peaceful state that you crave for." This helps the client feel understood and not scrutinized and judged.
- Amplified negative reflections are also used. It creates a paradoxical effect where the client starts to talk about the change. For example, "so we can say that there is absolutely no benefit in quitting drinking" statements like this often elicit response in favor of change.
- Double sided reflections are also used to address resistance.

- Sometimes helping the client come up with a menu of options or making them aware of the list of options is also helpful in addressing the resistance. For example, in case of client with obesity, options of indulging into alternatives such as fruits and artificial sweeteners can be either elicited or hinted to.

Role of 'Significant Others'

Studies have indicated that the involvement of the Significant Others (SO) have better treatment outcome. SOs are usually involved in the first two sessions of MI. However, if they are not involved in the first two sessions then they can be involved in the subsequent sessions. SOs are often invited in the first session and based on their involvement in the first session, decision to include them further is made. Advantages of engaging the SOs are discussed as below:

- The SOs are made more aware of the client's situation and about the problem in general. This helps them in empathizing better.
- SOs can help aid the process of recovery by providing the client the required support.
- Often, SOs' perspective of client's problem helps client in developing discrepancy e.g., a client reported that his drinking is not a problem. But when his wife was asked in front of the client about the effects it has on the family and she replied that she felt unloved and neglected. She went on to add that the kids who were teenagers now have started to resent their father because of his drinking. This led the client to develop a strong ambivalence which was further used to motivate him into reducing his intake.
- Therapist should elicit affirmative statements to help reinforce client's commitment to change.
- Therapist should also elicit self-motivational statements from the SO to help them play a significant role in helping the client bring about the change.

Care should be taken to prevent SOs from using too much of negative feedback, criticism, and complaints as this would prove to be detrimental for the therapy process. Reframing of negative instances presented should be done in order to use them as motivation for change. For example, if a SO complaint about persistent failure of the client in quitting alcohol, the situation should be reframed as the client putting constant effort to quit which highlights his sincerity towards his family. If the SO continues to remain hostile, critical, and uncaring about the client even after constant effort to navigate them towards being supportive, then a decision should be made to not include them in the therapy process.

Worksheets

As discussed above, the MI does not consist of specific techniques. It is a set of skills which the therapist needs to acquire. The entire therapy process is carried on the same principle. However, there are a few worksheets which can come handy. The Table 10.1 shows the Decisional Balance Sheet while The Table 10.2 shows the Change Plan Worksheet (adopted from Miller & Rollnick, 1995).

Table 10.1 Decisional balance sheet

	Disadvantages	Advantages
Change		
No change		

Table 10.2 Adopted from Miller and Rollnick (1995)

Change plan worksheet

Main Goals for Change

Reasons for Change

Action Required to achieve goals (with time)

People who can help

Ways in which they can help

Possible Hindrances

Ways to tackle the hindrances

Possible ways of knowing that the plan is working

Case Vignette (an Illustration for Describing the Process of Motivational Interviewing)

Following is an excerpt from the MI session of a 34 years old client, diagnosed with alcohol dependence and was brought-in for therapy by his wife.

Therapist: So, how may I help you?

Client: Well, my wife here, thinks I need help

T: Is that so?

C: Yeah, she thinks I am an alcoholic

T: I see, and what is your opinion about it?

C: I am not an alcoholic for sure! I do drink…quite frequently, but many people do that and I think that is okay

T: Right! Many people do drink frequently

C: Yeah, and they are absolutely fine. Like me!

T: Sure! You seem absolutely fine. I am sure there are absolutely no changes in your work life and relationships.

C: well yeah, almost

T: So, there are a few changes which are occurring?

C:Yeah, I mean, work is fine, but I do notice a few changes

T: Like?

C: Like in work, I am able to finish my work, but it gets very tiring. And sometimes I miss my deadlines. I tend to forget things too.

T: Forget things like how people usually do?

C: I will not say that, it is like nowadays I do not clearly remember client's information, my appointment details. Sometimes I miss out on my Boss's instructions too.

T: And was it like this always?

C: Oh no! I used to have a pretty sharp memory. I used to remember everything to the core. It kind of gave me an upper hand.

T: That's impressive! I am sure your people at work won't be minding the current changes

C: Well, as a matter of fact, they do. Few days back my boss gave pretty negative feedback…it was very unusual for me. I found it hard to handle

T: Negative feedbacks are heartbreaking. What did you go/do? in order to process it?

C: I had a couple of drink…it made me forget the pain I guess…at least for a while. I fell asleep

T: So how do you feel the next day?

C: Not so good. I do feel groggy. Maybe because of the hangover

T: Hangovers are pretty bad

C: Yeah, and then my wife starts cribbing

T: What does she crib about?

C: Usually about not giving her time

T: can you remember what she cribbed about the last time?

C: well, as far as I remember, it was 2 days back. I was supposed to take her and the kids out for dinner. Kids were asking for it since a couple of days. I had a bad day at work. So, I wanted to have a drink. And you know, feel at peace, before heading out. I had a couple of drinks. But she refused to go out after that. She said she did not want to go out with an alcoholic. We had a fight and then she slept off. I had a few more drinks before heading off to sleep

T: that must be pretty devastating for you. How did you feel

C: I was hurt. I am not an alcoholic.

T: it was pretty hurtful. It must have been disappointing for your family as well

C: yeah, kids were very upset. My wife too... she cried a lot. I love my wife and kids. It hurts me to see them in this state.

T: you do love your family a lot. You would perhaps do anything in your power to keep them happy

C: I would! Undoubtedly!

T: Sure enough

T: So, you said you had a drink after the fight, before falling off to sleep.

C: yeah…it helped. I mean it makes my mind calm and helps me sleep better

T: Alcohol tend to do that. It is a depressant. It slows down brain activities which creates a blur.

C: yeah, I guess I like that

T: It is tempting, especially when you are struggling with things and need peace

C: Yeah right! I usually do that often…I mean to find peace after a bad day. I mean I know I drink almost every day. But most of the time it is to forget a bad day and find some peace.

T: it makes sense to me. What are the things which make your day bad?

C: Well usually the work things, which I told you. And whenever I have arguments with my wife and friends.

T: the work problem, the changes which you reported…have you thought about the possible reasons?

C: well…yeah, I guess it can be due to age

T: possible. However, do you think 34 years is the age to suffer from these problems?

C: no…I guess, it can possibly be alcohol

T: what makes you think so?

C: well, for one, I do feel these more on the days when I have had too many drinks. And well…I have been told by a couple of people that alcohol could be behind this.

C: do you too think that I am an alcoholic?

T: 'alcoholic' is just a label. Labels are subjective. What I have here is your medical reports. What do you think about it?

C: the numbers are pretty high

T: they sure are. Do you think it is a matter of concern?

C: I guess. I mean my SGPT, SGOT levels are pretty high

T: and so is your bilirubin levels and uric acid. Do you know what it means?

C: yeah…my liver is not functioning properly

T: it looks like.

C: but I really don't feel a difference. I mean when I drink with my friends, they would usually puke after a couple of drinks. But I can tolerate my drinks pretty well. I don't feel a thing. In fact, I am popular amongst my friends because of this. I can drink like a fish!

T: you know this might not actually be a good thing. It is known as 'tolerance.' Your friend's' puking is a way in which their body deals with the alcohol. It is like an alarm system. When the alarm goes off body tries to eliminate alcohol from the body. Unfortunately, in case of tolerance, the alarm system stops working. So, the alcohol continues to damage the body.

C: but that doesn't make sense. I seriously don't feel a thing

T: well do you know that many cancer types or HIV virus do not manifest symptoms, or manifest it in a very later stage?

C: yeah. It's pretty bad

T: It is. If only the symptoms develop early…

C: it could be treated in the early stages and chances of survival would be high

T: exactly! But just because these symptoms are not present; do you think that they don't have cancer…or that they are not infected by HIV?

C: no. they are suffering…they are just not aware of it

T: absolutely! It is same with alcohol.

C: I wasn't aware. It's pretty alarming!

T: It sure is

T: I am glad that you could process this information. Now let me summarize what we have discussed so far. You were brought here by your wife who thinks that you need help. You, on the other hand did not find this as a matter of concern. I appreciate you coming here today despite feeling that you do not need help, on your wife's request. It shows how much you value your family. So, on one hand you do believe that you don't need to make any changes in your lifestyle as your drinking is pretty normal, and on the other hand, you did report facing issues at work along with your relationship. Your medical reports are pretty alarming too. You drink to find some solace. However, it looks like the problems for which you seek solace are somewhere linked to alcohol. Is there anything else?

C: No. you are right. It feels like I do have a problem. Alcohol is causing me problems. I should quit.

(The above excerpt highlights clients transition from precontemplation to contemplation stage).

Limitations of MI

Although motivational interviewing proved to be a significant gamechanger in the treatment of various types of addiction, it has certain limitations. Some clients are not ready to undergo MET. For such clients the therapist must schedule a referral when the client is ready. It also requires certain level of psychological sophistication in the client. It can be carried out properly only by a trained therapist as it is a skillful method.

Conclusion

Motivational interviewing is a set of skills rather than a technique which should be acquired by clinicians and counselors in order to deliver the desired therapeutic outcome effectively. The therapy employs ambivalence and discrepancy in order to motivate the client for change. The essence of MI is that the articulation about change is elicited from the client himself. The onus of bringing about the change is on client's shoulder and the therapy is collaborative. The therapy focuses on eliciting the motivation to change along with strengthening and maintaining the change. It is currently being used in adjunct to multiple modes of therapy in order to motivate the client and deal with their resistances.

Acknowledgements The authors would like to acknowledge that they have referred mainly the manuals written by Miller, W. R., & Rollnick, S.(2002) and Miller, W. R., Zweben, A., DiClemente, C. C., & Rychtarik, R. G. (1995) while writing the current chapter apart from other literature.

References

Arbuckle, M. R., Foster, F. P., Talley, R., Covell, N. H., & Essock, S. M. (2020). Applying motivational interviewing strategies to enhance organizational readiness and facilitate implementation efforts. *Quality Management in Health Care, 29*(1), 1.

Bassett, S. S., Delaney, D. J., Moore, A. M., Clair-Michaud, M., Clarke, J. G., & Stein, L. (2022). Motivational interviewing to reduce risky sexual behaviors among at-risk male youth: A randomized controlled pilot study. *Psychological Services, 19*(1), 167.

Bem, D. J. (1972). Self-perception theory Advances in experimental social psychology (Vol. 6, pp. 1–62): Elsevier.

Bien, T. H., Miller, W. R., & Tonigan, J. S. (1993). Brief interventions for alcohol problems: A review. *Addiction, 88*(3), 315–336.

Boom, S. M., Oberink, R., Zonneveld, A. J., van Dijk, N., & Visser, M. R. (2022). Implementation of motivational interviewing in the general practice setting: A qualitative study. *BMC Primary Care, 23*(1), 1–9.

Burke, B., & Arkowitz, H. (2003). Menchola. The efficacy of motivational interviewing: a meta-analysis of controlled clinical trials. *Journal of Consulting and Clinical Psychology, 71*(5), 843–861.

Hall, K., Gibbie, T., & Lubman, D. I. (2012). Motivational interviewing techniques - facilitating behaviour change in the general practice setting. *Australian Family Physician, 41*(9), 660–667.

Miller, W. R. (1992). Motivational enhancement therapy manual: A clinical research guide for therapists treating individuals with alcohol abuse and dependence (Vol. 2): US Department of Health and Human Services, Public Health Service, Alcohol ….

Miller, W. R., & Rollnick, S. (2012). *Motivational interviewing: Helping people change:* Guilford press.

Miller, W. R., & Rose, G. S. (2009). Toward a theory of motivational interviewing. *American Psychologist, 64*(6), 527.

Palacio, A., Garay, D., Langer, B., Taylor, J., Wood, B. A., & Tamariz, L. (2016). Motivational interviewing improves medication adherence: A systematic review and meta-analysis. *Journal of General Internal Medicine, 31*(8), 929–940.

Prochoska, J., & Velicer, W. (1997). The transtheoritical model of health behaviour change. *A Merical Jpurnal of Health Promotion, 12*, 38–48.

Rollnick, S., Miller, W. R., & Butler, C. (2008). Motivational interviewing in health care: helping patients change behavior: Guilford press.

Weiss, C. V., Mills, J. S., Westra, H. A., & Carter, J. C. (2013). A preliminary study of motivational interviewing as a prelude to intensive treatment for an eating disorder. *Journal of Eating Disorders, 1*(1), 1–10.

Yakovenko, I., Quigley, L., Hemmelgarn, B. R., Hodgins, D. C., & Ronksley, P. (2015). The efficacy of motivational interviewing for disordered gambling: Systematic review and meta-analysis. *Addictive Behaviours, 43*, 72–82.

Chapter 11
Practicing Social Skills Training in Mental Health

Pravin B. Yannawar

Abstract Social skills training is a collection of various techniques which includes instructions, modeling, behavior rehearsal, corrective feedback, social reinforcement, and selected cognitive restructuring which can be effectively utilized to modify the social behavior of person with a broad range of interpersonal difficulties. Persons recovering from long term mental disorders tend to lose social skills though they may have residual skills which the mental health professionals need to identify and work upon. However, application of social skills training and approaches to the treatment of major psychiatric disorders is a challenge to the professionals working in the field of mental health. The present chapter focuses on the vital areas where mental health professionals need to focus with regard to building social skills while working with the persons recovering from mental disorders. Elucidating the very nature of the technique, it seeks to present social skills training as an essential and viable alternative to pharmacological treatment for treatment of persons with long term psychiatric illnesses. Person with social skill deficits, like an inability to express thoughts, feelings and emotions, arising either as part of the illness, or due to restriction of learning new opportunities to acquire, the chapter highlights how the technique can help the persons in treatment gain new social skills. Through case illustrations that entail the adoption of social skills as a technique, it elaborates the usage of the technique in holistic attempts to rehabilitate the client back into the mainstream of society.

Keywords Social skill training · Psychosocial intervention · Rehabilitation

Introduction

Mental health has been one of the most neglected areas in the field of health sector in India. However, in the last two to three decades there has been paradigm shift as far as mental health and mental illness is concerned. By now, most of the health

P. B. Yannawar (✉)
Department of Psychiatric Social Work, Institute of Human Behaviour and Allied Sciences, New Delhi, India
e-mail: pravin007yann@gmail.com

M. Anand (ed.), *Mental Health Care Resource Book*,
https://doi.org/10.1007/978-981-97-1203-8_11

professionals started acknowledging the magnitude of the problem of mental illness, in particular the severe psychiatric illnesses like Schizophrenia and Bipolar Affective Disorder. The availability of the mental health services at district level as well as at peripheral areas have been one of the significant developments in the field of mental health.

One of the prominent features of Schizophrenia is severe impairment in social functioning. Deterioration of socialization or social withdrawal, or performance as major role in family setup has been listed as prominent prodromal and residual symptoms. It was observed in many research studies that there is relationship of cognitive deficits such as poor attention, incoherent speech, difficulty in learning and retaining information, to the social functioning of persons with mental illness. Schizophrenics can be expected to have marked difficulty in social interaction (Strauss et al., 1974).

Emphasizing the role of social skills training, it has been said "Social skills are important in the process of recovery and the training can help persons with social skill deficits to learn specific skills needed to live, learn and work in the community with minimum support. Addressing social skill deficits in persons with mental illness is an essential component in the treatment process" (Bhola, 2016).

The relationship of social behaviour to mental health and psychopathology was first stressed by the personality theories by Carl Jung, Alfred Adler, and Harry Stack Sullivan. Faulty interaction patterns were thought to result from problems in the personality structure e.g. repressed hostility and anxiety. A strikingly different perspective was explained by the pioneering work of Zigler, Phillips, and other researchers (Zigler et al 1986). First, they emphasized the concept of social competence, the notion that effective social functioning depends on set of cabilities, which some people warrant. Second, their work suggested that poor social functioning i.e. low competence could lead to psychopathology, rather than always resulting from it.

Wolpe & Lazarus have done wonderful work on primary stimulus for the behavioural interest in social functioning. They highlighted the importance of "assertiveness" in a variety of neurotic spectrum. Social skill training procedures have been well practiced or recommended for a wide range of dysfunctional areas including Schizophrenia, alcoholism, depression, marital conflict, juvenile delinquency and other psychiatric illnesses. Social skills training was developed to strengthen the communication and community survival skills of Schizophrenics who were at risk for relapse. Social Skills Training (SST) uses the principles of behavior therapy to teach communication skills, assertiveness skills, and other skills related to disease management and independent living. It has been shown to be effective for a number of mental illnesses, including serious mental illness.

Understanding of Social Skills Training

While working with persons from severe mental illnesses, one need to understand and differentiate between skills and abilities. Skills are basically based on the learning principles. Social skills training utilizes behaviour therapy principles and ways for tutoring existent to express their feeling and to achieve the goal and to meet their needs for developing relationship and perform the role which is required for independent living.

Social Skills Training (SST) is currently considered as "*the most potent intervention for helping individuals develop more rewarding and meaningful relationships, and for promoting social integration into the community*" (Mueser & Bellack, 2007). Social skills training can also be designated as a type of behavioral therapy used to advance social skills in people with mental disorders or developmental disabilities. SST can be used by eclectic range of practitioners including teachers, therapists, or other professionals to help those with anxiety disorders, mood disorders, personality disorders, and other diagnoses. It can be practiced either at individual level or in a group format, usually once or twice a week, and is often used as one constituent of a combined treatment program.

Social skill training is considered as one of the oldest and extensively studied approaches to psychiatric rehabilitation, which has more than fifty years of history. Mueser and Bellack (2007) allude:

> Social skills training involves the systematic teaching of interpersonal skills through the process of breaking complex behaviors into their constituent elements, demonstrating (modeling) those skills in role plays, engaging clients in role plays to work on those skills, providing positive and corrective feedback to ameliorate performance, additional role play practice, and developing assignments to practice those skills in naturally occurring interactions in clients' lives. With the roots of social skills training in conditioned reflex therapy (Salter, 1949), psychotherapy by reciprocal inhibition (Wolpe, 1958), and social learning theory (Bandura, 1969), social skills training was first packaged as "assertiveness training" for the general population, and was soon after applied to a broad range of clinical populations, including persons with severe mental illness (Mueser, 1998, as cited by Mueser & Bellack, 2007, pp.1).

Social skills training is an assemblage of techniques including instructions, modeling, behavior rehearsal, corrective feedback, social reinforcement, and selected cognitive restructuring techniques that have been successfully employed to amend the social behavior of clients with a comprehensive range of interpersonal difficulties. Social skills training has been pragmatic to the treatment of persons with major depressive episodes, and initial results suggest that it may be as effective in remediating depressive symptoms as some pharmacologically based treatment approaches (Bellack, Her-sen, & Himmelhoch, 1984; Hersen et al., 1984).

Many authors have explained about social skills training, however there seems to be no definition seems to be fully acceptable, but there is general agreement on certain issues:

1. Interpersonal behaviours consist of a set of learned performance abilities
2. Socially skilled behaviours like is situation specific. Both cultural and situational factors determine social norms
3. Another aspect of social skills involves the maximization of reinforcement (marriage, friendship, employment, service, personal rights, etc.).

Before moving to the various components of social skill training, lets us discuss the case vignette, based on the vignette the components incorporated in the particular case and in general other aspects can be discussed in the chapter.

Case Vignette 1

Mr. A was 25 year old unmarried middle class man who was diagnosed with Bi-Polar Affective Disorder. Patient was on regular treatment at the Psychiatric hospital over a period of 10 years, got admitted thrice during his symptomatic state. He was tried with multiple drugs and combination of psychosocial therapies. Patient was well supported by his parents, who used to bring him for outpatient department treatment and regular follow up.

Social skill training begins with an assessment of client's specific skill deficits and impairments. The process is structured, based on learning principles, as a ten-step model, which begins with Introduction, followed by Rationale, Instruction, Modeling, Review, Supervised Practice, Feedback, Problem solving ideas, Generalisation, and Independent practice of the skills. Here in this case initial couples of sessions were held with the family members, primarily parents so as to understand the skill deficits what they had observed in patient during the course of the illness. Later patient was helped to understand the deficits along with the parents and initiated the skill training.

Patient was lacking while taking initiative in the communication, he used avoid friends and relatives and use to confine to his bedroom. Patient was also shy and afraid of interacting with others due to his illness, he became introvert and prefers to speak less. Later after discussion, patient was giving specific instruction about improving his communication skills, under supervision and feedback from his parents. Patient was reassured about the proper outcome with the intervention and training. Gradually patient started gaining the confidence and worked upon improving those skills. Family was also counselled for creating conducive environment at home and not to be critical. Patient was well educated, having done diploma in engineering patient was helped to acknowledge his strength and also to cash on it while seeking the employment.

After sustainable intervention over a period of 3 month on the outpatient basis, at the follow up once in a week or two patient started showing improvement in his overall communication pattern, confidence was also increased and started well interacting with friends, relatives, and neighbours. With comprehensive treatment plan patient was well settled and managing well since last 7–8 years. He has been working in a private firm, mostly carry out the day time work, he has also been married and taking care of his family quiet well.

Case Vignette 2

Mr. N. was 35-year married male educated till higher secondary, from middle socio-economic status. He was diagnosed as a case of Schizo-affective disorder and had difficulty in handling the expressed emotions, as his father often used to be critical of him, wherein mother was over involved. Patient did not have good friend or did not get proper support from the other sibling as well. Patient had also low frustration tolerance and used to get agitated and throw tantrums. Family was called on regular basis for family sessions and were involved in dialogue and educated for working on the deficits, which mainly low self-esteem, pathological communication pattern, poor coping, difficulties in handling emotions.

Mr. N's family was called for the intervention, initial sessions were focused on understanding the skills deficits of the client. The patient and family members were helped in setting the goals for skill improvement and given its rational. The family was also demonstrated the role modeling and suggested to act at different situations at home and let the patient practice it. Parents were appreciated for their supervisory role and also suggested to give all the necessary feedback to patients at different point of time.

Mr. N was in need of constant motivation and reassurance. He has been on regular follow-up with the therapist. Focus was on to develop his confidence and also to work on his social and vocational skills. He was also referred to day care Centre and involved in trades of his liking and given the necessary training. Sessions were conducted over a period of 4–5 month, at the interval of once in a two week. Mr. N took his own time while attending the follow-up sessions independently, discussed about his apprehensions, guilt and shame related to his illness. After comprehensive psychosocial intervention, which were focused problem-solving skills, moral boosting, patient started working on it and managing to handle the stressful situations more efficiently.

Mr. N. was well treated for over a period of 17 years, earlier he was admitted for couple of occasion in the hospital, however maintaining well since last 3–4 years with the regular treatment, psychosocial intervention and having good compliance. Mr. N's family was also motivated to find out descent job and helped in gaining the much needed confidence. At present Mr. N is married, doing regular job in private firm to earn his livelihood and take care of the family.

Social Skill Training Techniques

Social skill training begins with a valuation of client's specific skill shortfalls and impairments. The therapist may ask regarding most challenging or difficult social interactions or the skills client feels could be improved. The purpose is to recognize the best targets for social skills training in the given context. Once specific target areas are acknowledged, techniques for refining social skills are introduced. Usually, changes are made in one area at a time to ensure the client does not get overwhelmed or stressed up.

A therapist may be in a better position to describe a particular skill, explain how to carry it out, and then model the behavior (Blote, 2010). Complex behaviors like how to carry on a conversation may be broken down into smaller pieces such as introducing oneself, making small talk, and leaving a conversation. Therapists will also discuss both verbal and nonverbal behaviors (Yen et al., 2012).

Social Skill Training Techniques can be described as below:

- Behavioural rehearsal: Role play which entails practicing new skills during therapy in simulated situations.
- Corrective feedback: Used to help enhance social skills during practice.
- Instruction: The educational component of SST that encompasses the modeling of appropriate social behaviours.
- Positive reinforcement: Used to reward improvement in social skills.
- Weekly homework assignments: Provide the opportunity to practice new social skills beyond the space of therapy.

Table 11.1 presents the learning based procedures that are used in the application of social skills training.

Table 11.2 presents the various types of social skills that are encouraged to be imbibed by the client.

Table 11.1 Learning-based procedures used in social skills training

"Problem identification" is made in collaboration with the patient in terms of obstacles that are barriers to a patient's personal goals in his/her current life
"Goal setting" creates short-term approximations to the patient's personal goals with specification of the social behavior that is needed for efficacious achievement of the short-term, incremental goals. The goal-setting attempt requires the therapist or trainer to elicit from the patient detailed descriptions of what communication skills are to be learned, with whom are they to be used, where, and when
Through "role plays" or "behavioral rehearsal," the client validates the verbal, nonverbal, and paralinguistic skills required for successful social interaction in the interpersonal situation set as the goal
"Positive" and "corrective feedback" is given to the client emphasizing on the quality of the behaviors exhibited in the role play
"Social modeling" is provided with a therapist or a peer signifying the desired interpersonal behaviors in a form that can be vicariously learned by the observing the client
"Behavioral practice" by the client is repeated until the communication reaches a level of quality tantamount to success in the real-life situation
"Positive social reinforcement" is given contingent on those behavioral skills that showed improvement
"Homework assignments" are given to motivate the client to implement the communication in real-life situations
"Positive reinforcement" and "problem solving" is provided at the next session based on the client 's experience using the skills

Table 11.2 Types of social skills as target behaviours for social skills training

Types of social skills	Examples/explanation
Social perception	Precise evaluation of emotional expressions from others
Processing of social information	Apposite construal of the meaning of expressions
Responding or sending skills	Functional use of verbal and nonverbal communication
Affiliative skills	Articulating affection to family and friends and using self-disclosure judiciously
Instrumental role skills	Purchasing food, renting an apartment, working on a job
Interactional skills	Initiating, maintaining and terminating a conversation
Behavior governed by social norms	Speaking politely to a policeman who has stopped the person for a traffic violation

Components of Social Skills

Social skill is a broad construct that incorporates a variety of interpersonal response dimensions, such as assertiveness, friendliness, warmth, conversational facility, and empathy. These can be divided into three categories.

A) Expressive elements:
1. Speech content
2. Paralinguistic elements
    - 1.Voice volume
    - 2.Pace
    - 3. Pitch
    - 4.Tone
3. Non-verbal behaviours
    - 1.Proxemics
    - 2.Kinesis
    - 3.Gaze
    - 4.Facial expression

B) Receptive element (Social perception):
- 1.Attention
- 2.Decoding
- 3.Social Intelligence

C) Interactive Balance:
- 1.Response timing
- 2.Turn talking

(A) Expressive elements comprise of those response parameters that communicate information to the interpersonal partner.

(1) Speech Content: What the person says—this element conveys the most information and is central factor in social skill.

(2) Paralinguistic elements consist of non-verbal aspects of speech that determine how things can be expressed or said viz. Humour, Sarcasm, joy, anger, or anxiety can all be transmitted by voice characteristics, even when the speech content presents an alternative meaning.

(3) Nonverbal behaviour includes the bodily movements and posture. Proxemics is, "manner in which indirect use physical space in their interactions with others and how physical space influences behaviour. The term kinesics subsumes a wide variety of body movements, including hand and arm gestures, head nods, and postures. Eye contact (gaze) involves how a person locks and what the person looks at, as well as eye contact. Facial expression also plays an important role in giving emphasis to and or qualifying speech content, it communicates affect.

(B) Receptive Element (Social perception): Involves a set of receptive features and comprise of the following:

   (1) Attention to the indications provided by interpersonal partner involves all of the expressive elements.
   (2) Decoding of perceived information is done. Here the cognitive element is obvious.
   (3) Social intelligence, involve wide-ranging knowledge about cultural moves and significance of a marvelous number of expressive cues and response patterns in diverse settings.

(C) Interactive Balance:—The final aspect of social skill is interactive balance, balance of time talking. This is not a definite response; it is a general parameter related to the flow of social encounters. Interpersonal behaviour is not static, it is interactive, and effective performance requires a delicate give- and -take, or meshing.

Assessment of Social Skills

(1) ***Interviewing***: Clinical interviews are probably the rifest employed technique. Client is the best person to describe about oneself, and the best source of information. Besides current functioning, the same also provides the interpersonal history and data through informal observation.
(2) ***Self-monitoring***: This has become one of the most extensively used behavioural assessment procedures. Generally, it is more unbiased, steadfast and valid than other types of self-report data, but it is subject to reactivity and inconsistency. With regard to the recording of interpersonal behaviour, it has distinct benefit of providing semi objective data on behaviours that are not otherwise open to direct observation.
(3) ***Self-report inventories***: Self report scales and inventories encompass the most widely employed assessment strategy.
(4) ***Behavioural observation***: One of tenants of behavioural assessment is that direct observation is the most valid and desirable strategies have been employed:

   (a) Observation in the natural environment: This has been considered as, most desirable strategy, however it is also most difficult to employ.
   (b) Staged naturalistic interactions: Attempts have been made to stage important interactions in the lab/clinic. Another variant of this technique-critical incidents,
   (c) Role-playing: Through this method, the interviewer or counsellor can help the patient in understanding, the ways of handling the emotions and its own behaviour. This technique also helps the patient in getting confidence and also helps in improving communication pattern.

Domains of Assessment of Social Skills

- Basic Conversation Skills
- Assertiveness Skills
- Conflict Management
- Anger Management
- Using Leisure and Recreation Time
- Prevocational Skills
- Vocational Maintenance
- Communal Living Skills
- Friendship Skills
- Familial Relationship Skills
- Coping with Substance Use
- HIV Prevention
- Developing Romantic/Intimate Relationships
- Health Maintenance
- Medication Management
- Managing Positive Symptoms

Steps of Basic Social Skills Training

1. ***Establishing rationale for the skill***
   (a) Produce reason for learning the skill from group participants
   (b) Recognize all contributions
   (c) Provide supplementary details not stated by group members.
2. ***Discussing the steps of the skill***
   (a) Break the skills down into three or four steps
   (b) Write the steps on a board or poster
   (c) Deliberate upon the reason for each step
   (d) Check for comprehension at each step
3. ***Modeling the skill in a role-play***
   (a) Elucidate how to validate the skill in a role-play.
   (b) Plan out the role-play in advance
   (c) Use two leaders to model the skill
   (d) Keep the role play modest
4. ***Reviewing the role-play with participants***
   (a) Converse whether each step of the skill was used in role play
   (b) Request the group members to appraise the efficacy of the role model
   (c) Keep the review concise and precise

5. ***Engaging the client in role play of the same situation***
   (a) Request the client to try the skill in a role play with one of the leaders
   (b) Request the client questions to make sure he/she understands the objective
   (c) Train the members to observe the client
   (d) Initiate with a client who is more skilled or is likely to be acquiescent
6. ***Providing positive feedback***
   (a) Elicit positive feedback from group members about the client's skills
   (b) Encourage feedback that is specific
   (c) Cut off any negative feedback
   (d) Commendation to all the attempts with tips provided to group members about good performance
7. ***Providing corrective feedback***
   (a) Elicit recommendations regarding enhancing the skills by the client
   (b) Restrict feedback to one or two suggestions
   (c) Endeavor to communicate the suggestions in a positive, upbeat manner
8. ***Engaging the client in another role play of the same situation***
   (a) Invite the client to change one behavior in the role play
   (b) Check by enquiring to ensure that the client understands the proposition
   (c) Attempt to work on behaviours that are easily changeable
9. ***Providing additional feedback***
   (a) Concentrate initially on the behaviour that the client was requested to change
   (b) Engross the client in two to four role-plays with feedback after each one
   (c) Utilize other behaviour shaping strategies to improve skills such as coaching, prompting, and supplemental modeling
   (d) Be plentiful but specific while giving positive feedback
10. ***Assigning homework***
    (a) Give an assignment to practice skill
    (b) Ask group members to recognize situations in which they could use the skill
    (c) When possible, tailor the assignment to each client's level of skill.

Persons with mental disorders may have many social skills deficits such as an inability to express thoughts or feelings and emotions appropriately. They may have these deficits or lacking the social skills, because of the very nature of illness, or because the early onset of the illness restricting the opportunities to learn new social skills, or use the skills that they have learned. It is also observed that, the person might have symptoms of the mental illness, such as anxiety, which can interfere with appropriate use of the skill.

There is a definite purpose to use the SST in persons with severe mental illnesses, which is based on multiple theoretical and empirical sources. Social skills and social aptitude can be viewed as protective factors in the vulnerability-stress–protective factors model of schizophrenia (Liberman et al., 2005).

In view of all these difficulties while dealing with the negative symptoms and other deficits in areas of social functioning, one of the most important approaches for improving social functioning and enhancing quality of life is social skills training (Bellack et al, 1978, Liberman et al., 1986).

Several studies support the efficacy of a hospital-based SST group protocol in enlightening the social performance of persons with severe mental illnesses. The study also demonstrated the probability of a multiple-stakeholder-involved program that can be implemented as part of routine clinical care and not just employed for research purposes. (Priyadarshini et al., 2022).

Conclusion

The comprehensive rehabilitation in management of persons with long term illness is equally important. Family member has to constantly involve in the treatment and rehabilitation process. Although, as literature suggests the recovery process is very slow, time consuming, but having followed the treatment plan, one can expect better treatment results. The negative symptoms, may take some time to disappear, but the constant and combined efforts put by the patient and family members can bring very encouraging results. The social skill training focusing on the deficits skills and subsequent intervention can take long way to the persons with long term illness in their recovery path.

There have been many success stories around, where despite the long-term illness, persons are able to earn and carry forward their personal, as well as professional life very successfully. However, one needs to constantly motivate them and give them much needed encouragement and positive reinforcement. It can be concluded that, social skills are nothing but, abilities that can be learned and are necessary to get along with others, and also to create and maintain satisfying relationships within the family, community, and society at large.

References

Bandura, A. (1969). *Principles of behavior modification.* Holt, Rinehart and Winston, Inc., New York 1969 [Google Scholar]

Bellack, A. (2004). Social skills training for people with severe mental illness. *Psychiatric Rehabilitation Journal, 27*, 375–391.

Bellack, A. S., Hersen, M., & Turner, S. M. (1978). Role-play tests for assessing social skills: Are they valid? *Behavior Therapy, 9*(3), 448–461. https://doi.org/10.1016/S0005-7894(78)80089-6.

Bhola, P. (2016). Understanding about Mental Health. Social Skills Training for Persons with Mental Illness. White Swan Foundation.

Blote, A. W., Duvekot, J., Schalk, R. D., Tuinenburg, E. M., & Westenberg, P. M. (2010). Nervousness and performance characteristics as predictors of peer behavior towards socially anxious adolescents. *Journal of Youth and Adolescence, 39*(12), 1498–1507. https://doi.org/10.1007/s10964-009-9463-3

Heinssen, R. K., Liberman, R. P., & Kopelowicz, A. (2000). Psychosocial skills training for schizophrenia: Lessons from the laboratory. *Schizophrenia Bulletin, 26*, 21–46.

Hersen, M., Bellack, A. S., Himmelhoch, J. M., & Thase, M. E. (1984). Effects of social skill training, amitriptyline, and psychotherapy in unipolar depressed women. *Behavior Therapy, 15*(1), 21–40.

Kim, T. M., & Bellack, A. S. (2007). Social skills training: Alive and well? *Journal of Mental Health, 16*(5), 549–552.

Kopelowicz, A., Liberman, R. P., & Zarate, R. (2006). Recent advances in social skills training for schizophrenia. *Schizophrenia Bulletin, Oct;32*(Suppl 1), S12–S23.

Liberman, R. P., Kopelowicz, A., & Silverstein, S. M. (2005). Psychiatric rehabilitation. In B. J. Sadock & V. A. Sadock (Eds.), *Comprehensive textbook of psychiatry* (pp. 3884–3930). Lippincott Williams & Wilkins.

Liberman, R. P., Mueser, K.T., Wallace, C. J. (1986). Social skills training for schizophrenic individuals at risk for relapse. *The American Journal of Psychiatry, 143*, 523–526.

Mueser, K. T. (1998). Social skill and problem solving. In A. S. Bellack & M. Hersen (Eds.), *Comprehensive clinical psychology, 6* (pp. 183–201). Pergamon.

Mueser, K. T., Bellack, A. S., Douglas, M. S., & Morrison, R. L. (1991). Prevalence and stability of social skill deficits in schizophrenia. *Schizophrenia Research, 5*, 167–176.

Mueser, K. T., & Bellack, A. S. (2007). Social skills training: Alive and well? *Journal of Mental Health, 16*(5), 549–552.

Priyadarshini, A., Thamarai, S. S., Srikrithika, S., Reema, S., & Jacob, K. S. (2022). Effectiveness of social skill training in groups with persons with severe mental illness: A pre post intervention study. *Indian Journal of Psychological Medicine, 44*(2), 114–119.

Salter, A. (1949). *Conditioned reflex therapy*. Farrar, Strauss. New York. [Google Scholar]

Strauss, J. S., & Carpenter, W. T. J. (1972). The prediction of outcome in schizophrenia I. Characteristics of outcome. *Archives of General Psychiatry, 27*, 739–746.

Wolpe, J. (1958). *Psychotherapy by reciprocal inhibition*. Stanford University Press. [Google Scholar]

Yen, J. Y., Yen, C. F., Chen, C. S., Wang, P. W., Chang, Y. H., & Ko, C. H. (2012). Social anxiety in online and real-life interaction and their associated factors. *Cyberpsychology, Behavior and Social Networking, 15*(1), 7–12.

Zigler, E., & Glick, M. (1986). *A developmental approach to adult psychopathology*. John Wiley & Sons.

Chapter 12
Group Therapy: Basic Concepts and Skills

Sangeetha Reddy Duvvur

Abstract Group therapy has a longstanding history of being an efficient modality of psychotherapy. In general, individual and group therapies are considered equally efficacious and often regarded as effective concomitant treatment modalities. Differing mainly in therapists' intent, processes, structure, and composition to meet client needs, group therapy broadly promotes preventive, remedial, educational, and skill acquisition functions through the lens of the interpersonal and interactional framework. Given the allowance of limiting the crucial aspects of group therapy to a chapter, the focus is on bringing together key ideas in group therapy. Learning group dynamics and the effect of influencing variables on the development and productivity of the group makes the foundational requisite for group therapy practitioners. This chapter highlights these select aspects from the vast and complex body of knowledge about group dynamics that have a significant impact on group therapy. Another closely related aspect central to group work is acquiring leadership skills. The style and skills a group leader displays have a direct impact on the behaviours of group members and the progress of a group. This chapter additionally focuses on effective leadership aspects, core and specific group skills, and strategies to navigate through certain challenging issues throughout group development. Core group skills as such are fundamentally group facilitation skills applicable to various group work settings—task, psychoeducational, crisis-intervention, therapy groups, and so on. Furthermore, practitioners will gain a brief understanding of ethical and professional issues of group practice, and the stages of group development (formation, initial, working, final, follow-up and evaluation). The main goal of the chapter is to introduce with conciseness a comprehensive body of text emphasizing the interpersonal and interactional underpinnings of group therapy. The chapter strives to achieve such a feat at different points through tangible and practical illustrations and case examples.

Keywords Concepts · Group dynamics · Skills · Leadership and facilitation skills

---

S. R. Duvvur (✉)
Trained Counselling Psychologist and Private Practitioner, Bengaluru, India
e-mail: sangz.dr@gmail.com

M. Anand (ed.), *Mental Health Care Resource Book*,
https://doi.org/10.1007/978-981-97-1203-8_12

We human beings are relationship-oriented beings. Arguably, humans by and large usually don't seek isolation. Humans are interestingly capable of creating relationships with people, places and things. We don't live in a vacuum or a sterile environment devoid of connections. We are dynamic, meaning making organisms connecting, interacting and evolving with our environment. We live in a matrix of relationships, co-creating our realities.

Throughout our lifespan we are inclined to many varied interpersonal experiences. These experiences can be positive, nurturing, or negative and in turn these experiences can impact the development of individual personalities. Harry Stack Sulivan (1953), a pioneer of a systemic theory of interpersonal relationships, suggests that psychological disturbance can result from experiences an individual had with others. He postulates that our behaviours are mostly motivated in our desire to reduce anxiety. According to him anxiety is rooted in interpersonal disapproval. This anxiety in interpersonal relations is the central organising influence of human behaviour. *For example, most people have pervasive anxiety rooted in the fear of being abandoned, rejected, and disapproved by others.*

Usually in groups, people are valued and included based on their accomplishments and abilities, often a deficit is considered unfavourable and can become the basis of exclusion. However, in psychotherapy groups this is not the case. Rudolph Dreikurs, an eminent psychiatrist, was among the first few to introduce the humanistic perspective to group psychotherapy. According to him, group psychotherapy perhaps is the only group that values the individual's deficits—members in group therapy are valued for who they are and not what they have accomplished (Fehr, 2018). For many people entering group therapy for the first time, this kind of acceptance and valuing based on one's human existence is probably an entirely new experience.

In this chapter, the group work presented is one of intense interpersonal oriented and interactive group therapy. Therapy groups are preventive, remedial and growth oriented. Typically, this kind of group work is conducted with a small number of people, usually between 7 and 10. Participation of members is highly valued and interactions among members is considered the fuel that drives therapeutic change. This kind of group work is suitable for both intense short term and long term outpatient therapy.

Representing the vast gamut of literature about group therapy into a comprehensible body of text demands for an elaborate undertaking. However, owing to the brevity this chapter offers mainly through a relational lens, the basic premise of group therapy, group leadership and foundational workings of interpersonal process-oriented group work. This intentionally measured approach allows for a relatively detailed showcasing of some vital mechanisms that every group therapist needs to have a sound grasp of for effective facilitation of group work.

Basic Premise of Group Therapy

Logically a rationale for group therapy should be understood clearly before practitioners attempt this approach. Let's commence with an understanding of a few basic premises about the nature of people's problems and the group format method to resolving these problems through the lens of the interpersonal approach to group work (Chen & Rybak, 2018).

Premise 1: Most Problems Are Interpersonal in Nature

According to Yalom and Leszcz (2005), most clients in therapy experience two common problems: low sense of personal worth and difficulties in establishing and maintaining relationships. As such, these difficulties are interpersonal in nature. Often people who seek therapy feel a chronic sense of isolation and depression. They are very likely to have problems in their relationships and require help in overcoming the challenges that keep them from living a more fulfilling life. The interpersonal process approach provides the exact medium to discover and learn new healthy perspectives of viewing oneself and replace impaired ways of relating to others. Consequently, through group participation and constructive feedback from others in the group, clients can increase their capacities to fulfilling relationships.

Premise 2: Family Experiences: The Primary Source of Interpersonal Process

Our family is the primary group and fundamental relational space, be it nurturing or wounding, we learn to relate with oneself and others through perceived family attachment patterns. Thus, family dynamics and patterns imprint our emotional identity and become interwoven into our sense of self. These core family patterns later tend to shape other relational interactions. As informed by many theoretical views, it's safe to say that many clients who are in therapy experience an unsatisfactory relationship with their primary group—their family. *Ex: Adults who have experienced severe emotional neglect in childhood experience devastating effects in adulthood, such as depression, chronic low self-esteem, dysphoria and even have trouble forming and maintaining relationships.*

Yalom and Leszcz (2005) indicate that therapy groups can resemble the family group in many aspects, and group members stand in consciously or unconsciously as symbolic family members. Clients who enter group therapy are offered the opportunities to relive, explore and work through themes and feelings related to paternal/authority figures, sibling/peer relationships, intimacy issues, core childhood experiences, familiar familial roles, and so on using the group members as symbolic representations.

Premise 3: Clients' Underlying Problems Will Be Played Out in the Group

One of the most fundamental and paramount phenomena of group therapy is the emergence of group members' true interpersonal style with its strengths and weaknesses. Yalom and Leszcz (2005) regard the group as a "social microcosm". The group setting offers a conducive and safe environment where over a period of time and group interactions, members' will inevitably in the group enact or create their maladaptive interpersonal patterns. *For example, the group will witness how members play out their interpersonal distortions, such as avoidance of intimacy, neediness, codependence, defiance of authority, impersonal communication styles, approval issues,* and in turn members realise how these affect their interpersonal problems. Rather than just talking about their problems, members will live out their problems in the group. Manifestation of this phenomena in the here-and-now in a group is particularly important as some of these patterns can be considered as blindspots, interwoven into a member's personality and often hard to self-disclose. Eventually group attention will be drawn to a particular member's interpersonal distortion and this gives the group a chance through constructive feedback to convey how a member affects others, experiment new behaviours and experience the possibility of change.

Premise 4: Group Offers Dynamic Pressure for Growth

In therapy groups often one can experience an inherent push to improve. There seems to be a systemic drive to encourage members to invest in personal growth. The interactive nature of group therapy provides member's opportunity to observe and give feedback to each other as the strengths and inadequacies in their self-image unravel. This growth promotive pressure, when devoid of undue coercive push or conformity, can be viewed as a creative and beneficial force that motivates members to move away from defensiveness and inertia toward more authentic sharing and openness to new ways of being.

Premise 5: Here-and-Now Can Bring About Change and Healing

In therapy groups, members are frequently presented with the immediate opportunity for learning new and more satisfying ways of relating with self and others. The here-and-now interactional process within a group provides personal and direct experience of ones' interpersonal fallacies. When members begin to feel like they belong in the group and are understood and accepted, they will attempt to share feelings at greater embodied levels and in effect be more open to move from fixed modes to more flexible ways of being. Thus the group serves as a reality testing relational field.

Premise 6: Group as a Safe and Supportive Container

In group therapy members often discover that their problems are not unique to themselves and begin to feel less dissimilar and alone. This in turn promotes a feeling of belonging in the group and members become less defensive and conspicuous as they perceive themselves to be less socially isolated. As members begin to feel more accepted and worthy, they readily immerse themselves in the group process and become more open to receive help, also in providing empathy and exhibit helping behaviours toward other members. In the context of this caring environment, as members' journey together, they form significant relationships with other members offering opportunities for corrective emotional integration.

The above premises strongly establish some beneficial viewpoints that confirm the uniquely therapeutic aspects of group therapy. Group practitioners need to integrate and work the above premises into their philosophy of practice.

Group Dynamics

Group dynamics can be explained as the forces that influence the relationship among members and ultimately affect the outcome of therapy. Essentially it includes phenomena that aids in creation and functioning of the group. A group therapist needs to be sensitive about group dynamics by being aware of the group as an entity on its own, also of individual members in the group and how they impact each other. To mention a few vital elements of group dynamics but not limited to such are, group process, group culture, members personality, power related issues, social situations, group development, member roles and norms.

It is crucial that group therapists understand the above-mentioned influences while planning and facilitating groups. Let's consider two such fundamental forces that underlay all types of group work throughout different developmental phases—group content and group process. Group content and process are closely entwined and yet should have clear boundaries. The appropriate balance of these basic elements determines the particular dynamics of that group.

Group Content—basically refers to "*what*" was discussed or said in the group. It's helpful to identify and understand the overt experience in the group, like the actual words, themes and information exchanged, and also the purpose of the group. *For example: Mary, a member who is unhappy and dejected about not getting the promotion she was due for 2 years in a row, shares her angst with the group. Another member, Thomas, launches into an advice of how the job situation is tricky in recent times and continues to encourage her to look at the positives of still holding a job. Mary remains silent.*

Here the content revolves around one member not getting promoted and the advice from another member as a way of coping with the situation.

Group Process—refers to "*how*" group members interact with each other. It is useful to understand what is not process; it does not include past narrative or sharing of what happened in the past, rather the focus centres on members' feelings and motives as they are talking about what happened.

Let's continue with the above exchange between the two members, at a process level, the leader can take note of how Mary was silent and said nothing when someone discounted her experience and on the other hand Thomas rationalising, speaks to his inability to stay with Mary on an emotional level. These are clues into a person's interpersonal styles. To further this, at a group level the leader needs to observe how this exchange impacted other members.

As mentioned earlier, for a group to function effectively it needs to cultivate healthy group dynamics. According to Donigian and Malnati (1997) a group is a system and is made up of 3 crucial parts: the group members, the group leader and the group as a whole. When viewed from a systemic perspective, achieving balance between content and process to create healthy group dynamics lies in the leader's skillful capacity to balance individual and collective needs as the group progresses.

Group Leadership

Often group leadership is considered challenging, many therapists find it daunting and shy away from this truly dynamic and powerful form of therapy. Facilitating groups is in essence an amalgamation of the artistic and scientific components of leadership. Mastery in facilitating group therapy is complex and requires gaining competence of various aspects - this segment focuses on the following five aspects of group leadership:

- Core attributes and personal development
- Knowledge base and sound conceptual understanding of groups
- Group leadership tasks and group development
- Group level skills
- Therapeutic factors of groups from a leadership focus

Core Attributes of a Group Therapist

Of all the above-mentioned aspects, self-development of the leader can be considered as pivotal to effective group therapy outcomes. Group therapy is a powerful therapeutic medium of healing and it is safe to operate on the premise that the leader's therapeutic presence is a vital component in the group. Logically so, when a therapist is open and receptive to personal growth and is committed to her own healing then she is less likely to carry negative impact from the past and shows up as therapeutically congruent.

Brown (2008) listed the following self-factors crucial for a group leader:

- Core attributes of being non-judgemental, genuineness, positive regard, warmth and caring are the recognised relational attributes for core conditions of therapy (Roger, 1951). These leadership qualities lend to the therapeutic presence of a therapist. Commitment to one's own personal growth is also viewed as allowing a greater capacity for presence. Bugental (1987) broadly describes presence as the intention for engagement. To quote Bugental "Presence is a quality of being in a situation or relationship in which one intends, at a deep level, to be as aware and as participative as one is able to". Imagine a leader who can learn all that she needs to learn about therapy and let it go to meet her client with genuine regard and warmth as fellow humans.

This state of evenly suspended attention suggests a broad detachment yet openness so that the therapist can pay attention in the moment to what they see and hear, without getting emotionally involved (Geller & Greenberg, 2012)

- Another attribute is tolerance of ambiguity and uncertainty. Especially in the beginning of groups, members are anxious and wary of participation. As members' anxiety runs high, leaders who can handle their personal anxiety can more readily be present for the group and show less need to assuage the group process to meet their own needs. They are able to model anxiety containment and are able to assure members of their ability as a leader to provide a safe and secure therapy environment.
- Additional elements of self factors mentioned are capacity for empathy, willingness to take risks, and self-reflection. Of particular importance is self-reflection, which refers to the therapist's ability to use their personal experience at a moment as a guide to intervene with the group and its members. When the leader uses their inner experiencing as a way to sense what is occurring in the group, they display great resonance to the group's needs and concerns at a particular moment and are able to engage the group with greater efficacy.

Knowledge Base of Group Theories

Considerable research shows that for effective group leadership, practitioners need to have strong knowledge base in the following areas—theoretical framework for group work; sound understanding of group dynamics and the factors that foster healthy progression of groups; supervised group leadership experiences; expertise in cultural and diversity issues; knowledge about effective communication, conflict resolution, resistance, reality testing, constructive feedback, and so on (Chen & Rybak, 2018).

Leadership Tasks and Stages of Group Development

Groups can be aliked to a physiological entity, from the point of creation it grows, stretches, contains, develops and inevitably terminates. Like all organisms, groups do go through this cycle of evolution experiencing different phases in its progression. Examining leadership tasks from the viewpoint of the developmental stages of a group and corresponding member issues is an attempt at deriving a more structured framework. This understanding can then reduce ambiguity and provide some guidance for suitable techniques and interventions.

In this segment we will consider the popular model of group development proposed by Tuckman (1965). This model categorises group development sequentially into 5 stages, namely, forming, storming, norming, performing and adjourning. Each of these stages along with member issues and leader tasks are explained below.

Stage 1—Forming

This stage is likened to infancy. Once physically the group is established and commenced the leader helps members navigate through the various degrees of implicit or explicit concerns they harbour. Understandably so, members experience the group as ambiguous and uncertain of what the group experience will be.

Central Member Issues

- Inclusion and dependency (Bion, 1969): Inclusion ties in with the fear of being judged or fear of being discovered, revealing parts of themselves that they rather hide from the group. As a result of these concerns and unknowns group members often exhibit high dependency on the leader for feeling secure and to establish a sense of equilibrium.
- Safety: Fear of being pressured or coerced to disclose, or losing control or even rejected by group members for having different opinions. Additionally, group members worry about confidentiality aspects.
- Personal gains (Brown, 2008): Questions about what will they benefit from group work?

Leader's Tasks

- The primary task is to establish trust and safety by addressing fears and feelings of ambivalence, promoting universality to foster inclusion and focusing on cohesion building exercises early into the process.

- Clarifying group's purpose and expectations, thereby the leader takes on an educative role about the aim and nature of the group work.
- Familiarising members to each other and facilitating member interactions.
- Establish collaborative goal setting.
- Structuring and directing—establishing open structure for proceedings of group sessions and helping members set some basic rules and regulations.

Stage 2—Storming

The next stage storming is characterised by competition and conflict in the relations being developed between group members and the group therapist. As group members begin to feel safe, asserting themselves and connecting with each other over similarities, experimentation of new behaviours and transparency begins to take stage. Members begin to depend less on the leader and gradually disagreements begin to emerge.

Central Member Issues

- Residual issues of 1st stage continue, members still grapple with doubts of how accepting the group will be if they differ from the rest.
- Disagreements and conflicts between members or hostility toward the leader emerge.
- Competition for the leader's attention can also occur.

Leader's Tasks

- The central task of the leader is to contain conflicts and teach conflict resolution to the members.
- Help members contain and regulate overwhelming emotions.
- The leader also has to block aggressive and attacking comments made by members.
- Be open to challenges or contradictions from members and display constructive ways of resolving differences and repair empathic failures.

Many theories of group development hold that these types of conflicts and tensions over authority and status are essential for the emergence of genuine cohesion and cooperation. (Bernard et al., 2008).

Stage 3—Norming

In the norming stage, there is greater sense of belonging and affinity between members, leading to the group being a remarkable space of mutual trust and cohesion. This phase is also marked by high engagement and self-disclosure fostering higher intimacy in the group, advertently building a healthy interpersonal feedback mechanism. Members are more accepting of individual differences, receiving and giving feedback.

Members Concerns

- Due to increased levels of cohesion members can suppress negative affect.

- Greater transference and projective identification can occur. However, this can provide greater opportunity for corrective emotional experiencing.

Leader's Tasks

- Refrain from taking an active role, model shared leadership and acceptance of members' independence.
- The primary role is to facilitate the working process around feedback, promoting insight and encouraging problem solving in an ongoing manner (Bernard et al., 2008).
- Assist and guide the group at maintenance tasks and norms.

Stage 4—Performing

Stage four is marked by interdependence in members' relationships, acceptance of individual differences and problem solving in the realm of task functions. It is at this stage the group should be most productive (Bernard et al., 2008). Group members experience the group as a caring, safe and accepting environment, members extend themselves in deeply trusting ways to forge interactions actively at deeper levels and focus on task and growth oriented goals.

Members Concerns

- To be responsible for continual involvement in maintenance of group proceedings.
- Members need to be highly committed to the process of collaborative work, yet being flexible and open to foster an atmosphere of aliveness and creativity.

Leader's Tasks

- Provide positive reinforcement and continue to practise shared leadership with as little direction as required.
- Share new information or perspectives when required.

Stage 5—Adjourning

Concluding the group can cause considerable distress and for some members can feel like a small crisis and loss of relationships, especially if the group was a source of psychological support to them.

Members Concerns

- Termination often represents fear of separation, loss of the deep relational bonds and support.
- Members need to arrive at acceptance that the group has to end and have to engage in the process of saying personal goodbyes.

Leader's Tasks

- The leader facilitates constructive practices for closure. Helps members express their feelings about the adjourning phase.
- Highlights and consolidates accomplishments and progress of members.

- Helps members formulate a plan to transfer their learnings to outside the group, promote discussion around on how members can continue to carry their growth, and if need be assess members for follow- up treatment.

Group Leadership Skills

Many novice group therapists will attempt at facilitating groups by attending to one individual at a time due lack of know-how of the perceptual shift needed to intervene in a group. This begs for the therapist to first use a different lens to facilitate groups. According to Brown (2008) a few central perceptual shifts include the following:

- The most crucial shift is to focus on the group as a whole. The leader has to have the ability to perceive interpersonal dynamics and view the group as a single functioning unit.
- The leader learns to observe and understand interactions among and between group members. What is of importance is not just the verbal content in addition the leader needs to take into account the timing and non-verbal aspects of the interaction. *For example, a reticent member, who usually refrains from providing validation or feedback to others sharing chooses to respond to a particular group member. This is of great significance as the member is not behaving as characteristically expected. An astute group therapist will take note of this change and explore the motivation underlying that interaction.*
- In groups the agent of change is the group.
- Effectiveness of the group therapist lies in her ability to promote emergence of therapeutic factors.
- Use group dynamics as a compass to inform and understand the process of group work.
- Leaders cannot be viewed as having favourites.
- Make group process commentary, to identify and remark on group themes and collective group states to help the group become aware and deepen their experiencing of groups needs and desires.
- Assume shared leadership roles, enable and empower members to share leadership as the group progresses.
- Balance between individual member needs and collective group needs.

Using the above guiding principles group therapists can apply fundamental communication skills and group level skills to conduct effective group work.

Group Level Skills

Considerable literature enlists different communication skills and group level skills a leader needs to master to competently lead a group. Several fundamental communication skills are common to individual and group therapy—such as listening, responding, questioning and reframing.

Group level skills are divided into two categories;

1. Specific group facilitation skill
2. Process oriented skills

Specific Group Facilitation Skills

The skills discussed in this segment are facilitation, blocking, linking, empathy, reality testing and immediacy.

Facilitation—Group leaders' foremost task is to be an interactional catalyst (Gladding, 2008). The leader facilitates interaction and open communication among group members. *Ex: After a member Ria takes initiative to share in the group, the leader can say, "How would the group like to respond to Ria?" Or addressing the group, "How does Ria's sharing make you feel?".*

Blocking—is used to protect members from attacks or from the group proceedings going in the wrong direction. Essentially used to keep potentially destructive processes from escalating. Leaders must consider using this skill in a tentative manner especially when members' emotions run high, as therapist intent can be misconstrued and members can end up feeling criticised. *For example, if a member displays intense anger during a conflict situation the leader needs to use blocking to keep the member from flying into rage.*

Linking—helps the leader string together themes, ideas, concepts, whose common thread may not be apparent easily. Linking is also used to highlight similarities in members sharing to bring about universality, resulting in members feeling they are not alone. Linking of the commonalities can occur over different sessions and hence requires leaders to be astutely attentive of group proceedings. *Ex: Leader's intervention in the initial stage—"Looks like many members in the group have a common concern of how to place your trust in each other. Perhaps we can spend time trying to explore ways to make the group a safe space."*

Empathy in groups—is a necessary condition for a therapist. However, in groups it's not just the leader who shares the responsibility, even members extend empathy to their fellow members.

In a group setting when a member shares, it can cause an emotional contagion, the leader needs to not only be empathetic to the person sharing, also to others who are impacted. This challenging feat requires the leader to tune into their own inner experiencing while remaining present centred and use active listening and sense the inner world of members. Resist the urge to attend to one member after the other and try to complete a round. Alternatively, try to see who jumps out the most to you in the focal field.

Reality testing—is used when a member makes a significant decision, the leader asks the group to give feedback to that member on how viable or realistic they think the decision is. *For example, if a member wants to change her job to an entirely different field and ask for group help, the leader can guide the group to give her concrete feedback as to their opinions and views on different aspects like viability of the change, skills needed, timing and purpose of the job change.*

Immediacy—is the skill of focusing and intervening to the here- and-now. This indicates that the leader makes a process comment to either the whole session, part of it or to a particular event, happening in the present. *Ex: Leader says, "I noticed that just after Jacob spoke the group went into a lull, silence of sorts. Can the members please help me understand what is happening here?"* The leader can proceed to process the group's responses to understand the group climate and facilitate crucial dialogue among members.

Confrontation—Oftentimes people think of confrontation as resulting in tension, conflict, or breaking of relationships. Even so, conflicts are inevitable in the interpersonal arena and when managed properly, becomes an opportunity for growth within the group. Chen and Rybak (2018) propose that group leaders need to consider two key steps when confronting:

- Timing—middle and later stages of group is considered good time for confrontation (Toth & Erwin, 1998)
- Every leader should equip themselves with a set of guiding principles for constructive confrontation.

Conflict management or the skill of confrontation is one of the most difficult aspects of group leadership. When confrontation is deployed as feedback, to invite members to examine their behaviours rather than as a corrective method, it can become a powerful catalyst for change.

Process Oriented Skills

Process commentary focuses on what is occurring between members, sub-groups and the group as a whole. Process commentary serves best to highlight the unspoken or unaware needs, desires of the group, such as, safety and trust issues, need for connection, resistance, exclusion, norms shaping and so on.

Let's first begin with understanding what processing is. Processing in a broad sense in small group work encompasses the leader helping the members identify and examine what transpired in the group. To hone process level skills the therapist needs to understand the mechanism of the here and now method.

The here and now method of communication is divided into content and process level. Furthering along this previously explained line of categorization, content level communication makes for less than 35% of the message and on the other hand process level sequence of communication conveys the other 65% of the message (Pease & Pease, 2006).

Yalom and Leszcz (2005) developed a refined 2 tier continuous, circular and fluid process of the 'Here and Now' technique:

- **Affect stimulation (experiencing the emotion)**
- **Process illumination (cognitive reflection)**

First Tier: Affect Stimulation

According to Yalom and Leszcz (2005), group leaders can achieve a level of emotional stimulation through here and now disclosure. Ex: *A group member, Jasmine is extremely helpful and polite. In group interaction it is observed that she has difficulty in saying anything negative to certain people and only gives positive feedback. She complains that her boss often takes advantage of her helpful nature as she can't say no, leaving her no time for her own work. Lately, she doesn't feel like going to work anymore.*

The therapist can dive into a here-and-now activation by first empathising with her and then addressing the group:

> *Seems like what Jasmine is telling us is that she finds it hard to say no to others and she can't confront people when she doesn't like something. I wonder who in the group Jasmine might find hard to confront?*

When the leader puts this out in the group to discuss, considerable commotion strikes, thereby more members get stirred up by the here-and-now activation. At this point the 2nd tier of process illumination takes off.

Second Tier: Process Illumination

This tier involves examining the process—cognitive reflection to help members understand what's going on internally for the members—intent and impact of their feelings and actions on others. Yalom and Leszcz (2005) explain this process as the group "performs a self- reflective loop and examines the here and now behaviour that has just occurred" (p. 142).

After a heated argument and many reactions surface, the leader's comments on wanting the group to talk about their observations:

(To the group): There seems to be a lot of important exchanges happening in the group right now. I wonder what the group is observing and what you think is going on here? (leader is trying to set forth cognitive reflection in the group).

Later after the group's reflections, the leader highlights the key aspects, with two other members Ria and Jacob.

(To Ria): Ria looks like the group is saying that when they pointed to Jacob as being the person Jasmine might have a problem confronting, you jumped in to protect him by using humour and narrating an incident not connected to the group. How do you think your behaviour impacted the group?

The leader continues this line of enquiry and wraps up the process illumination by saying:

(To the group): Ria's sharing shows that she can see her rescuing behaviour moved the members away from authentic dialogue and how it affected the group. I wonder if the group can see how Ria's behaviour of rescuing others and dissipating tension has any connection to what she disclosed about the role she played in her family when her parents were in conflict?

Later:

(Focusing on Jacob the leader asks the group): I can see Jacob is visibly disturbed. How is the group experiencing Jacob at this moment and can you explain the reason for making him the person Jasmine will have a problem confronting?

(To Jacob, who seems to be taking the group feedback and wrapping up process illumination with him.) Jacob, I can see you keenly listening to the group. I wonder where you are with all the feedback you have received? Can you tell us what feedback fits you and what doesn't?

Here Jacob learns how he perceives himself and how he comes across to others—what would he like to do with these revelations?

At some point the leader comes back to the first member who shared, Jasmine.

Jasmine, you seem to be aware that you find it especially hard to confront people who you perceive as having an aggressive tone or being stern and dominant in relationships. I wonder what this brings up for you?

Jasmine at this point is presented with the opportunity to work through her early childhood experiences and learn how she now perpetuates fixed childhood narratives in her adult life.

Chen and Rybak (2018) introduce the above complex skill of the here and now method as a concrete and comprehensive intervention, calling it *Zigzag the Hot Seat.* This method points to a non-linear strategy. In the above example, we can see that the sequence starts with a member who is on the *hot seat, this can be an intense experience* and so the leader shifts to the group. The group is looped in to create a possibility to activate multiple members in the here-and-now. The leader looks for opportunities to move the hot seat from member to member and creates a back and forth interaction loop—the Zigzag hot seat method. Through this method the whole group immerses in the interpersonal self-reflective loop (Yalom, 1995) and multiple members gain insight into their interpersonal distortions, and with group feedback relearn more adaptive interpersonal relating.

Therapeutic Factors of Groups and Leadership

Group leader's task, broadly speaking, is to therapeutically foster the emergence of favourable elements and to deter those elements that can deteriorate the group, such that the group is a safe space for members to trust and relate with each other, and progressively evolve as the main agent of change. Below is a highlight on a few therapeutic factors recommended by Yalom (1995), here the focus is on the rationale and strategy to assist leaders in the emergence of these positive elements.

- **Consensual validation**

Sullivan opines that interpersonal distortions can be modified through consensual validation. This is considered an important process by which group therapists guide a member to check his behaviour or perception of his experience with views of others in the group (Yalom and Leszcz, 2005). Group members often alter their perception after checking out other members' views of a significant incident. *For example, in group therapy, members can be questioned and confronted by others about their unhealthy self-talk and its impact on his/her feelings and behaviours. The group also comes to learn how common or unusual these self-evaluations can be and are challenged to adopt healthier ways.*

- **Instilling hope and altruism**

Hope is a vital component of therapy as many members in therapy can feel resigned to their struggles and leaders who focus on instilling a sense of hope are in effect infusing a sense of encouragement in members that their problems are resolvable. *Group leaders who recognize the importance of this, often get to work as early as the pre-meeting phase, by sharing testimonials of previously helped members and their own strong convictions about the benefit of group work.*

Additionally in group therapy members are at different points along the coping and collapse continuum (Yalom and Leszcz, 2005). *Group leaders, rather than give his expert advice, can initiate members to learn from others who have struggled the same and are now able to cope better or overcome their challenges, they feel a real sense of hope and resolve.*

Interestingly, a reciprocal effect sets about when a member selflessly helps other members, they feel they are needed and worthy. This altruistic involvement advertently helps members who have feelings of low self-worth, to not just be always in a position of receiving help but also to be in one of giving help. *Group therapists can highlight these positive reciprocal outcomes of sharing to deepen belongingness among the group members.*

- **Promoting universality and cohesion**

Members find great comfort and experience a sense of belonging when they learn that other members within a group experience similar feelings and struggles. *Group therapists need to link similarities among members and also interactions that promote universality early in the group's development.* This process invariably will enhance cohesion building in the group, which in turn makes the group open for experimentation and interpersonal learning.

- **Imparting information**

Information imparting as an educational leadership task is usually implicit in interactional group work. However, many group therapy models have formal psychoeducational goals integrated into process work groups. *For example, members of an anxiety management group can greatly benefit from gaining knowledge about misconceptions, cognitive distortions and insight into how panic attacks can be managed.*

- **Interpersonal learning**

Yalom asserts interpersonal learning is the mechanism that mediates therapeutic change in group therapy. Previous sections on the premise of group therapy and process oriented skills cover elaborate explanations on interpersonal learning.

Interpersonal learning also encapsulates learning socialisation techniques, proven to be particularly helpful to reduce or eliminate isolation and alienation. Members through sharing and feedback can learn healthier ways of alleviating relational and social disconnect—*To exemplify, when a member keeps rambling and is overly descriptive in his sharing, in a way keeping him from being in touch with his emotions and inadvertently at a risk of potentially losing the group's attention, the leader can intervene in this situation and ask the group for feedback.*

Ethics in Group Therapy

Although, in our country there is no professional governing body for group work that has a framework of safe practices and ethics, group practitioners must adhere to ethical decision making and practice as it is the cornerstone to effective group practice. Adherence to ethics shows the group members that the group leader will maintain integrity and safety as primary responsibility. Group practitioners can look to international associations to abide by, to name a few, American Group Psychotherapy Association, Association for specialists in group work and so on.

Conclusion

In closing, group therapy works magnificently for a whole range of psychological and social issues and it is considered the treatment for certain problems. The interpersonal approach presented in this chapter is the very fabric of therapy groups. Every seemingly ordinary interaction that transpires has a world of interpersonal dynamics and an astute group therapist knows to harness this alchemy.

References

Bernard, H., Burlingame, G., Flores, P., Greene, L., Joyce, A., et al. (2008). Clinical practice guidelines for group psychotherapy. *International Journal of Group Psychotherapy, 58*, 455–542.

Bion, W. R. (1969). *Experiences in groups and other papers* (1st ed.). London: Routledge.

Brown, N. W. (2008). *Becoming a group leader* (1st ed.). Allyn & Bacon.

Bugental, J. F. T. (1987). *The art of the psychotherapist*. W W Norton & Co.

Chen, M., & Rybak, C. J. (2018). *Group leadership skills* (2nd ed.). Sage Publications.

Donigian, J., & Malnati, R. (1997). *Systemic group therapy: A triadic model.* Pacific Grove, CA: Brooks/ Cole Pub. Co.

Fehr, S. S. (2018). *Introduction to group therapy: A practical guide* (3rd ed.). New York: Routledge Press.

Geller, S. M., & Greenberg, L. S. (2012). *Therapeutic presence: A mindful approach to effective therapy*. American Psychological Association.

Gladding, S. T. (2008). *Groups: A counseling speciality* (5th ed.). Pearson.

Pease, A., & Pease, B. (2006). *The definitive book of body language.* New York: Bantam Books.

Roger, C. R. (1951). *Client entered Therapy, Its current practice, implications and theory*. Houghton: Muffin.

Sullivan, H. S. (1953). *The interpersonal theory of psychiatry*. New York: Norton.

Toth, P. L., & Erwin, W. J. (1998). Applying skill-based curriculum to teach feedback in groups: an evaluation study. *Journal of Counseling & Development, 76*(3), 294–301.

Tuckman, B. W. (1965). Developmental sequence in small groups. *Psychological Bulletin, 63*(6), 384–399.

Yalom, I. D. (1995). *The theory and practice of group psychotherapy* (4th ed.). Basic Books.

Yalom, I. D., & Leszcz, M. (2005). *Theory and practice of group psychotherapy* (5th ed.). Basic Books.

Chapter 13
Integrating 'Spirituality' in Social Work—Challenges and Opportunities

R. Srinivasa Murthy

Abstract The existence of spirituality throughout human history and in all the communities calls for serious examination of its value for the mental health of the population in general and social work practice in particular. There is a major rethink in the broad area of mental health towards the need to think of mental health and not only mental illnesses; interventions in terms of addressing the larger social determinants and; to utilise fully the community-level resources for the mental health of the population. In this context, there has been a growing recognition of social, religious and spiritual factors that contribute to the mental health of individuals, families and communities. The growing evidence for the importance of spirituality has implications for social work practice. This can be seen at four levels. Firstly, people with spiritual practices are known to live longer and have better quality of life. Secondly, in the face of adverse life situations like exposure to conflicts/disasters, living with life-threatening illnesses like cancer, chronic heart and kidney diseases, ageing, loneliness, refugee status, people with spiritual orientation respond with greater resilience. Thirdly, caregiving, a growing need all over the world, benefits from spirituality. Fourthly, in mental disorders treatment spirituality has importance both as part of the treatment and associated with better treatment acceptance and outcomes. Based on the currently available evidence, there is value in integrating spirituality for the benefit of the mental health of individuals, families and communities. All of these aspects of spirituality are in line with social work practice, which recognises the value of community resources for mental health. The current chapter examines this issue from the following aspects: (i) research evidence of spirituality and health/mental health; (ii) research on spirituality and serious medical illnesses; (iii) spirituality and suicide; (iv) spirituality and HIV/AIDS; (v) spirituality and loneliness; (vi) experiences of application of spirituality in cancer care; (vii) caregivers of special children. Last but not the least, the chapter explicates the implications of these developments for social workers' training and practice.

Keywords Social work · Spirituality · Cancer · AIDS

R. Srinivasa Murthy (✉)
Professor of Psychiatry, NIMHANS (Retired), Bangaluru, India
e-mail: smurthy030@gmail.com

M. Anand (ed.), *Mental Health Care Resource Book*,
https://doi.org/10.1007/978-981-97-1203-8_13

Introduction

Spirituality in different forms has been a vital part of human history. Religion, medicine, and health care have been related in one way or the other across all population groups since the beginning of recorded history. Only in recent times, during the last few centuries, have these systems of healing been separated, and this separation has occurred largely in highly developed nations; in many developing countries, there is little or no such separation (Harrington, 2008; Koenig et al., 2012; Pulla, 2014). The existence of spirituality throughout human history and in all the communities calls for serious examination of its value for the mental health of the population in general and social work practice in particular.

The link between spirituality and social work has been effectively recognised in social work literature. For example, Pulla (2013, 2014) has observed that spirituality is one of the very important tools that help social work to be more connected to people. He recognises that every person and community has their own perspective to understand the concept of spirituality and calls for social worker practitioners to be open with their own transformation to be able to develop their own worldview of spirituality. Donaldson (2018) in her editorial of a special issue of 'Journal of Spirituality in Social work: Social thought' under the broad theme 'The importance of religion and spirituality in social work practice to strengthen practitioners, communities, couples, and individuals and in the cultivation of a praxis of love' brings together five articles and three book reviews. In more recent times, Dombo (2023) in the editorial of the special issue of the same journal, recognises the scope of spirituality as follows: '*social work educators have a unique opportunity to influence what issues the next generation of professionals choose to address in practice and explore in their research*'. The 'Handbook of Religion and Spirituality in Social Work Practice and Research' edited by Loue (2017) is a rich resource in this field. Loue observes, '*Religion and spirituality constitute but one facet of each individual, yet it is often an important one. Our religious and spiritual views provide insight into how we view the world and our place and roles within it, and how we treat others and wish to be treated ourselves*'. The book is a rich resource (having four parts with 22 chapters) for social work practitioners as it comprehensively covers the subject. Part one of the book has seven chapters covering the topics related to definitions of religion and spirituality; religious underpinnings of social work; cultural competence role of rituals in families; assessment/screening; and the importance of life cycles. Part two has six chapters covering various healing traditions, mental illness, coping, death and dying, and mourning practices. Part three has seven chapters covering forgiveness; community worship; inclusion/exclusion in religious groups; and distortion by political forces. There are three chapters in Part four focussing on social work research, in terms of methodology; relationship with religious leaders; and ethical aspects.

Mental health is the defining public health challenge of our times (Office of Surgeon General, 2023). There is a major rethink in the broad area of mental health, as reviewed in the chapter on 'Understanding mental disorders, mental health and well-being' (Murthy, 2023, 2024; Chap. 2 of this book). The mental health of the total population and not only mental illnesses affect about 10% of the population. Interventions in terms of addressing the larger social determinants of mental health/illnesses are needed to utilise fully the individual, family and community-level resources for enabling mental health of the population. In this context, there is a growing recognition of social, religious and spiritual factors that contribute to the mental health of the individuals, families and communities and their value in addressing the adversities of life.

The chapter examines this issue from the following aspects: (i) research evidence of spirituality and health/mental health; (ii) research on spirituality and serious medical illnesses; (iii) spirituality and suicide; (iv) spirituality and HIV/AIDS; (v) spirituality and loneliness; (vi) experiences of application of spirituality in cancer care; (vii) caregivers of special children; and (viii) implications of these developments for social workers training and practice.

Research Evidence of Spirituality and Health/Mental Health

Koenig (2012) has extensively reviewed the evidence and presented the research and clinical implications of religion, spirituality and health in the review article covering 602 references (Table 13.1). The handbook of religion, spirituality, health (Koenig et al., 2012) is another resource covering the same subject. In September 2023, An updated 3rd edition is published in (Koenig et al, 2024).

Koenig (2012) outlines the clinical implications in terms of the rationale for integrating spirituality in health care in general and mental health care in particular and the ways to integrate spirituality in patient care (Koenig, 2013). Under the rationale, he recognises that many patients have spiritual needs in relation to their medical and psychiatric illnesses. R/S influences the patient's ability to cope with illness. R/S beliefs affect patients' medical decisions. Physicians' belief of R/S often influences medical care. R/S is associated with both mental and physical health and likely to affect medical outcomes. R/S influences the kind of support and care received on returning home. Failure to address patients' spiritual needs can increase health costs, especially toward the end of life.

Research on Spirituality and Serious Medical Illnesses

A recent review of 371 articles (Balboni et al, 2022) presents evidence concerning spirituality in serious illness and health and to identify implications for patient care and health outcomes. The Delphi panel review yielded 8 evidence statements supported by evidence categorized as strong and proposed 3 top-ranked implications of this evidence for serious illness, namely, (i) incorporate spiritual care into care for patients with serious illness; (ii) incorporate spiritual care education into training of interdisciplinary teams caring for persons with serious illness; and (iii) include

Table 13.1 Religion, spirituality and health (Koenig et al., 2012) summary of evidence

• Approximately 80% of research on religion/spirituality (R/S) and health involves studies on mental health. • Majority of studies show R/S to be helpful in coping with adversities like living with medical illnesses, pain, caregiver burden, end-of-life issues, bereavement, natural disasters and adverse life situations. • Positive association between R/S and well-being. • Hope, optimism, meaning and purpose, self-esteem, sense of control is positively associated with health and mental health. • Greater R/S predicted lower levels of depression or faster remission of depression. • Inverse relationship between R/S and suicide. • R/S predicted lower level of anxiety and R/S reduced anxiety more than standard interventions. • R/S predict better outcomes in psychotic disorders. • R/S have inverse relationship with substance abuse. • R/S has inverse relationship with delinquency/crime. • R/S is related to greater marital stability. • R/S is associated with greater social support. • R/S is related to greater social capital.
Health behaviours and R/S
• Positive correlation with exercise and physical activity. • Inverse relationship with cigarette smoking. • Healthier and better diet. • Inverse relationship with risky sexual behaviours.
Physical health and R/S
• Inverse relationship with coronary heart disease. • Lower blood pressure. • Lower risk for stroke. • Better cognitive functioning. • Lower infection rates and viral loads. • Better immunity. • Lower risk of cancer and better prognosis. • Better self-rated health. • Lower levels of pain and better response to interventions. • Longer life-span.

speciality practitioners of spiritual care in the care of patients with serious illness. Further, from the 215 health outcomes articles, the Delphi panel review yielded 8 evidence statements supported by evidence categorized as strong and proposed 3 top-ranked implications of this evidence for health outcomes:

(i) Incorporate patient-centred and evidence-based approaches regarding associations of spiritual community with improved patient and population health outcomes.
(ii) Increase awareness among health professionals of evidence for protective health associations of spiritual community.
(iii) Recognize spirituality as a social factor associated with health in research, community assessments, and program implementation.

Based on this extensive review, authors emphasise the need for recognition of spirituality in serious illness and health outcomes as part of person-centred, value-sensitive care.

Spirituality and Suicide

Social and spirituality roots of suicide have been well recognised following the pathbreaking research of Emily Durkheim during the nineteenth century (1897). He concluded 'Suicide is individual action based on social factors' on the basis of study of church records and suicides in persons of subgroups of Christianity, and the association of social factors and rates of suicide.

Koenig (2012) reviewing 141 studies examining the relationship between R/S and suicide variables, found that 75% of studies reported inverse relationships and 3% positive relationships. Of the 49 studies with the highest methodological rigour, 80% reported less suicide, fewer suicide attempts and more negative attitudes towards suicide among the more spiritual individuals.

It is important to recognise the continuing importance of spirituality in suicidology and suicide prevention. In the second edition of the 'Oxford Textbook of Suicidology and Suicide Prevention' (Wasserman, 2021) containing 96 chapters and 15 sections, the first section is on 'Religion and suicide' having 11 chapters. The titles of the chapters illustrate the importance of spirituality in suicide, namely, (i) religion, more than just protective; (ii) role of religion in suicide prevention; (iii) Confucianism, Taoism, and suicide; (iv) Hindu religion and suicide in India; (v) Buddhist perspective om suicide; (vi) Shinto Religion and suicide in Japan; (vii) Suicide in Jewish scriptures; (viii) Suicide and Islam; (ix) Christianity and suicide; (x) Religion and suicide prevention in Uganda; and (xi) Maya Religion influencing suicide prevention in Mexico.

Spirituality and HIV/AIDS

Persons living with AIDS (PLWAIDS) face many challenges from the time of diagnosis and throughout their life. These relate to the questions relating to *why me*? (accidental infection or risky behaviour), stigmatisation from the community, need for lifelong treatment, restrictions in personal, family and community life. This group has been studied extensively, as interventions that influence immunological status can either facilitate or adversely affect the outcome. Koenig (2012) reports that in 56% of the 27 studies, there is a positive relationship between R/S and immune functions. He further reports that 67% of twelve studies of the viral load had significantly lower viral loads in those who were more R/S. Dalmida et al. (2015) report negative religious coping, religious attendance, religiousness, and social support satisfaction significantly predicted quality of life. Depressive symptoms, positive religious coping and social support satisfaction significantly predicted quality of life. Participants who were females, prayed less than daily, attended religious services less than weekly or who were non/less religious had significantly poorer quality of life. The authors conclude that their findings confirm the importance of religion, mental health, medication adherence and social support in the quality of life of PLWAIDS and further suggest that spirituality should be routinely assessed by clinicians.

Spirituality and Loneliness

There is a growing recognition of the importance of loneliness for health in general and mental health in particular. On 3 May 2023, Dr. Vivek Murthy, Surgeon General of the United States of America, releasing the Report 'Our Epidemic of Loneliness and Isolation 2023' observed 'Loneliness and isolation represent profound threats to our health and well-being. But we have the power to respond by taking small steps every day to strengthen our relationships, and by supporting community efforts to rebuild social connection, we can rise to meet this moment together' (Office of the Surgeon General, 2023).

During the recent COVID-19 pandemic, the importance of social determinants has come to the forefront (Murthy, 2020a, b). In a study across the U.S. and European populations, the differences in loneliness before and after the pandemic were found to be small. One meta-analysis published this year by the American Psychological Association analyzed 34 studies conducted before and during the pandemic that were focused on loneliness, an emotional state distinct from anxiety or depression that signals when social needs aren't being met. Researchers found about a 5% increase in loneliness during the pandemic (Law, 2022).

There is a need for thinking the issue of loneliness in innovative ways (Murthy and Banerjee, 2021; Office of the Surgeon General, 2023). For example, the traditional practices of India have a special relevance to address the loneliness issues relating to old age. The view of focussing on 'continued normalcy' misses the complimentary view of considering aging not as 'loss' but as a 'transition' in life. This is the essence of the spiritual approach to aging as reflected in the 'Ashrama' system of India (Wig, 1990, 2010). The focus is to move from loneliness to solitude that is filled with tranquillity and peace. Instead of considering it as a 'separate pathological entity' that deserves a 'special treatment', to deal with it as part of aging by 'letting go when it's time'. The above approach forms the very foundation of the Hindu philosophy. The central theme of all Indian or Eastern religions, Hindu, Buddhist or Jain is the idea of *Tyaga* or renunciation. This has been a powerful concept that has withstood civilizations for years. It has been linked to the last two Ashramas (stages of life) according to Hinduism, i.e., *Vaanaprasth*a (Forest Dweller) and Sanyas (Ascetic). Wig (1990, 2010) has written about the applicability of *Vaanaprastha i*n modern society. The literal translation of living in the forest definitely does not hold true in today's socio-economic context but rather refers to acceptance, wisdom, maturity, and solitude as a person ages. *Manusmriti* also describes how Eastern traditions aim for being with oneself (oneliness instead of loneliness), optimism and hope which are associated with letting go of one's abilities in a graded yet respectful manner rather than lamenting for the loss. This concept of living in old age is fully developed in the '*Sadhana Panchakam*' of Sri Adi Shankara. The five shlokas present forty tips to guide a person in his spiritual unfoldment making it a practicable approach to old age in general and loneliness in particular. Wig (2010) has synthesized it as follows: (i) voluntary withdrawal from the routine hustle of life and trying to unify emotionally with nature, (ii) deliberately attempting to reduce one's needs to maintain a balance with the available resources, (iii) acceptance of aging and associated limitations, enjoying the positive constructs and wisdom of age, reduced need to be in control, (iv) contribution to the society and focusing on social welfare to the extent possible, and (v) pursuit of spirituality.

The path-analysis model based on a study from Portugal showed the mediating effect of spiritual practices between aging and perceived social connectedness as well as life satisfaction. A pragmatic group intervention trial in the senior housing communities of the U.S. involved savouring, acceptance, gratitude, and engagement in value-based activities to improve resilience and reduce loneliness. The systematization and making it an activity incorporated in the daily lifestyle of the older age population could be the greatest gift of all religions to humanity towards the challenges of aging.

Experiences of Application of Spirituality in Cancer Care and Caregivers' Support

The following two experiences of the author illustrates the importance of spirituality in two care-providing situations, both to understand the role of spirituality in understanding the coping approaches of Indians and the scope for utilising spirituality in the support programmes for better physical and emotional health.

Cancer Care and Spirituality

The diagnosis of cancer is a life-changing experience for the affected individual and their families. A wide range of supports are needed by the patient and the family. Ms. Harmala Gupta, founder of 'CANSUPPORT' in Delhi, has written her experiences ('Cancer, the life changer') in the book, 'Life After Cancer' published by the Indian Cancer Society as follows: '*There is no getting back to the way as it was, for you and the members of the family*' (Govil, 2013; Gupta, 2013) It is significant that she utilised the pain of her personal journey, to establish the biggest free home care palliative care programme in Delhi. Similar are other experiences: 'Suddenly at [age] 35, I get this stage 4 cancer diagnosis, and it's just like a bomb went off and everything around me is debris'. 'But you are immobilised with uncertainty. It takes a long, long time to push despair away and bring hope back into your life. I will miss a whole bunch of things that I love. But that is what dying is all about. You get one life, you enjoy it as responsibly as you can, and then you die'.

Scientific Evidence of Relationship Between Cancer and Spirituality

Koenig (2012) reports 29 studies relating to cancer and spirituality to the relationship between religion/spirituality (R/S) and either the onset or outcome of cancer, including cancer mortality. Of those, 16 studies (55%) found that those who are more R/S had a lower risk of cancer or a better prognosis, although two studies (7%) reported a significantly worse prognosis. Of the 20 methodologically most rigorous studies, 12 (60%) found an association between R/S and lower risk or better outcomes and none reported worse risks or outcomes. The results from some of these studies can be partially explained by better health behaviours (less cigarette smoking, alcohol, abuse etc.) but not all effects are explained by better health behaviours and could be explained by lower stress levels and higher social supports in those who are more R/S. Although cancer is not thought to be as sensitive as cardio-vascular disorders to show psychosocial stressors, psychosocial influences in cancer incidence and outcome are present.

There is growing evidence that support of different varieties of psychosocial interventions can alleviate the distress and, in some cases, improve the survival time. However, there are two challenges in receiving/providing emotional support to persons living with a diagnosis of cancer. There is an urgent need to not only think of services and supports but also strengthen the individuals living with a diagnosis of cancer and their caregivers, by harnessing the resources within. It is for all of these reasons of the great need and difficulties of providing the needed emotional care, measures to address the need through 'self-care' becomes urgent.

In India, one of the pre-existing sources of support is the spiritual resource. Spirituality in all religions addresses the problems faced by a person experiencing pain, suffering, fear of death and to find the meaning of life during adverse life situations (Ahmadi & Ahmadi, 2018). As noted earlier, the diagnosis of cancer is a life-changing situation and is eminently suited for spiritual support.

The following sections present the importance of spirituality in cancer and the scope for social work through two aspects. Firstly, the review of literature about cancer and spirituality. Secondly, the personal experiences of the author in providing emotional support to persons living with a diagnosis of cancer and their caregivers, as part of total cancer care in a hospital for cancer care.

Epidemiological studies have shown that persons living with a diagnosis of cancer have higher rates of emotional disorders in all countries (Holland, 2001; Koenig et al., 2012; Murthy & Alexander, 2019). Indian research in the area of psycho-oncology has addressed the prevalence of emotional health problems (Alexander et al., 2019, 2020; Chaturvedi, 2015; Mehrotra, 2008), needs for assessment of needs (Chittem et al., 2012; Saxena et al., 2018), importance of family (Alexander et al., 2019) issue of suicide (Mohandoss & Thavarajah, 2016), need for emotional support (Ghosal et al., 2016; Barthakur et al., 2016) and the importance of communication in cancer care (Chaturvedi et al., 2014). A special area of studies has been in spirituality (Kandaswamy et al., 2011; Shukla & Rishi, 2014; Chaturvedi, 2022a, b). Gielin et al. (2017) report that more than half of the Indian cancer patients need spiritual care. An Indian measurement has been developed to measure spirituality and its utility has been evaluated (Bhatnagar et al., 2016; Gielin et al., 2022). Value of yoga too has been reported (Agarwal & Marako-Afeq, 2018). Another area of recent interest is the scope for post-traumatic growth in cancer experiences (Tandon & Mehrotra, 2017).

A recent publication from Iran (Ahmadi & Ahmadi, 2018; Ahmadi et al., 2022) with 27 participants with various kinds of cancer and meaning making found, nine secular existential meaning-making coping strategies. These coping methods included ignorance of the illness, distraction, altruism, encounter with others, nature, discourse of the self, visualization, positive solitude and positive thinking and transformational orientation. It seems that using these strategies, the sample of Iranian cancer patients/survivors were denying/ignoring their illness, and/or empowering themselves. Authors also emphasise the potential influence of cultural elements, including Iranian Islam, Persian mysticism and Persian literature, on the selection of the coping strategies. The study contributes to the understanding of coping via elucidating how seriously ill individuals in Iran try to manage the challenges caused by a health crisis.

One of the important developments in the disaster mental health field is the possibility of post-traumatic growth. This is reported to occur in about one-third of survivors. There is growing literature on PTG in cancer survivors (Tandon & Mehrotra, 2017). Some examples will illustrate this aspect. 'I feel a sense of purpose I didn't have when I was 22 and totally adrift. There's also a richness to be excavated; in fact, those transitional moments have ultimately been the most powerful and pivotal of my life' (Parker-Pope, 2022); 'This ordeal taught me to cherish life and its simple joys that we all take for granted. More so, I started looking at my relationships in a new light. I started loving those relationships, my friendships that I had often taken for granted' (Bhattacharjee & Nazier, 2022).

Personal Experiences in a Cancer Hospital

Following my life journey with cancer (Murthy, 2016a, b) I wanted to utilise the personal/family experiences and mental health professional expertise to assist people living with cancer. These experiences have close similarity to the work undertaken by the social workers. I worked as a volunteer psychiatrist at the Sri Shankara Cancer Hospital (SSCH), Bangalore for about two years. The experiences described below provide the foundation for examining the importance of spirituality in cancer care. When I started working at the SSCH in 2015, there was already a professional social worker with decades of cancer care experience, and a senior and experienced psychiatrist providing psychosocial care. When I met them for the first time, both of them said to me, 'why are you coming, patients do not come even when they are referred by the oncologists'. Further, about spirituality, social worker said: 'the topic is of interest to me but I am a little curious/apprehensive to know if people would be open to talk about spirituality…or perceive it to be private personal affair'.

These responses puzzled me, as it was contrary to my personal experience. However, I went on to work there and found their conclusions were not correct. I understood the reason for the situation, as the two professionals were using the referral and specialist approach rather than working to empower the people/families living with a cancer diagnosis. For the first few months, I worked with all patients receiving chemotherapy. The focus of my interaction was to understand their experiences, their needs and the ways they were addressing the challenges of diagnosis, treatment procedures, the side effects, cost of care, interpersonal relationships within the families, uncertainties of life and the resources they were utilising to address these needs. Unexpectedly, during these open-ended conversations to understand the cancer journey, I understood that persons living with cancer and their caregivers were most often utilising their spiritual resources, to cope with the multiple challenges.

Few examples will support this conclusion. A few examples will illustrate the same:

1. One person on chemotherapy, shared what helped her: 'I have read somewhere that When Shri Raman Maharshi was enduring the pain of osteocarcinoma, someone asked him 'Swamyji, is it not painful?' to which he answered, 'It's not 'me' but it is 'the body' which is undergoing the pain. I am aware of the pain'. These words appealed to her greatly during the chemotherapy days and she would repeatedly tell her mind that 'it's my "body" not "me" who is undergoing the pain. The spiritual story provided a role model to address a life challenge'.
2. Elderly lady with terminal cancer was calm about her life situation and the uncertain future. On enquiry about what helped her in the challenging life situation, she said: 'doctor, I read everyday *Sunderakanda* for about 90 min and it gives me peace' On further enquiry, she said: 'In *Sunderakanda* Matha Sita is in Ashokvana and for all practical purposes there was no hope. However, she maintained hope and a solution came. I believe something similar will happen in my life'. I saw how comparing personal life situation to a spiritual situation helped navigate the uncertainties of future.
3. One of the fears of persons living with cancer during the recovery face is the 'fear of recurrence' During my work with a 35 years old lady with triple negative breast cancer, I enquired about how she addresses this challenge. She narrated the story from Mahabharata. She said, 'Faith and Fear can't co-exist'. The story was that of Krishna and Balarama walking through the forest and meeting a demon. The fear of Balaram makes the demon huge while the faith of Krishna reduces the demon to a puppet.

4. During the last one year I was partner in the end-of-life journey of a senior psychiatrist and a dear friend (Gupta, 2023). We examined the issues of end-of-life situation, from both the personal and professional viewpoints. It was a rich learning experience for me and taught me that it is possible to face death positively, as my friend did. One interaction stays in my mind forever. In one of the conversations, in response to issue of death, he said, 'How hard one may strive, death is a reality. Even *Hiranyakasyap* and *Ravana,* who were blessed with immortality had to die. Death is a blessing. It creates space for new viable life'. Looking at this interaction of many sessions/hours, I can say that my friend found more solace from spirituality than my professional skills.
5. Different people use spirituality differently. A senior academician with multiple recurrences of breast cancer and in an end-of-life situation, shared how reading *Bhagavatham* helped her. She said: 'Every evening my husband and myself read the book for about an hour. It gives me peace of mind' When I asked to give an example, she related the story of *Parikshith.* 'Parikshith, facing death within one week, chose to leave his kingdom and move to live in Varanasi with the sages and devote time in spiritual practices'. She whispered to me, 'doctor do not feel bad if I tell you, in my current life situation, my spirituality is greater value than medical help!'.
6. During the last few years, I am coordinating a WhatsApp group of persons living with a diagnosis of cancer and their caregivers. Group members have been sharing the value of the four 'pillars' of cancer care, namely, medical care; psychological support; social support and spirituality. In a situation of uncertainty like the diagnosis of cancer enters life, the past is largely irrelevant, the future is vague and the present becomes the only thing to hold on to. However, all of our life we have not learnt to live in the present, in the truest sense. Learning to live in the present, often referred to as mindful living, has to be learnt, along with putting the past and the future in the back burner.

These professional interactions have taught me that spirituality is a resource people harness when they have medical challenges in general and cancer in particular.

The above experiences have taught me that, cancer changes life like no other experience of life. There is need for utilisation of all the resources to find relief from 'distress' and strengthen persons living with a diagnosis of cancer. However, as noted by my social worker colleague, there is a considerable ambivalence in the caregiving professions about the best way to integrate spirituality in their work. Developing practical ways of strengthening the spiritual resources is a task for all professionals in general and social workers in particular.

Caregiving of Special Children and Spirituality

Throughout history of India, caregiving is a commitment that the family members of persons with special needs take by choice (Murthy, 2021). Caregiving for a family member with special needs challenges the economic, physical, emotional, interpersonal, and intrapersonal relationship and spiritual aspects of the caregivers. Caregiving brings to the family life, a new way of living. In the Indian context and culture, mothers are more involved in the caregiving- rearing, and educating the child with special needs along with taking care of the needs of other family members and the responsibilities of running the home. In more than two dozen studies from India, these added efforts and responsibilities and associated increased emotional distress have been documented. (Nischitha et al., 2023).

Spirituality is one resource that helps to meet the challenges of caregiving. As noted earlier, spirituality is that aspect in everyone's life which individuals utilise in order to make sense of experiences of life in relationship with a 'higher power'.

The Association for Mentally Challenged (AMC), Bangalore, under project ENRICH (Empowering families to fulfil their Needs and Rebuild families through Information, and Skills of Caregiving towards Holistic development of the families), one of the areas explored with the caregivers of children with special needs has been the place of spirituality in their lives. Interviews with parents explored the spiritual experiences of caregivers and understanding of spirituality as a part of caregiving experiences. The sample for the qualitative explorative study was conducted with 20 caregivers of the beneficiaries of AMC. All the parents were approached through phone. Each interview took around 15 to 30 min. The interviews were transcribed and were manually read through many times to identify the themes and sub-themes. All the participants were informed about the study and consent was taken to audio record the interview for research purposes. The families interviewed were practitioners of Hinduism, Islam, and Christianity. The study identified seven themes.

Theme 1: Meaning and relationship with god

All the parents in the interviews shared their belief that 'God is present', a higher power who is protecting all and guiding everyone in life. Each of them understood this belief in different ways, level of beliefs, rituals and philosophies. One parent is a working woman and a mother of two children in a nuclear family. Her younger son who is 17 years old, is a special child. She said that God according to her is a belief, and a source of strength, and hope. 'Every time I step out of the house or make any decision I first pray and ask for strength to do that. I put 100% effort and put all my beliefs in God to help me with it'. With all the distress in her life, she believes that God is present for her to hold her hands at the time of difficulties and looks forward to the guidance of God to cope with that situation. Similarly, three other parents expressed their thoughts on the similar lines. Other parents shared the following: 'God to me is a "Belief". I believe in God to be like a friend with whom I can confide anything and everything. I believe that God guides me in the course of life'.

'God is *bhakti,* doing pooja and telling all her difficulties to the god, 'talking to god makes me feel good and relaxed'. 'God is '*Bhakti*/Devotion' we have to pray with devotion and anything will happen.

Theme 2: Spirituality as a coping tool

Parents were consciously or unconsciously using spirituality to help them cope with the challenges of having a special child and other life challenges. Here are a few examples:

> I was very sad in a way that I got the feeling of not wanting this life at all, I felt why me? Sometimes I get the feeling that it might be due to the karma of my past. I had many questions when I think about it and it stresses me a lot but I can't leave my child. This is my responsibility as a mother so I will do until I can. I pray to God every day to give me more strength to care for them.
>
> Since last night I got a very severe headache because of my son. I was not able to handle him, help him calm down. Sometimes nothing works, all we can do to wait for him to calm down by himself and keep trying all the things that we can. I believe Allah is there for us. We live because we believe in Allah, actually, he gave us a special child but at the same time he gave us strength to look after this child, he gave us patience, he knows that we can bear this child that's why he gave us. Not everyone can bear this child. We are alive because of Allah. Without him, nothing is there. He has planned everything in our life even if it is in small aspects, he has planned.

Theme 3: Rituals to connect with god

Rituals are one way to connect with God. It gives caregivers a chance to introspect on the changes that have happened in life and engage with the larger community that has similar beliefs. Most of the parents are practicing rituals that are part of their family, community, culture or religious beliefs. Parents belonging to different religion and cultures shared the practices of visiting temples/church/mosque, lighting lamps/candles, performing prayers more than one time a day, chanting mantras/prayers from their religious texts, fasting on special occasions, and other rituals regularly. Here are some examples:

> My sister suggested to start writing 'Sri Rama Jayam' as a part of my spiritual routine. Without fail every day I write. When I am in distress, I tend to write two more extra pages than usual. In the beginning it was difficult. But with practice, I started to like writing it. Writing 'Sri Rama Jayam' gave me a lot of calmness'. 'When I pray it feels like I have hugged my God and is letting go of all my miseries. God talks with me in the verses in Bible. The Verse says 'You are in a difficult time now, but don't lose hope on God, he will always be by your side'. These verses are like the hands that hold me tightly when in need. 'Belonging to Islamic community, we all do namaz five times a day and also read Holy Quran. Sometimes on special occasions we go to *Dargah* too. Following and practicing these rituals gives me calmness and I feel things will get better and Allah will lead my way.

Theme 4: God's connection with self

Practicing spirituality has not only connected the parents towards the higher power but they also have a belief that God/higher power will reach out to them at the time of distress in many ways. A lot of parents believe that in every difficult situation, God will send them a person to help these people and will decrease their difficulties. This gives them hope to continue their life. 'We didn't have a single penny for his operations. It is still a miracle, I don't know how, people we know from church, school, our relatives came to help. Over all we got 1 lakh cash in our hands within 24 h and with that amount we were able to spend for the three surgeries. Doctors also gave the concessions after we let them know our condition. People who don't know us were supporting us'. Other parents shared: 'I usually get help through my mother-in-law and my sister-in-law, like whenever I ask help they will always be there. So, I see God in them, I feel God is helping me through them, I get strength and comfort from them. Sometimes things don't go as I hoped for, but there are times it goes well and I am thankful for that. My family is always there for me and I feel they are my God'. 'God cannot be present everywhere, so he gives a heart for people to help others and I don't follow any rituals, or I don't have any discrimination between Hindu, Muslim, Christian. All I know is people who follow kindness, forgiveness, service to others, being selfless, helpful, and showing gratitude, where there is no greed then, God will be present, that's all I believe and I would tell other peoples to do the same'.

Theme 5: Spiritual practices

Taking on the responsibility of caregiving has widened the scope of spiritual practices by the caregivers. 'Instead of saying thank you, we do services to the residents of old age homes and other ashrama people. For example, on his birthday or any other occasion, instead of celebrating by spending money with the family, I give that money to ashrama people so that they can get a day's food for those in need and they give blessings to us. That's enough for us and that's how we say thanks to God. I think forgiveness is also a good thing. After having a special child my life totally has changed. I used to be so stubborn and angry but now I don't show any anger to anyone. Even for the people, who I don't like, if they come now home, I just say let's forget the old things that happened, let's have a good relationship'. 'Forgiveness is a trait that Allah likes a lot. We as his worshippers, should inculcate that to please Allah. If there is someone who has hurt you, it will be Allah's decision to protect or punish him, we are no one to judge, talk bad about others and hurt them with words'.

Theme 6: Understanding the special child through spirituality

Making sense of what is happening in life can give direction and acceptance of the situation.

Parents who believed in the concept of 'Karma' feel that it is the deeds in the previous life of the child or the parents is why they have a child with special needs. Some examples: 'When I got a special child–I was very upset, got angry towards God, thinking why me and what did I do to have a special child? Nobody in our family had a special child. Why did God give it to me? Then I thought it might be mine or my husband's sins, from the past life. to have a special child'. 'Looking after my brother with special needs was never a burden. When I was young, I was very angry because I had a brother with special needs and he was not mingling with people. Then my elder sister got married and things changed, mom also was saying I should stay independent. I am used to having him around and caring for him. Maybe that is why he was made to stay with me forever now'. 'I think our special child is a god gift and God gave us because he knows that we have enough strength to take care and I think because it's a god gift we need to take care of him with all the love and joy'. 'I went to our guruji to ask why I was blessed with a child who has special needs? He said 'it is God's gift. In this world children like these are born because Allah is blessing you a paradise for your afterlife through them.' The rule to serve the needy has been fulfilled through my son which will make Allah bless us'.

Theme 7: Finding meaning through spirituality

All of us have an inherent capacity (mental-emotional-physical) for negotiating the meaning of life through spirituality. In the context of special children, spirituality has given the opportunity for the parents to look at the life situation in a different way and find meaning/purpose within themselves. The belief in the higher power, practice of rituals, their life situations, the understanding of their religious texts have helped the caregivers to make sense of their journey as a parent/family member/caregiver of a person with special needs. Some examples: 'There still are things that make me worry at times. But still, somehow everything is in order even when we are in a chaos. We are paying the bills and his treatment is still continuing, I have the hope my son will get better in the course of time. We have to go to hospital every other day for his dressing and other things. No one in our house is earning. But still, everything is going on, life is going on. It feels like there is nothing for me to be worried about. Difficulties are man-made, but only God can save us from all the misshapes we have bought on ourselves'. 'I think this was all God planned, because every day I used to pray when I was in a joint family that I needed peace from all these problems. Why are there so many difficulties for me? Now I think God gave me an answer by helping me to coming out of the joint family. He gave me relief'. I think our special child is a gift of God and God gave us because he knows that we have enough strength to take care and I think because it's God's gift we need to take care of him with all the love and joy.

Spirituality is considered the master key of the Indian mind (Murthy, 2010; Mehra, 2015). This was succinctly expressed by one caregiver, 'My faith has become stronger'. In this explorative study, it is seen that the parents/caregivers of people with special needs are utilising spirituality to understand the loss and love their children and using it as a source of growth. The above two examples from clinical situations illustrate the need and scope to integrate spirituality in clinical situations.

To summarise, there is a growing evidence for the importance of spirituality social work practice. This can be seen at four levels. Firstly, people with spiritual practices are known to live longer and have better quality of life. Secondly, in the face of adverse life situations like exposure to conflicts/disasters, living with life-threatening illnesses like cancer, chronic illnesses, ageing, loneliness, refugee status, people with spiritual orientation respond with greater resilience. Thirdly, caregiving, a growing need all over the world, benefits from spirituality. Fourthly, in mental disorders treatment spirituality has importance understanding of clients, as part of the treatment and associated with better treatment acceptance and outcomes.

Challenges to Integration of Spirituality into Care Programmes

Historically, especially in the Western countries, there is separation of the body-mind. There are many reasons for this development. The philosopher, Descartes is a significant personality in this story. For example, Thomas (1997) and Harrington (2008) relate the separation as follows: 'One morning, so the story goes, the seventeenth-century philosopher/scientist awoke from a dream, inspired to pursue the study of metaphysics. The culmination of this study was his conclusion that body and mind were separate entities. At that point he and the Roman Catholic Church struck a deal: As a man of science, Descartes would restrict himself to the study of human anatomy, leaving the mind and soul to the care of the church. From that time on, studies of mind and body have for the most part remained two distinct and separate fields. Scientists endeavoured to stay within the realm of the observable and strictly quantifiable. Meanwhile, those in the religious life lifted thought, reason, and emotion out of the body, into the realms of the spiritual'. Even now, in the Western countries, there are strict boundaries in dealing the spiritual matters even in medical settings only by the religious leaders. This is not so in the Eastern cultures, where there is greater openness to utilise spiritual resources by a wide range of community members. The second aspect is the politicisation of the religion in many ways. Issues of abortion rights, food habits, same sex marriage, personal laws are becoming the battleground between opposing political groups and this makes looking at spirituality in a neutral and personal manner difficult. Thirdly, religious/spiritual practices have been largely rooted in the local communities and thus there are no standardised way of applying the interventions. Fourthly, the creation of strong evidence of effectiveness (Table 13.2) (Modified from Murthy & Banerjee, 2021).

There are positive developments to include spirituality in health settings and develop methods of practicing the same.

'The recurring central theme of human life on this planet appear to be one of coping, and resilience and that of relying on one's own inner strength. The world is also witnessing increased number of people that are able to cope, hope, act, anticipate,

Table 13.2 Approaches to develop practice of spirituality and evaluate its impact

- Examination of the concepts and practices in different religions.
- Adaptation of the concepts/practices to modern societal realities living in rural, urban, and other settings and different population groups.
- The development of case studies of persons utilizing these measures and finding meaning of life Preparing people, as they age, (from 50 years on) to include this in their overall life plans.
- Case control studies of people in society with varying degrees of spirituality.
- Longitudinal studies in the specific population groups (elderly, adolescents, persons with chronic illnesses, disabilities, etc.), to understand the value of spirituality in promoting QOL, mental wellness, preventing depression, dementia, etc., and coping better with adverse life situations of disease, grief, etc.
- Standardization of spiritual practices as applicable to all groups, for wider dissemination in the society QOL: Quality of life.

prevent, promote and transcend. There is an assumption that these pointers suggest a growing awareness of religion and spirituality as two important sources of inner and outer strengths to deal with adversities, illness, ageing and disability. In many Western nations, the notion of spirituality is not embedded within the definitions of mainstream, 'culture' and with much sadness, we admit that social work practice has also remained aloof and cold to this vital and positive force of spirituality in our societies despite its assistance to human coping and human resilience. (Further he) argues for an appropriate client centered service to ethnic groups, in multicultural nations and societies and for this to happen social workers need to deal with their own reticence and prejudices at tacking the client's beliefs. This is both a challenge and an innovative opportunity for modern work' (Pulla, 2014).

Koenig (2012, 2013) also outlines the following approaches to integrate spirituality in patient care. All health professionals should take spiritual history. The beliefs of clients should be always respected. Interventions should be always patient-centred and patient desired. Health professionals' beliefs should not influence the medical care. Health professionals should learn about the R/S beliefs and practices of different religious traditions that relate to health care, practiced by the clients of the practice area. Spiritual practitioners like chaplains in Christianity should be utilised in patient care as and when appropriate.

Chaturvedi (2022a, b) has outlined a seven-step process of spiritual assessment in clinical settings (Table 13.3).

He has outlined the need to create a suitable atmosphere in care settings, as follow: 'All health care settings must have a cordial and welcoming spiritual atmosphere. It should comprise of an environment that encourages listening to each other, and people with similar spiritual wavelengths working together in an atmosphere of warmth, caring and kindness'.

Further, spiritual intervention should focus on strengthening the faith and reducing the feelings of hopelessness and abandonment. He calls for anonymity of the care provider's beliefs as follows: 'The staff and health care professionals should maintain spiritual and religious anonymity, i.e., the patient should/need not know their beliefs, values, and attitudes and these should also not be imposed onto them. The patient's caregivers must also be taken care of. The most important issue is that we should

Table 13.3 Spiritual assessment (Chaturvedi, 2022a, b)

Step 1: Elicit spiritual history, including information about spiritual practices and beliefs that exist within the patient's family.
Step 2: Elicit spiritual concerns, problems, and challenges.
Step 3: Assess Spiritual pain (meaning, believing in God and practicing religious activity, purpose, hope, legacy, values, attachment and detachment, faith, acceptance of reality, transcendence, relationships, forgiveness, losses, etc.).
Step 4: Spiritual distress.
Step 5: Assessment of spiritual strength and weaknesses.
Step 6: Spiritual Quotient.
Step 7: Spiritual sensitivity.

understand each other's spirituality and enhance spiritual satisfaction' (Chaturvedi, 2022a, b).

Looking Ahead

India is the spiritual capital of the world. Sri Aurobindo in his essay 'The renaissance in India' described the Indian mind as 'Spirituality is indeed the master key of the Indian mind; the sense of the infinite is native to it' (Mehra, 2015). Indian spiritual contributions have influenced the world through leaders like Sri Adi Shankaracharya of the twentieth century, Swami Ramakrishna and Swami Vivekananda of the nineteenth century, Sri Aurobindo and Swami Chinmaya of the twentieth century. In the current times leaders like Sri Ravi Shankar, Guru Jaggi Vasudev and others are spreading the spiritual wisdom of India as it is relevant to the current times of the world. In addition, in the twenty-first century, yoga, meditation and other spiritual practices in a wide range of forms have been accepted as an important part of life all over the world (McCall, 2007; Chopra, 2013; Gangadhr & Verambally, 2015; Kapur, 2020). All over the world, there is a recognition of 'mental health epidemic' and the need to move from mental illness to mental health (Insel, 2022). Further, many of the mental health issues that the current population are facing like disaster mental health (Murthy, 2014), child trauma and its mental health consequences (Murthy, 2024), domestic violence, addiction, loneliness (Law, 2022; Murthy & Banerjee, 2021) and living with chronic illnesses like heart, kidney disease and cancer do not have pure medical solutions.

At the international level issues of 'addiction epidemic' (Smith, 2021; Westhoff, 2019; Kala, 2023), adolescent suicides (Twenge, 2023), 'loneliness epidemic' (Law, 2022), 'gun violence' (Dioeden, 2019) 'conflicts' (Murthy, 2016a, b, 2018) and other societal issues need solutions beyond modern medicine. There is a need for rethink as noted by Klineman (2009) 'The moral failure of humanity in the past does not mean we must tolerate this failure any longer'. There is a need for a wider framework to understand/meaning making and accept pain, suffering, disability and death (Ahmadi & Ahmadi, 2018).

It is in this space that spirituality has a vital role. Can we work together to find the spiritual resources that can address these human issues, very much similar to the way yoga, meditation and mindfulness have come to be seen as an important part of physical and mental health? For this to happen systematic efforts are needed (Table 13.4). Social work is specially placed for this transformation of humanity.

The following are the implications of these developments for social workers training and practice. As noted in the second chapter of this book (Murthy, 2023, 2024), there is a widening of the understanding of mental health from the bio-psycho-social-spiritual basis, and the current approach to care in not only medical but the full utilisation of all the resources at the personal, family, community and governmental levels.

Table 13.4 Priority areas for action to bring spirituality in social work practice

1.	Need to define the boundaries between religion and spirituality.
2.	Development and standardisation of measurement tools for spirituality.
3.	Development of specific interventions and measurement of outcomes.
4.	Models for collaboration to provide the spiritual care with spiritual leaders.
5.	Need for skills training of the social workers at all levels.
6.	Addressing the possible negative effects of some of the interventions.
7.	The need for a larger consensus on spirituality in individual and public lives at the societal and political levels.

It is against this background, based on the currently available evidence (reviewed in the earlier sections), the value of integrating spirituality for the benefit of the mental health of individuals, families and communities. All of these aspects of spirituality are in line with social work practice, which recognises the value of mobilising all levels of resources for promoting mental health and mental health care. However, the aspects need attention towards integration of spirituality in social work (Table 13.4).

Here lies the challenges and opportunities for Indian social work to fully utilise the benefits of spirituality. This could be the greatest contribution of India to humanity.

Acknowledgements My heartfelt thanks and sincere appreciation to all the caregivers of persons with developmental disorders and those living with a diagnosis of cancer, for sharing their personal journeys. My thanks to Ms. Divya B and Ms. Nischitha S, members of the ENRICH project team, for their interviews and the rich contribution to my understanding of the spirituality aspects of caregiving of persons with developmental disorders. I also thank Mr. Joseph George, a practicing clinical pastoral counsellor with 30 plus years of experience and the current President of MPA, Dr. Usha Ramanathan, New Delhi, Ms. Suman Chandra, psychiatric social worker and counsellor, Chandigarh, for their valuable suggestions on the draft of the book chapter which has enriched the chapter.

References

Agarwal, R. P., & Maroko-afek, A. (2018). Yoga into cancer care: A review of the evidence-based research. *International Journal of Yoga, 11*, 3–29.

Ahmadi, F., & Ahmadi, N. (2018). *Meaning making methods for coping with serious illness*. Routledge.

Ahmadi, F., Khodayarifard, M., Rabbani, M., Zandi, S., & Sabzevari, M. (2022). Existential meaning-making coping in iran: A qualitative study among patients with Cancer. *Social Sciences, 11*, 80. https://doi.org/10.3390/socsci11020080.

Alexander, A., & Murthy, R. S. (2020). Living with cancer: Urgent need for emotional health support. *Indian Journal of Cancer, 57*, 360–362.

Alexander, A., Kaluve, R., Prabhu, J. S., Korlimarla, A., Srinath, B. S., Manjunath, S., et al. (2019). The impact of breast cancer on the patient and the family in Indian perspective. *Indian Journal of Palliative Care, 25*, 66–72.

Alexander, A., Sreenath, K., & Murthy, R. S. (2020). Beyond numbers–recent understanding of emotional needs of persons diagnosed with cancer 2007–2018. *Indian Journal of Palliative Care, 26*, 120–128.

Balboni, T. A., VanderWeele, T. J., Doan-Soares, S. D., et al. (2022). Spirituality in serious illness and health. *JAMA, 328*(2), 184–197. https://doi.org/10.1001/jama.2022.11086.

Barthakur, M. S., Sharma, M. P., Chaturvedi, S. K., & Manjunath, S. K. (2016). Experiences of breast cancer survivors with oncology settings in urban India: Qualitative findings. *Indian Journal of Surgical Oncology, 7*, 392–396.

Bhat, M. (2022). *Diary of a cancer patient.* The Beacon.

Bhatnagar, B., Noble, S., Chaturvedi, S. K., & Gielen, J. (2016). Development and psychometric assessment of a spirituality questionnaire for indian palliative care patients. *Indian Journal of Palliative Care, 22*, 9–18.

Bhattacharjee, D., & Nazir, T. (2022). (Digital Journalist). *The Logical Indian.*

Bowler, K. (2021). *No cure for being human.* Penguin.

Chaturvedi, S. (1991). What is important to Indians when they have cancer? *Social Science and Medicine, 33*, 91–94.

Chaturvedi, S. (2018). Hand of god in psychosocial rehabilitation. Psychosocial rehabilitation. *Journal of Psychosocial Rehabilitation in Mental Health, 5*, 1–3.

Chaturvedi, S. K. (2022a). The spiritual satisfaction. *Journal of Psychosocial Rehabilitation in Mental Health, 9*, 125–126.

Chaturvedi, S. (2022b). Spirituality in the air. *Journal of Psychosocial Rehabilitation in Mental Health, 9*, 347–350.

Chaturvedi, S. K., Strohschein, F. J., Saraf, G., Loisell,e C. G. (2014). Communication in cancer care: Psycho-social, interactional, and cultural issues. A general overview and the example of India. *Frontiers in Psychology*, 5, 1332.

Chaturvedi, S. K. (2015). Psycho-oncology: Indian experiences and research. In: S. Malhotra, S. Chakrabarti (Eds.) *Development of psychiatry in India* (pp. 2–11). New Delhi: Springer India.

Chittem, M., Norman, P., & Harris, P. R. (2012). Relationships between perceived diagnostic disclosure, patient characteristics, psychological distress and illness perceptions in Indian cancer patients. *Psycho-Oncology, 22*, 1375–1380.

Chopra, D. (2013), *Brotherhood: Dharma, destiny and the American dream.* Tranquebar, New Delhi.

Dalmida, S. G., Koenig, H. G., Holstad, M. M., Thomas, T. L. (2015). Religious and psychosocial covariates of health-related quality of life in people living with HIV/AIDS. *HIV/AIDS Res Treatment,* 1(1). https://doi.org/10.17140/HARTOJ-1-101.

Divya, B., Nischitha, S., & Murthy, R. S. (2023). *Caregivers and spirituality.* (Under publication)

Doeden, M. (2019). *Gun violence: Fighting for our lives and our rights.* Twenty First Century Books.

Dombo, E. A. (2023). Why it matters: Teaching about religion and spirituality leads to research on religion and spirituality. *Journal of Religion and Spirituality in Social Work: Social Thought, 42*, 1–2.

Donaldson, L. P. (2018). The importance of religion and spirituality in social work practice to strengthen practitioners, communities, couples, and individuals and in the cultivation of a praxis of love. *Journal of Religion and Spirituality in Social Work: Social Thought, 37*, 329–330. https://doi.org/10.1080/15426432.2018.1529927.

Durkheim, E. (1987/1951). *Suicide.* Free Press. New York.

Gangadhr, B. N., & Verambally, B. S. (2015). Integrating yoga in mental health services. *Indian Journal of Medical Research, 141*, 741–742.

Ghoshal, S., Miriyala, R., Elangovan, A., & Rai, B. (2016). Why newly diagnosed cancer patients require supportive care? An audit from a regional cancer center in India. *Indian Journal of Palliative Care, 22*, 326–330.

Gielen, J., Bhatnagar, B., & Chaturvedi, S. K. (2017). Prevalence and nature of spiritual distress among palliative care patients in India. *Journal of Religion and Health., 56*, 530–544.

Gielen, J., Kashyap, K., Singh, S. P., Bhatnagar, S., & Chaturvedi, S. K. (2022). Psychometric assessment of SpiDiscI: Spiritual distress scale for palliative care patients in india. *Indian Journal of Palliative Care, 28*, 13–20.

Govil, J. (2013). *There is life after Cancer*. Indian Cancer Society.
Gupta, H. (2013). Cancer the Life changer, In Govil J. (Ed.) *There is life after cancer.* New Delhi: Vitasta, pp. 39–44.
Gupta, R. (2023). Psycho-oncology: Caring, sharing and being connected–what matters when facing uncertainties of life. In R. Srinivsa Murthy, & N. Gupta (Eds.), *Leadership in Indian psychiatry*. Department of Psychiatry, Chandigarh Medical College, Chandigarh.
Harrington, A. (2008). *The cure within- a history of mind-body medicine*. Norton.
Holland, J. C. (2001). Lewis S. *The human side of cancer*. New York. Harper.
Insel, T. (2022). *Healing: Our path from mental illness to mental health*. Penguin Press.
Kala, A. (2023). *Most of what you want to knout addiction*. Speaking Tiger. New Delhi.
Kandasamy, A., Chaturvedi, S. K., & Desai, G. (2011). Spirituality, distress, depression, anxiety, and quality of life in patients with advanced cancer. *Indian Journal of Cancer., 48*, 55–59.
Kapur, M. (2020). *It is okay: To reach out for help*. Vitasta Publishing.
Klineman, A. (2009). Global mental health: A failure of humanity. *The Lancet, 374*, 603–604.
Koenig, H. G., et al., (2012). Religion, spirituality and health: The research and clinical implications. *ISRN Psychiatry*. https://doi.org/10.5402/2012/278730.33pages.
Koenig, H. G. (2013). *Spirituality in patient care*. Templeton, Conshohocken, 3rd Edition.
Koenig, H. G., et al. (2024). *Handbook of religion and Spirituality*. OUP.
Law, T. (2022). *Loneliness is a public health emergency*. The Time, June 1,2022.
Loue, S. (2017). *Handbook of religion and spirituality in social work practice and research*. Springer.
McCall, T. (2007). *Yoga as medicine: The yogic prescription for health and healing*. Bantam.
Mehra, B. (2015). *The thinking Indian: Essays on Indian socio-cultural matters in the light of Sri. Aurobindo*. Mantriwords, Pondicherry.
Mehrotra, S. (2008). Psycho-oncology research in India: Current status and future directions. *J Indian Academy of Applied Psychology, 34*, 7–18.
Mohandoss, A. A., & Thavarajah, R. (2016). A study on suicide among Indians living with cancer during 2001–2014. *Indian Journal of Cancer, 53*, 435–440.
Murthy, R. S. (2014). Mental health of survivors of 1984 Bhopal disaster: A continuing challenge. *Indian Psychiatry Journal, 23*, 86–93.
Murthy, R. S. (2015). Impact of child neglect and abuse on adult mental health. *Institutionalised Children Explorations and Beyond, 1*, 150–162.
Murthy, R. S. (2016a). Lessons of being a patient–Personal thoughts about psycho-oncology in India. *Mens Sana Monographs, 14*, 171–186.
Murthy, R. S. (2016b). Psychosocial and behavioral aspects of populations affected by humanitarian emergencies: Recent developments. *Current Opinion in Psychiatry, 29*(5), 280–285.
Murthy, R. S. (2018). Disaster mental health and social psychiatry: Challenges and opportunities. *Indian Journal of Social Psychiatry, 34*, 324–327.
Murthy, V. H. (2020a). *Together: The healing power of human connection in a sometimes lonely world*. Harper Collins.
Murthy, R. S. (2020b). COVID-19 pandemic and emotional health- social psychiatry perspective. *Indian Journal of Social Psychiatry, 36*, S24-42.
Murthy, R. S., & Alexander, A. (2019). Progress in psycho-oncology with special reference to developing countries. *Current Opinion in Psychiatry, 32*, 442–450.
Murthy, R. S., & Banerjee, D. (2021). Loneliness in older people: From analysis to action. *World Social Psychiatry, 3*, 120–122.
Murthy, R. S., & Gupta, N. (2023). *Leadership in Indian psychiatry*. Chandigarh: Department of Psychiatry, Chandigarh Medical College.
Murthy, R. S. (2010). Hinduism and mental health. In: P.J. Verhagen, H. M. Van Praag, J. J. Lopez-Ibor, J. L. Cox, & D. Moussaoui (Eds.), *Religion and psychiatry: Beyond boundaries* (pp. 159–179). USA: John Wiley and Sons.
Murthy, R. S. (2021). Overview (of Disability in India). In B. S. Chavan, W. Ahmad, & R. K. Gupta (Eds.), *Comprehensive textbook on disability* (pp. XXVII–XXXI). Jaypee. New Delhi Pages

Murthy, R. S. (2023) Concept of Mental disorders, mental health and Well-being. In M. Anand (Ed.), *Mental health care resource book: Concept and praxis for social workers and mental health professionals.* Singapore: Springer (Forthcoming).

Murthy, R. S. (2024). Cancer and spirituality: Underutilised resource for cancer care in India. *Indian Journal of Medicine Paediatric Oncology* (In Press).

Nischitha, S., Divya, B., Murthy, R. S. (2023). Caregivers emotional health: a priority. In R. Srinivasa Murthy, & N. Gupta (Eds.) *Leadership in Indian psychiatry.* Chandigarh: Department of Psychiatry, Chandigarh Medical College.

Office of the Surgeon General. (2023). Our epidemic of loneliness and isolation: The U.S. surgeon general's advisory on the healing effects of social connection and community. Government of U.S.A.Washington.

Parker-Pope, T. (2022). Interrupted, Again: Suleika Jaouad on cancer and healing the second time around New York Times, Mar 29, 2022.

Pulla, V., & Salagame, K. K. K. (2018). Wellbeing: Through the lens of Indian traditional conceptualisations. *International Journal of Social Work and Human Services Practice, 6*, 94–100.

Pulla, V. (2013). Coping and resilience: People's innovative solutions. *International Journal of Innovation, Creativity, and Change,* 1(1).

Pulla, V. (2014). Spirituality sensitive social work: The road worth taking. Chapter 11. In B. R. Raju, & Z. A. Hatta (Eds.), *Social work education and practice: Scholarship and innovations in the Asia Pacific* (pp. 182–200). Primrose Hall Australia.

Saxena, P. P. U., Kulkarni, V., Thapar, R., Pai, K., Gupta, A., & Kotian, H. (2018). Assessment of spectrum of mental disorders in cancer patients. *Journal of Cancer Research and Therapeutics, 14*, 1312–1315.

Sharma, A. (2009). *Spirituality and mental health.* Indian Psychiatric Society in association with Rajayoga Education and Research Foundation.

Shukla, P., & Rishi, P. A. (2014). Correlational study of psychosocial and spiritual well being and death anxiety among advanced stage cancer patients. *American Journal of Applied Psychology, 2*, 59–65.

Smith, E. (2021). The opioid epidemic and the addiction crisis. Lerner.Minneapolis.

Tandon, S., & Mehrotra, S. (2017). Posttraumatic growth and its correlates in an Indian setting posttraumatic growth and its correlates in an Indian setting. *International Journal of Indian Psychology, 4*, 101–119.

Thomas, K. Q. (1997). The Mind-BODY connection: Granny was right, after all. *Rochester Review,* 59(3). https://www.rochester.edu/pr/Review/V59N3/feature2.html.

Twenge, J. M. (2023). *Generations.* Atria.

Wasserman, D. (2021). *Oxford textbook of suicidology and suicide prevention* (2nd ed.). Oxford University Press.

Westoff, B. (2019). Fentanyl Inc. Scribe. London.

Wig, N. N. (1990). The Indian concept of mental health and their impact on the care of the mentally ill. *International Journal of Mental Health, 18*, 71–80.

Wig, N. N. (2010). The relevance of Vanaprastha ashram in modern times. In *The joy of mental health* (151–157). Chandigarh: Servants of the People Society.

Part III
Experiential Insights from Praxis

Chapter 14
The Banyan Journey: A Continuum in Community Mental Health Care

M. Namrata Rao, A. Lakshmi Ravikanth, Lakshmi Sankaran, Palaakshee Bansal, and Rima Chowdhury

I was out in the heat, The Banyan gave a shade to me
—A client at The Banyan

Abstract The Banyan, a mental health service organisation, came into fruition in 1993 in response to complex problems surrounding the mental health of ultra-vulnerable populations. They offer comprehensive mental health and social care solutions for persons who are homeless and living in poverty with severe mental disorders. Whilst the services are social justice-centred and promote community inclusion; the need to build culturally specific, diverse and scalable models that address care gaps is of vital importance. Over the years, they have worked towards reframing mental health solutions using a person-centred, cross-sectoral and trans-disciplinary approach, in line with variegated socio-political and cultural contexts. In this chapter, some of The Banyan's flagship programmes such as its hospital-based services (Emergency Care and Recovery Centres), inclusive living options (Home Again) and mental health and social care units (NALAM) are explored. For stake-holder responsibility and partnership for sustainability, they collaborate with multiple government and non-government agencies, and global partners with a common vision and values.

Keywords The banyan · Service users · Homeless · Mental health · Research · Education · ECRC · Home again · NALAM

M. Namrata Rao (✉) · L. Sankaran · P. Bansal · R. Chowdhury
Centre for Trauma Studies and Innovation, Banyan Academy of Leadership in Mental Health, Chennai, India
e-mail: banyan.mis@thebanyan.org

A. Lakshmi Ravikanth
Banyan Academy of Leadership in Mental Health, Chennai, India

M. Anand (ed.), *Mental Health Care Resource Book*,
https://doi.org/10.1007/978-981-97-1203-8_14

The Banyan's Origin

The Banyan came into being on 27 August 27 1993 in Chennai, as a registered NGO, in response to the gaps in mental health services particularly for the ultra-vulnerable population in India. They envisioned a safe place for homeless women with mental illnesses. Over the last 29 years, the organisation has created, validated and scaled models of care. Today, The Banyan offers comprehensive mental health solutions and supports a million service users across the country through its hospital-based services, inclusive living options and community mental health outreach programmes. It focuses on service users living at the intersectionality of poverty, homelessness, gender and mental illness. It has partnered nationally and internationally with civil society organisations, user-caregiver groups, Governments and academic institutions. These innovative, time-tested and flagship models have established The Banyan as a unique entity, owing to the determination, and confidence of the founders. This chapter will elucidate the journey of The Banyan.

The Banyan's Vision

The **biopsychosocial model** of care is followed across all services provided by The Banyan. Adhering to the belief that mental illness and its intersectionalities are intertwined and must be addressed—the chapter will present these facets through its various programmes.

Value-based care[1]: The Banyan adopts facets of a 'value-based care' approach, in terms of promoting a collaborative environment, focusing on client satisfaction, and optimising the use of all available resources—expanding beyond the economic model, to assimilate the social and developmental perspectives of value. Innovation and creativity are encouraged in line with a commitment to the organisation's core values and culture. The foundational principles assisting the articulation of vision and values into mental health practices are as follows:

- ***Wellness, 'open dialogues' and agency***: Driven by the belief that clients and service users define their own path to recovery, The Banyan healthcare models weave in processes which translate this belief into practice at each step of their journey. Irrespective of their health status, the users not only engage with but contribute in shaping an environment fostering growth, decision-making, dialogue, and respect.

[1] The phrase "value-based care" by Prof. Michael Porter refers to, "a care model in which incentivisation, efficacy and effectiveness of programmes are measured based on patient health outcomes. The 'value' in value-based care is derived from measuring health results that matter for a patient's condition across the care cycle, as against the costs of care for a patient's condition over the care cycle."

- ***Collaborative care plans***: This means that, unless the patient poses a threat to their own or others' safety, treatment decisions are reached by consensus with the patient's agreement, caregivers' input, and support from the community (Seshadri, 2021).
- ***Promoting inclusion, social justice and recovery***: Taking into account the socio-economic deterrents to a healthy life helps in contextualising interventions, and being sensitive to the needs of the ultra-vulnerable population. Being presented with opportunities to work and make a difference also helps the clients in their journey forward.
- ***Interdisciplinary approaches to care***: The Banyan uses a transdisciplinary framework for all of its services, incorporating interventions from several fields such as social welfare and disability departments. The many objectives of recovery, such as instilling a positive outlook, participation in work and sociocultural life, or influencing legislation, are equally dependent on the service user (client). The care teams constitute community health professionals, social workers, counsellors, clinical psychologists, psychiatrists, nurses, and others.
- ***Advocacy***: The Banyan also advocates for the rights of people with mental illnesses; leading mental illness to be recognised in the Disability Act, allowing eligible people to avail the benefits of the same. Maintaining focus on social inclusion and participation, the organisation also assists clients in issuance of essential documents and IDs like bank accounts, Aadhaar cards and Voter ID cards. Possessing Voter IDs helped the residents of The Banyan vote in the Tamil Nadu assembly elections in 2021 (Sheshadri, 2021). The citizen rights accompanied with this give a sense of agency and choice via advocacy to reconnect with the voices of the invisibilized mentally ill population.

With a commitment to serve low-income households and homeless people, The Banyan offers comprehensive mental health services in a range of institutional and community settings which include: hospital-based care, housing in rural and urban neighbourhoods, and community, clinic-based mental health solutions, in different parts of the country.

The Banyan's Models of Mental Health Care

1. Emergency Care and Recovery Centres (ECRCs)

The ECRC and shelter-based services of The Banyan resulted from consumer feedback to improve upon a care model that is a unique **amalgamation of clinical and social interventions**. ECRCs offer person-centred, hospital-based care for homeless people with mental health issues to recover and re-enter stable housing and community living arrangements where they may pursue fulfilling lives. ECRCs offer access to a range of facilities that best suit a client's individual needs like Critical

Time Intervention (CTI) and admission to The Banyan's In-Patient (IP) services, pharmacological and therapeutic interventions, and recreational and referral services.

As of 2022, there are 13 ECRCs. Four of them are run directly by The Banyan (2 in Chennai, 1 in Chengalpet and 1 in Kerala. The remaining are run in partnership with the state Government (National Health Mission Tamil Nadu) and NGOs in Tamil Nadu.

Unique Features

- ***Person-centred care***: Operating with a firm belief in the clients' right to choose makes them active participants in the process of recovery and rehabilitation. To maintain and ensure this, The Banyan periodically carries out internal reviews based on the service user's feedback. These reviews serve a two-fold purpose of enhancing the quality of their services, and adding on to the available literature on human rights in institutional settings. Further, every resident at the centre has 24*7 access to a human rights, grievance and legal aid cell, along with the ability to self-discharge when they deem fit.
- ***Support groups***: Therapeutic group sessions (involving creative arts, drama, and dance), movie screenings, peer discussions, and information dissemination sessions on crucial themes, such as caring for self, skill enhancement, and career counselling, are an integral part of the clients' lives at the centre.
- ***Sense of responsibility***: Residents are also encouraged to treat the recovery centre as their home. They take responsibility for maintaining surrounding spaces, get employed (running stores, cafes), look after their pets, and design a timetable collaboratively for cooking, cleaning, washing, purchasing groceries from nearby stores, and money management—also aiding in enhancing functionality.
- ***Creative living spaces***: The facility offers clients the option of residing in different spaces depending on their levels of functionality and makes smooth transitions amongst them. Interaction between residents is encouraged, and those with higher levels of wellness and independence act as *'agents of change'*, instilling a sense of hope amongst others.
- ***Social role value***: An essential component of the care model is the emphasis on the client's social well-being and participation (through the promotion of work participation, employment assistance; recreational activities: music, theatre; setting up support groups), as well as the facilitation of socio-economic welfare benefits (Aadhar cards, Voter ID cards, etc.) through liaisons with government.

- ***Skilled, non-technical workforce***: Given the severe human resource crunch in social and mental health sectors, the trained healthcare and community workers are not only their backbone but also contribute to the organisation's capacity building and self-reliance[2]—accounting for 60% of their staff strength.
- ***Recovery Hub***: The growth labs, social skills, vocational skills hubs, and multipurpose spaces that host support group meetings and peer support opportunities are an essential part of the client's ECRC experience.
- ***Livelihood***: The meaning of employment in the clients' lives is worth noting as expressed in Singh's Evaluation Report (2019)—'*The pride you get while working is different*', '*Mind doesn't wander. You can concentrate and focus when you work*', and '*Job uplifts you*'. The ECRC model enables livelihoods and assists in poverty reduction by creating job opportunities like selling hand-made baskets, block printing products, offering lunch services, running cafes, and the like.
- ***Continued care***: Contact and engagement with care providers reduces the rate of readmission and prevents collapse into a state of ill-health and/or homelessness again. The Banyan ensures that the client has continued access to care, by means of individualised aftercare plans and follow-up services (to support them upon their return to family or transition to other living arrangements).

Table 14.1 presents an overview of the ECRC structure and processes[3] (from rescuing an individual to their discharge from the facility[4]).

Case Vignette: Reintegration of Prerna[5]

How the ECRC Programme of The Banyan helps their service users find their families, after being separated due to consequences of mental illness:

> Within months of arriving at The Banyan, Prerna (name changed) yearned to find her family that she had left behind inadvertently in the unfortunate haze of her illness. Armed with asymmetrical memories of her past, she strung together her life before The Banyan in effusive Telugu. Based on hunches, directions and re-directions with just a single clue in hand, we traced Prerna's son. A video call was initiated on the spot, but Prerna could not recognise her son - the adult, when all she remembered was the little boy she left behind. The scene shifted quickly to her older sister's home nearby and once the latter's face filled the screen, Prerna burst out into tears but did not derail and started calling out for her akka. After the call was done, it was reiterated to her that her relatives would be coming for her, soon. And that's exactly what happened, with the visit of her husband, who filled her in on how their daughter is already married and that she doesn't have to do anything but come home; and that her life and lives of the multiple others would become better in an instant.

---

[2] Healthcare and community workers are trained to identify mental health issues, ease referral pathways, facilitate socio-economic entitlements, and engage with clients to help them navigate the challenges of managing their illness and achieve their own subjective notions of wellness.

[3] Source: Vaidyanathan et al. (2018).

[4] These phases happen organically at each client's pace and readiness.

[5] Source: The Banyan Annual Report 2016–17.

Table 14.1 ECRC phases and processes

Phase 1 CTI, Safety planning	Phase 2 Welcoming the client	Phase 3 Engagement with client	Phase 4 Pre-discharge and transition
Crisis team is called all for support leading to action Individual safety is of utmost importance, assessment and understanding of the nature of distress Trust building to encourage effective help-seeking pathways, and peer users to share lived experiences Community education and creation of support networks Filing individual details as per MHCA (2017)	Introductions (to the facility, staff, and professionals) Offering of food, clothing, accommodation, and rest (safety) Showing them around the facility when ready Emphasising freedom, and choice of the client Validating their distress Information sharing (no matter how mentally ill one may be)	Orientation to services; general and psychiatric health reviews Assignment of a care team[6] Formulating individual care plans: triggers, conflicts, strengths, recovery goals-worked on collaboratively with the client Focus on self-awareness, resilience training, and self-directed care Understanding socio-economic profile and self-reliance: vocational, social skills training Referral to a pre-discharge hub (going home or transition to HA[7])	Client's narration of journey so far (open dialogue, user focus on strengths, etc.) Assess preparedness and readiness in functional domains (social functioning scale & discharge tool used) Addressing apprehensions—pre-discharge planning Revisiting domains of independence, self-awareness, building resilience and effective coping strategies Simulate real-world challenges in recovery hubs Fulfilling goals, aspirations, meaning and purpose

The Figs. 14.1 and 14.2 show the ECRC locations (2022) and ECRC locations in Tamil Nadu (2022) respectively.

2. **Reintegration and Aftercare Services**

The Banyan strives to create an environment that promotes personal recovery, and its reintegration and aftercare services can be best understood as an extension of the ECRC model itself. In order to enable the well-being of its residents, the organisation has a structured flow and protocols in place (refer Table 14.2) for considering pre-discharge assessments, the reintegration process and the appropriate aftercare needs of the clients. Before formally leaving the facility, the residents go through a screening

[6] Care team comprises case manager, program manager, nurse, psychiatrist and other professionals.

[7] HA - Home Again.

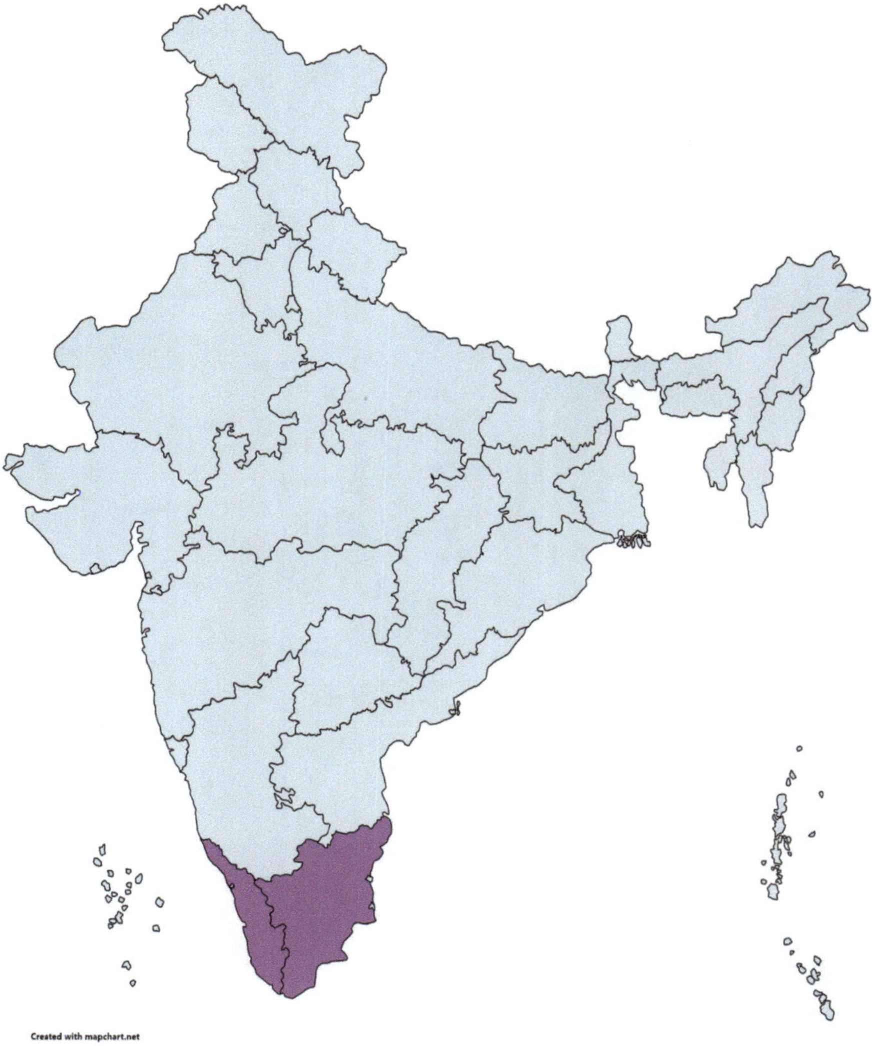

Fig. 14.1 ECRC locations (2022)

procedure which assesses their readiness to re-enter the community and reconnect with their family or move to inclusive living options, such as Home Again (HA).

Table 14.2 presents an overview of the reintegration process.[8]

[8] Source: Vaidyanathan et al. (2018).

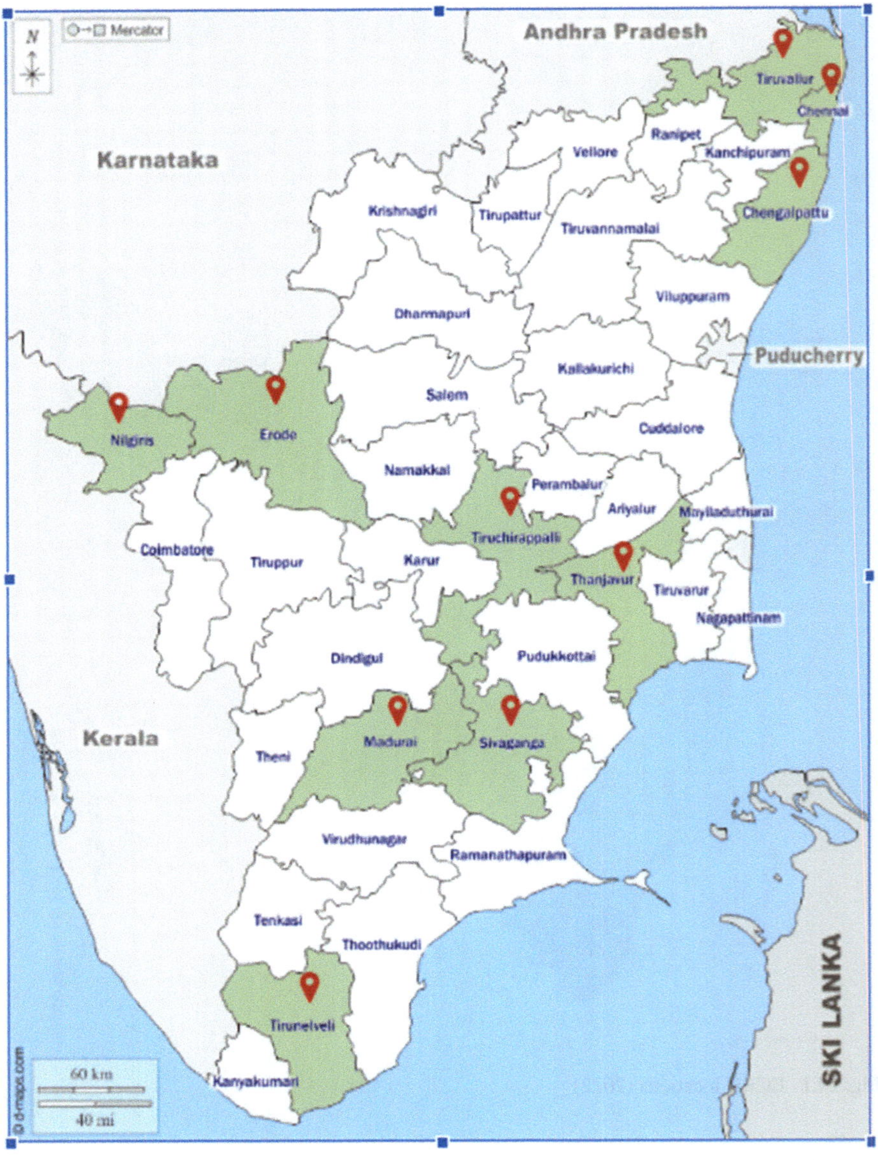

Fig. 14.2 ECRC locations in Tamil Nadu (2022)

Table 14.2 Steps involved in reintegration

Step	Description
Information dissemination	Sharing information about reintegration and aftercare with residents and care staff in group meetings held at the institutional facility
Discharge readiness screening	Screening entails one-on-one conversations with residents regarding their life (prior to the hospital, recollections of how they came there, the prospect of moving back home, known family, and relationships) and what they seek to reconnect with from the past life A ***screening form*** assesses the clinical status, expressed intent and ethical considerations, social capital/resources available, safety planning, and organisational capacity to carry out the clients' discharge and reintegration process
Pre-discharge (working towards independence and social inclusion)	About a month is aimed at helping residents retain skills, build on and/or acquire new skills for independent living. Residents are assisted in identifying anticipated challenges in the home environment and preparing for them (like, self-care, home management, economic transactions, and stress coping strategies) Meanwhile, networks are formed with the nearest police station/local government/NGO in the location (indicated by the client), requesting them to identify family and connect them where possible
Preparing discharge summary	This includes the known history of the client (onset of illness, homelessness, critical incidents), treatment during stay, current client status, level of support required to be offered by/to the family for community re-entry through reintegration with family, and their proposed living arrangements and aftercare plan
Reintegration	It is a highly client-centred process, which focuses on assessing any challenges the client might face in their life outside of The Banyan and how to equip them/their family to deal with them The reintegration process includes: – Identifying and reconnecting the client with their family, and planning a reintegration trip – Connecting them (family and client) with nearby resources (like, a physician and psychiatrist) and explaining the client's history, treatment and medication requirements to the family (to the extent the client is comfortable with) – Figuring out logistics and living arrangements – Observing the client in their home setting (for few days) – Offering solutions for any problems they encounter
Aftercare packages	The appropriate package to maintain continuity of care post a client's discharge from the facility is based upon their pre-discharge screenings' consolidated score The Banyan reintegration team regularly follows up with the discharged clients via phone calls and home visits by their NALAM mobilizers to reinforce the client's strengths, skills and build on their resources (frequency of contact depends on the level of support needed by the client)

Case Vignette: A New Beginning[9]

***Homelessness can hinder one's life and growth in ways unimaginable, however, support from the community can do wonders*:**

Running away from her home, a second time - without her children, Sunitha (name changed) ended up being homeless. She was eventually offered support by an actor and began working in his house. But the baggage of the past - a life of hardship and uncertainty had taken its toll. She began to slip away from reality and was soon brought to The Banyan. A course of treatment helped her reintegrate with reality and her family of origin, but her husband refused to accept her. After the demise of her parents, Sunitha eventually returned to The Banyan and moved to the **Clustered Group Homes** (CGH) in Thiruvidanthai, on the outskirts of Chennai. Sunitha found some joy in cooking for her fellow residents who occupy the cottages in this sheltered community and makes excellent Chicken curry. Her close and enduring relationship with the actor who continued to support her for some years, earned her the tag 'Actor' Rani.

Rani hadn't seen her children in over 12 years, but in February, following a sudden urge to speak to her husband and try to reunite once more, a re-integration trip was planned, and Rani's husband visited her at The Banyan's Clustered Group Homes. On seeing her, and how well she was doing, her husband felt extremely emotional, disappointed in himself, and wanted her to come back home with him. Sunitha has now left The Banyan, and has gone back to her marital home, and is doing well and is happy. Her husband is not a chronic drinker anymore, and The Banyan team is in touch with her regularly to check on her status.

The Impact

Overall, across all ECRC sites[10] there have been 3,023 admissions with 65.3% (1,975) cases of reintegrations to date (1993–2022). The Banyan continues to ensure that people living with mental health conditions in homelessness make journeys back to families and communities of choice, re-enter work, reclaim social relationships and pursue lives of their choosing. As of July 2022, 651 clients have been availing of The Banyan's aftercare services from all over India[11] (Fig. 14.3[12]).

3. **Inclusive Living Options**

Usually when an individual shows progress and achieves a state of recovery over the course of their stay at The Banyan, their homes are traced and plans are made to facilitate community reintegration and social inclusion. However, when individuals

[9] Source: Singh (2019) Evaluation Report of The Banyan for Azim Premji Philanthropic Initiatives.

[10] Mogappair, KK Nagar, Kovalam, Guruvayur; and Replication sites: Sivagangai, Erode, Tanjore, Tirunelveli, Nilgiris, Madurai, Trichy, Tiruvallur, and Gunaseelam.

[11] The Banyan has also been catering to the aftercare needs of some clients from neighbouring countries of Nepal and Bangladesh.

[12] Source: M&E team, The Banyan (17 August 2022). *Note*: Facts are dynamic, and the data reported pertains to the time of writing.

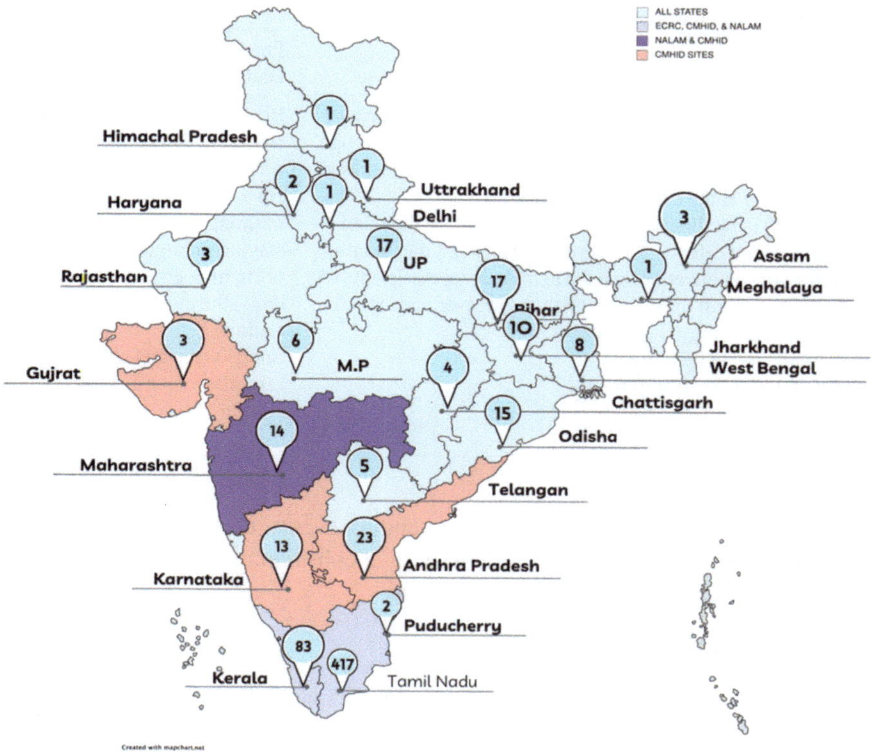

Fig. 14.3 Active aftercare service users (2022)

do not recall address details or their families are unwilling/not able to care, or if they choose to stay at The Banyan and not return home—in such circumstances, the resident is given an option of moving out of the ECRC, to graded forms of supported living. **These alternatives entitle individuals to experience a sense of agency and make a choice** for themselves.

a. Clustered Group Homes (CGH)

CGH (now ECRC Kovalam) was an inclusive housing programme that provided housing assistance to women with severe mental illness requiring long-term care. It was a semi-institutional facility that offered residents the opportunity to pursue meaningful goals whilst achieving personal recovery. ***Livelihood opportunities, skills training, and financial management skills*** were introduced to her CGH resident in a care package to emphasise development of agency, identity, and self-improvement. It is worth noting that the CGH campus was co-located with The Banyan Academy of Leadership in Mental Health (BALM), creating an ecosystem in which diverse actors (postgraduate students, faculty, researchers, clients, and mental health professionals) co-existed, establishing a strong sense of belongingness. Everyday rituals, no matter

Table 14.3 Client transition to HA

Phase 1 Pre-engagement	Phase 2 Setting up a home	Phase 3 Daily activities
Introducing client to the HA approach The process is participatory, with the client at the centre The process is facilitated with utmost care and offers flexibility to suit client needs Conversations with those already living in the programme might be initiated, a brief stay at a home and/or weighing the pros-cons could help facilitate the process	Encouraging the resident to express themselves (through photos and decorative pieces, gifts, etc.) Creating a space they find comforting and meaningful Their Personal Assistant (PA) helps wherever needed	Residents engage in their routine activities like self-care activities and spiritual rituals Having breakfast in the morning, leaving for work, staying in or going for a walk, or running errands for the next day—the clients design their routine Social visits and celebrations take place occasionally

how big or small, (like eating together, attending events, celebrating festivals and social interactions, etc.) contributed to a sense of cohesion that was mutual, and left a positive imprint on the residents' well-being.

b. **Home Again (HA)**

The Home Again innovation offers inclusive living spaces through clustered or scattered homes in rural or urban neighbourhoods, with a range of supportive services for users who opt to transition from the institutional facilities. The home environment ***fosters shared responsibility, equal opportunity, organic relationships, development of life skills, and social inclusion***. The programme also ensures frequent home visits by the care team at scheduled time intervals to discuss and review the residents' health status and concerns. Records are maintained and reports are filed with the project team (refer Table 14.3[13]).

True to its name, the Home Again programme brings one back home as expressed by Ms. Kavitha (name changed), a HA beneficiary[14]:

> Moving into this house reminds me of all the positive times I had with my mother and father as I was growing up. We had a house that was our own, with four rooms. We all had lunch together, then I would go play outside, as my father went to work, and my mother was inside making a healthy meal. I can practically smell her sambhar and oh, the jasmine flowers on her hair - this feels just like that - like I'm home

[13] Source: Vaidyanathan et al. (2018).

[14] Source: Vaidyanathan et al. (2018).

The Impact

Till date, the Home Again model has successfully aided 524 clients[15] across six states (refer Fig. 14.4) at different Banyan sites[16] in community reintegration. HA has also been extremely influential in decreasing the rate of disability and has empowered clients (Narasimhan et al., 2019).

Case Vignette: Being a Family[17]

Read this heartwarming tale about how Karuna aunty not only supports others who use The Banyan's services, but lives a life she loves through the Home Again Programme:

> Karuna (name changed) aunty defines herself through the food she cooks. On a typical day, one can find her leading a group of users to execute an elaborately planned menu in a home in the community that she shares with four other women like her. Women from the ECRC in Mogappair who are ready to leave to their families, spend the days before making this journey in Karuna aunty's home relearning and reconnecting with household tasks, adherence towards medication and managing goals and expectations of self and carers.
>
> Women identify with Karuna aunty as they would with the elderly matriarch in the family, their adoptive motherly figure if you will. And they do so because of Aunty's experiences - a failed marriage and domestic violence precipitated her mental illness and homelessness. Abandoned by her family, forced to part with her two young sons and having to witness her husband's remarriage without her consent, exacerbated Aunty's condition, rendering her homeless, desperately ill and in need of care. Aunty has been at The Banyan for close to two decades now. She has made peace to the extent possible with her fractured family - she is on talking terms with her husband who helps her out financially and is known, visited and acknowledged by her two sons – grown up and married now.
>
> Aunty's narrative resembles every user, here and there, in some form or the other. Except for one difference – she has been in this for longer years than them and continues to navigate the system undeterred. Perhaps, this is why conflict resolution and addressing interpersonal dynamics comes naturally to Aunty. She is widely accepted and the go-to confidante in the house and beyond. Aunty says, 'Some years back, my family called me back to live with them. I rejected that and chose to live alone and rented a house in Kovalam and worked to meet my expenses. Living alone was contagiously comforting – I could engage and disengage as per my emotional needs and preferences. However, when the Wardha Floods damaged the house along with all my belongings, I decided to return to living with The Banyan. Shared homes as part of Home Again have been an extension of the life I was getting used to. I get to live life on my terms, with support being available when required".

---

[15] Source: M&E team, The Banyan (19 July 2022). *Note*: Facts are dynamic, and the data reported pertains to the time of writing.

[16] Tamil Nadu (Chennai, Chengalpattu, Trichy, Villupuram), Kerala (Malappuram, Kozhikode, Thrissur, Ernakulam, Alappuzha), Maharashtra (Ratnagiri, Thane), Andhra Pradesh (Visakhapatnam), Gujarat (Mehsana), Karnataka (Mysore).

[17] The Banyan Annual Report 2017–18.

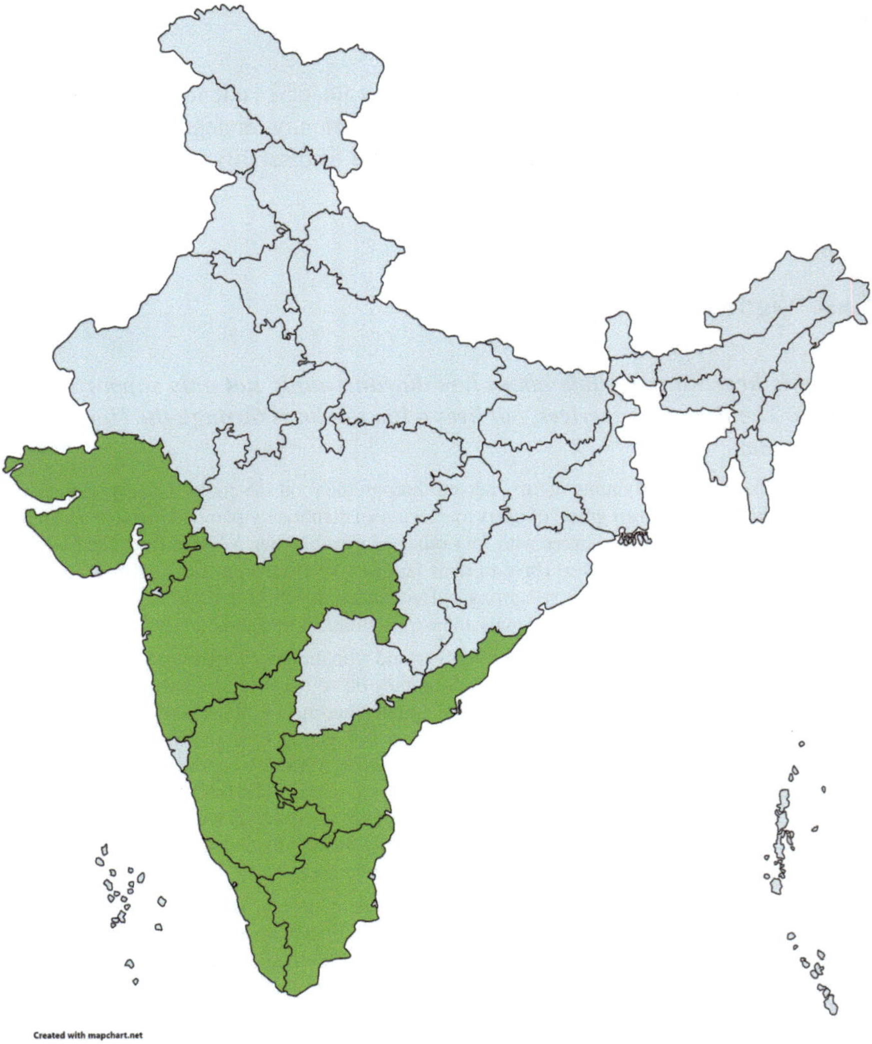

Fig. 14.4 Active HA locations (2022)

c. **Independent Living**

This is an option for those who choose to live independently in shared housing or women's hostels. These individuals can find work, rent housing, and become financially independent whilst still having access to the Banyan outpatient and social care. In times of economic or social crises, the Banyan provides livelihood opportunities, financial aid for specific purposes (building a house, starting a business, etc.) and in many cases, supports the education of children in the household.

As the above narratives indicate, the option of returning home to one's family might not be available or chosen by an individual after being homeless and/or institutionalised for a period of time. However, choices prevail and are discussed based on which individuals can choose to live in community-based settings.

4. **NALAM**

Gaps in Care

Even though the state fares quite well in multiple socio-demographic areas, information from the National Mental Health Survey 2015–16 revealed the prevalence of mood disorders (4.6%) and schizophrenia (0.5%) was comparatively high in Tamil Nadu. Moreover, the rural population of the state experiences higher vulnerabilities than the urban population (NIMHANS, 2016), whilst there is a paucity of mental health professionals to service multiple vulnerable groups. This pointed to the need for expanding the availability of mental health services in the community. Thus, Banyan's NALAM came to be.

The Main Components of NALAM

The NALAM programme,[18] quite aptly named in Tamil, has focused on the 'wellness of people'. This recasting of mental health programmes to the varied needs of the local population such as education of children, access to government benefits, employment and livelihood and mental health services represents a deeper engagement with the community. It works towards the following:

- Community awareness programmes related to Mental health and allied themes
- Identification of vulnerable populations in the community
- Identification of persons with mental health issues
- Referral for treatment
- Referral for welfare entitlement and social care. For example—the NALAM mobilizers help members of their community in seeking Social Entitlement Facilitation like ration cards or Disability assistance
- Employment facilitation and daycare centre
- Clinical services
- Follow-up care
- Networking with stakeholders. NALAM mobilizers have not only connected with various members of their community to assist them but have also helped improve communication amongst them. It has led to them being more aware of the world today and demanding rights for themselves

[18] NALAM means "wellness" in Tamizh.

- Training of staff
- After school services and stipends for children
- Advocacy.

NALAM's Backbone

This multi-interventional approach is delivered by **lay workers, known as NALAM mobilisers** and supported by clinical services to improve mental health and well-being. The NALAM workforce consists largely of middle-aged women aged between 30 and 44 years (61.5%) who belong to the community worker cadre. The majority of the NALAM mobilisers (80.2%) graduated from the Banyan Academy of Leadership in Mental Health (BALM's) diploma course on **Community Mental Health Care** (7 batches to date). Most of them had found the course to be useful in gaining knowledge about mental illness and identification of persons with mental illness (Balagopal & Vivek, 2019).

One of the major conduits of the wellness approach is these trained NALAM mobilisers. They interact closely with the clients at home and in the clinic to understand their mental health status, treatment compliance as well as socio-economic problems and facilitate access to social care. In addition to clients with mental health issues, the mobilisers are also expected to identify persons with social and economic vulnerabilities and respond to their needs.

According to a client,

> It was staff visiting that gave me something to look forward to. I was happy that someone cared enough about me to come all the way to my home to ask me about how I was doing and spoke to me so kindly. Maybe if the staff hadn't come home regularly and checked on me, I might have not had the strength to face challenges.

The NALAM programme operates both in rural and urban areas.

a. **NALAM-Rural** offers inpatient and outpatient programmes that address the clinical and social care needs of vulnerable groups. Outreach clinics are operated at The Banyan's Health Centre at Kovalam in Thiruporur block and are co-located with government-run spaces. It has one vocational training centre at Kovalam Health Centre. Clients who cannot come to the centre are trained and given options to make products like baskets and bags from their homes with raw materials provided by The Banyan.
b. **NALAM-Urban** serves predominantly low-income areas in Chennai City and serves wards in Mogappair, Padi, Padiputhunagar, KK Nagar, Jafarkhanpet, West Saidapet, Choolaimedu, Santhome and Teynampet. There are 3 daycare centres, as well as a vocational training centre at Emergency Care and Recovery Service Centre at Mogappair.

Most rural and urban programmes have an active follow-up plan to ensure that there is continuity of care. The NALAM mobilisers play an important role in this. After 2015, the community programmes have included interventions that have an approach that addresses deprivations. Whilst the share of dropout clients was higher in urban than rural areas in both time periods, there has been a small increase in dropouts in rural areas across time. This could also be due to the expanding footprint of clinical services in difficult-to-reach rural areas, where challenges in encouraging clients to continue with care are more difficult.

The Impact

Till date, more than 9000 clients have registered for NALAM services since 1998, and 1392 of them are being actively served by NALAM as of July 2022.[19] Working at The Banyan has positively affected the majority of NALAM mobilisers, which alludes to personal empowerment. Whilst the majority reported that they developed confidence, 7.7% said that the work gave them happiness. According to a mobiliser,

> I feel relieved to know that I am not the only one with problems when I see people with more serious problems than me. So that gives me strength.

Some also spoke about receiving blessings from caregivers.

The Banyan established the NALAM cafe which is run by some of the service users. Uma Devi, who works at the cafe lost her job and became homeless soon after she was diagnosed with schizophrenia.

> After I began working at the cafe, I started interacting with the public, gained financial stability and am now saving up to buy a house, she says (Aditi, 2021).

In an audit, clients were asked about what contributed to social and economic distress[20] after using services at The Banyan. It was found that, whilst rural society is known to be more socially stratified with caste-based discrimination, persons with mental illness in rural areas face more social problems—these are not easily amenable to change. This also makes the job of NALAM mobilisers working in rural areas much more challenging. There was a slight improvement in social distress amongst a majority of clients, which suggests that the care package provided by The Banyan was effective.

According to a client,

> I used to have frequent thoughts of dying by suicide. After taking treatment at The Banyan, these thoughts have gone away. Now I feel interested in life and like gossiping with my friends and playing with my grandchild. After NALAM mobilisers discussed my illness with my husband, he became very supportive towards me. He also gave up alcohol consumption on the Nalam staff's advice.

[19] Source: M&E team, The Banyan (19 July 2022). *Note*: Facts are dynamic, and the data reported pertains to the time of writing.

[20] Social distress includes social boycott, family conflicts, inability to have social interaction, facing ridicule from neighbours, loneliness, neglect by children and reduced access to education. Economic distress included loss of livelihood, low or no access to pensions, being terminated from employment etc.

Regarding the change in economic distress, nearly one-fourth experienced medium improvement. The rural–urban distinction persists with regard to economic distress. A client from the urban site spoke about how treatment at The Banyan has controlled his illness (epilepsy). He stated.

> After I took treatment here my fits stopped. Initially, I worked as a community health worker in The Banyan. I enjoyed the work, as I like working with communities. I am a political party worker too. After I got confidence working at The Banyan, I started a tiffin centre with my wife. The business is doing well and we earn enough to run our house. Now I want The Banyan's help to organise community programmes on drug abuse for youth who live in slums.

Case Vignette: Support After Adversities[21]

How the NALAM Programme supported communities, including the Irula tribe following the 2016 floods:

> The NALAM Community Mental Health Programme in Thiruporur Taluk initiated a Housing Support intervention following the floods as several clients registered with the outpatient clinics were living in poor housing conditions. In addition, the programme engages with the Irulas, an ethnic minority, facing ongoing oppression, discrimination and poor access to resources, 30 households with homes made predominantly with dry grass and with a person with mental illness were supported to renovate their homes and undertake urgent repairs. 24 households in the Irular section of Kottamedu Panchayat were identified for the construction of new homes. Through a partnership with Nivasa, a low-cost housing social enterprise, we have rolled out a participatory approach to home ownership where the local community contributes to the building of their homes by making bricks and in the process acquiring a skill to enhance their livelihood.

For a detailed view of the impact made by The Banyan programmes till date, refer Table 14.4.

'I Exist, Therefore I Am'

The Banyan includes individuals from all walks of life in its organisational structure and encourages them to be involved in the innovation process. They value the strength of persistence and resilience—and believe every individual is capable of it, with a little bit of support. In a nutshell, motivating clients to face their distress, overcome challenging barriers, and persist through the difficulties experienced externally and internally is what they stand for, which has led to the creation of a unique social care model particularly to address the mental healthcare needs of the ultra-vulnerable community. The ECRC model combines clinical solutions with collaborative, person-centred care to facilitate their journey towards health and wellness. The Home Again

[21] Source: The Banyan Annual Report 2016–17.

Table 14.4 The Banyan's reach in the three models of care

Care model	Programme site	Clients served[22]
ECRC (1993–2022)	Mogappair	2059
	KK Nagar	432
	Kovalam	137
	Kerala	28
	Sivagangai	58
	Erode	38
	Tanjore	54
	Tirunelveli	35
	Nilgiris	36
	Madurai	45
	Gunaseelam	32
	NULM Trichy	54
	Tiruvallur	15
	Total	**3023**
Reintegrations	Mogappair	1559
	KK Nagar	195
	Kovalam	68
	Kerala	9
	Sivagangai	33
	Erode	13
	Tanjore	25
	Tirunelveli	11
	Nilgiris	15
	Madurai	16
	Gunaseelam	17
	NULM Trichy	10
	Tiruvallur	4
	Total	**1975**
Home again (2014–2022)	Chennai	108
	Chengalpattu	96
	Trichy	60
	Ratnagiri	31
	Thane	29
	Kerala	116

(continued)

[22] *Source:* M&E team, The Banyan. *Note:* These figures indicate the number of unique clients served by various programmes as of 19 July 2022. The facts are dynamic and pertain to the time of writing.

Table 14.4 (continued)

Care model	Programme site	Clients served
	Visakhapatnam	21
	Mehsana	22
	Mysore	27
	Alappuzha	4
	Villupuram	10
	Total	**524**
NALAM (Total registrations) (1998–2022)	Chennai	5083
	Chengalpattu	3533
	Maharashtra	387
	Kerala	25
	Total	**9028**
NALAM (Active registrations in July 2022)	Chennai	407
	Chengalpattu	621
	Maharashtra	347
	Kerala	17
	Total	**1392**
Aftercare (Active clients in July 2022)	Mogappair	219
	KK nagar	99
	Kovalam	51
	Kerala	145
	Replication sites	137
	Total	**651**

(HA) programme encourages agency and inclusion by assisting clients in setting up their homes within the community and facilitates their growth; with regular check-ins from The Banyan team. Lastly, the NALAM programme attempts to strengthen the community itself, by training individuals to be community mental health workers and serve as the 'aerial roots' of the organisation. The NALAM mobilizers ensure that everyone in their community receives the help they deserve with their assistance. The Banyan Academy of Leadership in Mental Health (BALM) not only aims at providing training and education to NALAM mobilizers, and other care providers but also designs internships at various Banyan sites to engage students of social work and mental health to give them hands-on, empathetic training experience in the field of homelessness and mental illness.

They have succeeded in achieving their mission through transformative social justice. Gaining credibility both nationally and internationally, their models are being talked about highly with great value to replicate in many other places in India and elsewhere. True to their name, which is that of an eternal tree, the organisation indeed has been spreading its healing shoots wherever it reaches. To ensure that their services can be replicated and the government can be involved in the development, The Banyan has strived to work towards policy change, to increase sustainability. Multiple stakeholders of the organisation ranging from service users and peer advocates of The Banyan to their co-founder and director have been involved in creating guidelines and protocols for the 'Tamil Nadu State Policy to Address the Needs of Homeless Persons with Mental Health Issues'. The MHCA of 2017 speaks of mental health rights for everyone but fails at an implementation level. They strive to bridge that gap. Along with training other organisations and increasing services across the country and neighbouring countries, they have replicated projects providing services both in rural and urban areas to address the needs of homeless individuals with psychological and social needs.

Moving forward: The Banyan aims to scale up their flagship social care models and periodically audit to cater to contextual needs. Their focus is to create replicable, scalable and sustainable models of change, particularly in the field of community mental health. This is possible through partnerships with local state, central government and non-government organisations and their global partners. They plan to partner with various central and state government and non-government bodies (as it has done in the past) to launch projects and programmes that will help individuals from marginalised groups to access affordable mental health solutions. The Banyan will strive to create acceptance of mental health issues as something solvable, instead of a deterrent. The Banyan's core effort based on its value system is to promote equity, justice, non-discrimination and seamless community inclusion of persons living with mental illness. This aspiration is a continuous process led by all stakeholders, peer advocates in the society. Hence The Banyan is a people's movement to make mental illness actively accepted and addressed.

Like the Banyan tree and roots that give shelter and shade to many, the organisation similarly embodies this via the continuum in mental health care models.

References

Aditi, R. (2021). *Helping people heal & breaking stigmas, one cafe at a time.* The Times of India. https://timesofindia.indiatimes.com/city/chennai/helping-people-heal-breaking-stigmas-one-cafe-at-a-time/articleshow/84519235.cms.

About Us. (n.d.). https://thebanyan.org/aboutus/.

Balagopal, G., & Vivek N. (2019). *An evaluation of the wellness-centered NALAM programme of the banyan.* A Report.

Monitoring and Evaluation (M&E) team, The Banyan. (2022). Data on programs impact. A report.

Narasimhan, L., Mehta, S. M., Ram, K., Gangadhar, B. N., Thirthalli, J., Thanapal, S., Desai, N., Gajendragad, J., Yannawar, P., Goswami, M., Sharma, C., Ray, R., Talapatra, S., Chauhan, A., Bhatt, D., Neuville, E., Kumar, K. V. K., Parasuraman, S., Gopikumar, V., and NILMH Collaborators Group. (2019). *National strategy for inclusive and community based living for persons with mental health issues.* New Delhi: The Hans Foundation. A Report.

Seshadri, H. (2021). Mental health care: The Banyan shows the way forward. The Week. https://www.theweek.in/leisure/society/2021/03/21/mental-health-care-the-banyan-shows-the-way-forward.html.

Singh, I. P. (2019). *evaluation report of the banyan for Azim Premji philanthropic initiatives*. A Report.

Vaidyanathan, A., Ravi, M., Narasimhan, L., Vinayak, N., Padmakar, A., Krishnadas, P., Easwaran, K., Philip, L., Abigail, S., Anand, R., Joseph, T., Priyanka M., Kumar, K. V. K., Jayakumar, V., Gopikumar, V. (2018). *Structure, process and outcomes. The banyan*. A Report.

Chapter 15
The Indian Family Caregivers of Persons with Mental Illness—PwMI: Large Canvas, Beyond Family

Amrit Bakhshy

Abstract Mental health care is a challenge all over the world. There are acute limitations in the resources to meet the care needs of persons with mental illness. Countries like India, with limited infrastructure and resources for mental health care, largely depend on the traditional strengths of the families for care. Family caregivers are the bedrock of care of PwMI in India. This important role of the family caregivers needs to be recognized for its value and strengthened. Unfortunately, there is lack of appreciation of family caregivers' role and contribution. Indian Family Caregivers are a link between the patients and the mental health professionals and a source through which treatment and recovery are channelized. The current chapter focuses on the Indian family caregivers of the PwMI who form a unique unpaid workforce, providing services out of love and bonding at the cost of their own health and well-being. Recovery rate of persons with mental illness is reported to be higher in India than in the developed countries where much better infrastructure exists for their therapy and treatment, which is attributed to family caregiving. They suffer as much as their dear ones do and need support from the State and the community to provide better care to their dear ones. The chapter also covers mental health needs of India, challenges of caregiving, various acts and provisions related to mental health care. One of the most unique aspects of this chapter is the coverage of unique countrywide initiatives by some of the caregivers who have come forward to start NGOs, for families with one or more members living with mental illness, with focus on creating awareness, promoting peer support groups, running residential and day rehabilitation centres, rescuing and rehabilitating mentally distressed wanderers and an active role in advocacy.

Keywords Family · Caregivers · Resources · Challenges · Mental illness · Awareness · Support · Opportunity

---

A. Bakhshy (✉)
Schizophrenia Awareness Association, Pune, India
e-mail: akbmail@gmail.com

M. Anand (ed.), *Mental Health Care Resource Book*,
https://doi.org/10.1007/978-981-97-1203-8_15

Introduction

In India, care for persons with mental illness (PwMI) is provided practically in their homes by the family caregivers. More than 90% of patients with chronic mental illnesses live with their families. The Indian family caregivers of PwMI who play a critical role in the caregiving process are spouses, parents, siblings, other family members or even friends. Generally, when the illness strikes, a family member takes over the caregiving responsibility, as a part of the family duty without knowing anything about the mental illness and without realising the enormity of the caregiving burden. No one else can take care of the PwMI as their family can. While the family support is a blessing for the PwMI, it is an enormous challenge for the family caregivers (cost, impact on their health, distress, burnout, worry about the future, stigma, etc.). (Narayanan & Reddy, 1968; Kapoor, 1994; Janardhan et al., 2015; Chaddha, 2014; Seshadri et al., 2019).

There are changes happening in the Indian society which have an impact on the caregiving by families, e.g., the breakup of the joint families, increase in number of women working outside their homes, urbanization, migration of young persons, awareness about human rights of PwMI etc., which affects the role of family members as the primary caregivers. Thus, there is a need for a "larger canvas" for family caregivers to plan services/supports to PwMI and for socially oriented family caregivers, who can spare time and resources, to provide help and support to the community of family caregivers.

The present chapter covers: (i) mental health needs in India; (ii) inadequate infrastructure; (iii) family involvement; (iv) trials of caregiving; (v) challenges of caregiving and burnout; (vi) Mental Healthcare Act 2017; (vii) Tele Manas; (viii) international support for caregivers; (ix) advocacy initiatives of family caregivers; (x) promotion of peer support groups; (xi) WhatsApp groups; (xii) NGOs run by family caregivers; (xiii) looking ahead and (x) Conclusion.

Enormity of Need for Mental Health Care

As per WHO, one in four persons suffers from mental illness sometime in their life (WHO, 2022). Recent surveys in India also report similar needs (Gururaj et al., 2016). The Indian Psychiatric Society, in a survey soon after the first wave of the pandemic, found that there was a 20% increase in mental illness, which means every household has some family member or some relative or friend or a neighbour or a colleague who has lived with mental illness at some stage in life. This makes the PwMI and their family members a huge vote bank. The political parties need to be made aware of it by the activist caregivers. In the 2019 general elections, one of the organizations supporting the cause of mental illness through partners attempted to convince the all-India political parties to include in their manifesto the implementation of the Mental Health Care Act 2017, MHCA 2017. Only two of the nine, all India parties obliged.

An Act passed by both the Houses of the Indian Parliament, received the President's assent, was duly notified, and yet there seems to be hesitancy to commit to meet the state obligations as provided in the Act (Bakhshy, 2021).

Inadequate Infrastructure

The number of psychiatrists in India is only about 10,000; the number of psychiatric nurses and clinical psychologists, who have completed their Masters in Philosophy and registered with RCI is about 3000. The number of psychiatric social workers with MPhil in Psychiatry is also very small and the number of beds is about 50,000 for over 200 million severely ill PwMI. The role of family caregivers as a consequence becomes important in the light of a small number of professionals and inadequate rehabilitation facilities. The charges in a private residential establishment for a dormitory bed are mostly Rs. 25,000, which is exclusive of the cost of medicines, visiting psychiatrist fees, laundry, activity charges and other personal expenses which range between Rs 5000 and 10,000. As a result, families bear the brunt of providing care to more than 90% of the PwMI, with high symptoms, mostly without any proper professional care or medical treatment.

Family Involvement in Mental Health Care

Indian psychiatrists recognized the importance of families and caregivers, even when the rest of the world was treating the family as "toxic." The most notable of these was the initiative of Dr. Vidyasagar of Government Mental Hospital Amritsar in the 1950s, who encouraged the relatives to stay with the patient during the treatment period. He also encouraged them to participate in the daily nursing care of the patients and by doing this, to learn about managing medication and caring skills (Murthy, 2016). The Mental Health Centre, Vellore, from 1958, made it a policy to admit patients along with a relative: "*The close participation of the relatives in the treatment of the patient provides an opportunity to give them a better understanding of the peculiarities of the individual case*". Through spread of this knowledge into wider circles of the public, a general education in the matters of mental health is affected (Kholmeyer et al., 1963). Similar was the focus of starting of family ward at NIMHANS, Bangalore, "*Our experience of treating patients in the Family Ward has been very gratifying. Treatment of the patient in the family unit prevents the separation of patient from his family during therapy, prevents chronicity, lessens the length of stay of the patient in the hospital, and helps in lessening the stigma attached to mental illness*" (Narayanan & Reddy, 1968).

Late Prof. G. G. Prabhu, former Professor of Clinical Psychology, NIMHANS, Bangalore wrote about the importance of family in mental health care in the 1960s in the Indian Journal of Mental Retardation. He observed 30 years later, in 1995, "*It is high time that one evaluates the strengths and weaknesses of the oriental family and its ability to care for the mentally disabled persons*" (Prabhu, 1995). Similarly, Radha Shankar observed in 1994,

> There is limited holistic understanding of both the difficult circumstances under which relatives look after persons with serious mental illness, as also the emotional and practical challenges they face through the different phases of the illness. Consequently, families receive limited support and guidance from professionals, suggesting that mental health establishment often regards family members as low cost, plentiful resource in the community, who are required to offset the limitations of a poorly funded mental health system. However, if these primary care providers have to offer long term sustainable care, it is both ethical and imperative that their needs are understood and addressed in a systematic manner. ...family caregivers need to be supported and nurtured through programmes of information and guidance and practical assistance (Radha Shankar, 1994).

The situation in 2023 remains largely the same, as evident from the caregivers' stories in the book "The Indian Family Caregivers of Persons with Mental Illness" (Bakhshy, 2022).

Trials and Tribulations of Caregiving

Family caregivers are not the "Sons of God" but their sufferings are no less. At times, those who are caregivers of family members with severe positive symptoms, get assaulted at vulnerable spots, threatened with butcher's knife, abused, insulted and humiliated by their care receivers. Injuries and bruises are common occurrences. Risk to life looms large. They sacrifice golden years of their lives for their dear ones. There are no holidays for them, no outings, no socialization, no visits from friends and relatives as they fear visiting. Neighbours resent shouts and screams coming from their homes at odd hours. Most of the Indian family caregivers continue to suffer till their final call comes. While the family caregivers have a demanding role in the treatment and care of their dear ones, they get no support or acknowledgement from any agency, leave alone any appreciation from the State or the society for the challenging services they render. Unless the difficult role of family caregivers is recognized and supported, this valuable resource may slowly start drying up to the detriment of millions of those who suffer from mental illnesses.

Caregiving of someone with a physical ailment is not so arduous as the patient cooperates. The family caregivers of PwMI mostly lack awareness about the mental illnesses. They face difficulties in arranging treatment and providing care for their care receivers as usually such patients neither accept their illness nor cooperate in their treatment. They resist meeting a psychiatrist and taking medicines. If it is a severe mental disorder, one of the parents is required to assume the role of a full-time caregiver. In cases where the affected family member is married, the spouse may take that role. If the parents are too old, a sibling may come forward to take the responsibility of a part time caregiver. Trained, paid caregivers of mentally ill are not easily available in India. There are agencies in large towns with experienced professional caregivers on their roll but they generally have experience in attending to the elderly patients needing palliative care. They lack experience in providing care to the persons with severe mental health disorders. Most of the families cannot afford to pay for their services. RCI recently approved a certificate course in caregiving of persons with mental illness. Gradually, a cadre of qualified professional caregivers of PwMI should be available to relieve family caregivers in exigencies. Professional caregivers, however, cannot fully replace the family caregivers as the care provided by the family caregivers is based on love and bonding and therefore, more effective than the paid care.

Neglect of Self-care and Burnouts

Arrival of a severe mental disorder in the family brings about a major change in priorities as the lifestyle is changed; financial worries start, confusion and dilemmas prevail, earnings come down; expenses mount up, exchange of pleasantries stop among family members; gloom sets in. There is a feeling of guilt and shame. (Bakhshy, 2022; Murthy et al., 2023a, 2023b). Caregivers' careers too suffer and self-care often becomes a casualty since there is hardly any time for hobbies, personal pursuits and other chores. There is also social ostracization that happens as a result of which the feeling of helplessness sets in when they see that the illness is not getting cured despite their best care and treatment. Caregivers need guidance to decide about the treatment during high support needs and in many other caregiving responsibilities such as obtaining disability certificate, approaching court for granting guardianship and in other treatment-related issues.

The PwMI are not able to manage their affairs especially the financial affairs. Their caregivers remain worried about who would take their care, especially in cases where there are no other family members who are available to provide support after their demise. There is little chance of their marriage and even if a marriage is arranged, it is unlikely to last long. India has very few long-stay facilities at a reasonable cost for PwMI. As the life span has increased for PwMI, so has the span of care providing for the caregivers. Demands of caregiving are also indeed very overwhelming with varied uncontrollable situations that may surface unannounced. Caregiving for a PwMI has many stressors including the changes in family dynamics, disruptions in set routines and sheer exertion- both mental as well as physical. As the stressors pile up, frustration sets in and burnout happens. In this regard, the recent initiative of The Association for the Mentally Challenged (AMC), Bangalore to develop self-care for emotional health of caregivers under the project "ENRICH" is a welcome initiative (Srinivasa Murthy et al., 2023a, 2023b)).

Mental Health Care Act 2017 (MHCA 2017): Disappointing for Caregivers

Passing of the MHCA 2017 was a milestone in the history of India (Bakhshy, 2021). However, the Mental Healthcare Act, 2017 was a disappointment for family caregivers. As there was no separate act for caregivers to provide any relief to them in their caregiving duties, the expectation was that some respite would come to them in the new Act to make their caregiving role less arduous. However, the Act had nothing to offer to them. The stark answer given for ignoring the family caregivers was that the Act was for PwMI and not for their family caregivers.

There are provisions within the Act regarding "Advance Directive" (Chapter III) and "Nominated Representative" (Chapter IV) and about admission in a mental health establishment (Section 89) which are based on alien concepts and adversely affect the family caregivers in their caregiving roles. The Act provides that any person can write an advance directive and get it registered, stating that how they want to be treated or not treated. The implication is that the treatment given to a patient will be, as the patient wants and not as is required and prescribed by a mental health professional. In such cases, the patients may not recover and the burden of family caregivers will remain the same or might increase due to illness not treated as per a professional's advice. The Act gives a person a right to appoint a nominated representative. The person so appointed is expected to provide support to the PwMI in taking treatment-related decisions. This provision can create a piquant situation, when the family caregivers bear the treatment-related expenses of their dear ones but the decisions regarding treatment are taken by a third person.

There are various provisions in the Act, which give certain rights to PwMI, such as the right to access mental health care, free/affordable services, to get quality services, to get free essential medicines, to community living, to get insurance cover for mental illness at par with other illnesses, community-based rehabilitation and services (18.4d), to get integrated mental health services as a part of general health care services (18.5a), to get treatment which enables their living in the community and with their families (18.5b) etc. The State is also obliged under the Act to provide acute mental health care services, outpatients and inpatients (18.4a), provide halfway homes, sheltered accommodation, supported accommodation (18.4 b), to facilitate home-based rehabilitation (18.4c), community-based treatment in a non-government health establishment if the state-run mental health services are not available within a district (18.5 f). If such rights and services are made available to PwMI, then indirectly it will be a relief to the family caregivers. But unfortunately, the government has hardly done anything so far to provide such services which is their duty under the Act (Chapter VI). The hardships faced by the family caregivers consequently remain unaddressed by the State.

National Tele Mental Health Programme (Tele-Manas)

On February 1, 2022, the Finance Minister of Government of India, announced in the budget speech that "*to better the access to quality mental health counselling and care services, a National Tele Mental Health program will be launched—51 nodal centres for telemedical mental health will be operated, with NIMHANS serving as the nodal centre. The International Institute of Information Technology, Bengaluru will provide technical support.*" The Government of India followed it up by forming three sub-committees of experts in April 2022. The author was given the opportunity to serve on the Tele Manas Sub Committee on Health Systems. Tele Mental Health Assistance and Networking Across States (Tele-MANAS) was formally launched on 10th October 2022, the World Mental Health Day (https://telemanas.mohfw.gov.in/). It is a comprehensive mental health care service, which can be availed by dialling the toll-free numbers. This initiative focuses on population-level interventions by a decentralized approach to care rather than only a clinic-based intervention. It is yet to be seen to what extent the mental health needs of the PwMI are met by this programme and whether it provides some relief to the family caregivers.

International Recognition of Caregivers

Caregiving is receiving a lot of attention all over the world. It is challenging at many levels (WFMH, 2013; WHO, 2001; Gangler & Kane, 2015; WHO, 2020; WHO, 2022). "Recognize, Assist, Include, Support, and Engage Family Caregivers Act of 2017" of USA is a milestone in this field. On November 18, 2020, the Family Caregiving Advisory Council constituted under the Act adopted 26 recommendations aimed at establishing a national approach to addressing the needs of family caregivers of all ages and circumstances. They addressed critical priority areas including awareness and outreach to family caregivers and their engagement as key partners in healthcare delivery and long-term services and supports; strengthening community-based supports for family caregivers; ensuring financial security for family caregivers (RAISE, 2018 and 2021). One of the recent initiatives of the WHO's Department of Mental Health and Substance Abuse is the Caregiver Skills Training for caregivers of developmental disabilities (Salamone et al., 2021; Sengupta et al., 2021). The course contains journal exercises that will help caregivers to plan and practise the strategies at home with their dear one. During the last few years, it has been implemented in 30 countries.

UNICEF too has developed a "Caring for the Caregiver" (CFC) training module consisting of (i) Participants Manual (60 pages); (ii) Facilitators Manual (78 pages) and (iii) Implementers Manual (31 pages). The above three examples illustrate the recognition of the importance of support to caregivers and ways by which the caregivers' needs can be addressed. As noted, earlier, another important development of the last two decades is the growing evidence for individual actions for "Self Care for Emotional Health" (Murthy, 2016).

Advocacy Initiatives by Family Caregivers

When the severity of the symptoms comes down, and the remission is nearing, or when the realization comes that whatever was possible, by way of treatment, therapy and care has been done for the dear one, some enlightened family caregivers take to volunteering and advocacy related work to help the community of family caregivers. Advocacy by family caregivers includes increasing awareness about family caregiving issues, pleading, supporting, arguing and espousing the cause of the families of PwMI and improving their quality of life. Local-level advocacy by individuals or group of family caregivers can be effective to seek better care and treatment for their family members with mental illness. Organized advocacy and activism by family caregivers can help to make the society and the state aware of the contribution of the family caregivers towards maintaining the well-being of all those they care for and seeking implementation of the laws and the policies framed for their benefit.

It is observed that activist caregivers often acquire information about the mental illness, their family members are suffering from, by attending awareness-related webinars, participating in caregivers' online peer group meetings, joining caregivers' organizations, getting information from the media and internet. Some of the caregivers also liaise with local people's representatives to seek their support. Many family caregivers involved in advocacy work, get in to statutory bodies constituted under the Mental Healthcare Act 2017, Rights of Persons with Disability Act, 2016 and the National Trust Act, 1999 as caregiver representatives or as representatives of the organizations of caregivers at local levels, state level and national level. For advocacy work and to know what rights are available to the persons with mental disability under the law, the caregiver activists need to find time to get fully familiar with the provisions of the above three acts.

There have been few recent successful examples of advocacy by family caregivers. In the Union Territory of Chandigarh, family caregivers joined hands in demanding from the "Chandigarh Administration," a home for the PwMI and their caregivers within the community. They approached the administration directly, through the Ministry of Health and Family Welfare and the Ministry of Social Justice and Empowerment. Through various press conferences, they sought the participation from media to give coverage to their demands, which was indeed met. The Administration agreed to build a home for them. This has been a good example of what the family caregivers can achieve through advocacy, lobbying and liaison with the press. Similarly, Dr. Nirmala Srinivasan, an activist from Bengaluru, succeeded in getting ambulatory services for PwMI needing hospitalization. Her recent initiative is the start of assisted home care services in the city of Bangalore.

When the MHCA 2017 was being drafted, the author tried for total ban on lobotomy, a primitive irreversible procedure, banned by many countries. However, lobotomy was retained with some safeguards. When the rules were being drafted by the committee of experts formed by the concerned ministry, the author, as a member of the committee could convince the other expert members to add such stringent conditions that getting permission for performing lobotomy becomes very difficult. Thus, it may be noted that the family caregivers who get into advocacy, not only advocate for the needs of the caregivers, but also put forth their strong/united voice on the behalf of other caregivers, to seek the much-needed changes in the mental health laws and policies.

Peer Support Groups

Peer Support Groups initiated by active family caregivers play an important role in providing relief to the family caregivers. In many countries, peer support groups of families, with a family member living with mental illness are doing very well. They often have large number of paid members spread over many cities. In India, however, initiatives taken by some family caregivers in their personal capacity or on behalf of caregivers' organizations have not been successful. When a Peer Support Group is formed by them, a few caregivers may turnup as a novelty. As their expectations are high and they do not find miracales happening, they lose interest and slowly stop participating.

Family caregivers and volunteers associated with Schizophrenia Awareness Association (SAA), Pune, which works for families of PwMI, were running four such groups in Pune and had also setup such groups in other cities of Maharashtra with the hope of identification of local anchor caregivers to take over the running of the peer support groups. It was seen that as long as the facilitators from Pune were going to those locations to conduct meetings, few caregivers would turn up for the meetings but after the facilitators handed over the charge of running of the groups to the local caregivers, the attendance fell down and the groups became non-functional. It was observed that the caregivers who had been identified as anchor persons were not able to retain families for group meetings. In Gujarat too, as a part of the Quality Rights Project, such peer support groups were formed by the author where the project team members had been working. However, it was seen that once the project got over, the support groups gradually stopped functioning.

During the phase of COVID-19 lockdown, caregiver office bearers of SAA and the staff mooted the idea of SAA starting an online peer support group for family members on second and fourth Saturdays. As the number of participants from family was small, it was decided to open the group to the family caregivers from outside Maharashtra and the language of conversation, which was only Marathi, was changed to English or Hindi. The group has survived and has been running fairly well. The second Saturday is kept for experience sharing and on the fourth Saturday a guest speaker is invited. As no travel is involved, caregivers find it convenient to participate from their homes. The talks by the guest speakers have been found to be more popular.

Why Peer support groups are functioning so well in Western countries, but not in Global south is an interesting subject matter for the researchers to find out.

WhatsApp Groups

In a recent experiment, the author started a WhatsApp Group of family caregivers, "MISSION" with an objective to provide a platform to the caregivers to share their experiences, chat with each other, talk about new developments related to the treatment, care and other significant subjects. The group has gained unexpected popularity. There are nearly 350 caregiver members in the group with day-to-day educative and helpful conversations. The same shows that family caregivers do wish to interact with each other, have conversations among themselves and learn from each other. Contributory factors for the success of this WhatsApp group can be attributed to the flexibility of time and the familiarity/trust/comfort of all members on the group administrator with whom they had discussed their problems over messages/mails with him to seek his help and guidance whenever needed.

NGOs Formed and Run by Family Caregivers

As the State has not been able to meet its statutory obligations towards the PwMI and their families, quite a few activist caregivers have come forward to start NGOs to render the needed services to them. The focus of such NGOs is on creating awareness, promoting peer support groups, running residential and day rehab centres, rescuing, and rehabilitating mentally ill wanderers, and an active role in advocacy. Presented below is the brief about the work being done by such NGOs started by family caregivers and the important role they play in providing relief to the persons with mental illness and their families.

Ashadeep, Gauhati: Mukul Goswami and his wife Anjana Goswami from Gauhati, while struggling to provide care and treatment to a family member with schizophrenia, realized that there were many families like them who faced challenges while looking after a mentally disabled family member. They decided to support such family caregivers and facilitate clinical rehabilitation of PwMI in the North-East Region (NER). Ashadeep has done pioneering work in rescuing female wanderers, treating them for their mental illness and for physical injuries and brutalities they were subjected to and rehabilitating them and uniting them with their families. The Government of Assam has collaborated with Ashadeep for establishing a rehabilitation home for homeless men with mental illness. Ashadeep runs an OPD in Guwahati and has set up mental health camps in eight remote regions of Assam and Bodo Territory.

Aasha and Atmanirbhar, Chennai: Ratna Chibber took over the responsibility of her brother living with schizophrenia as his primary caregiver as her parents were old and did not understand what mental illness was. Her daughter Tanya is now the secondary caregiver to her uncle.

Aasha, a caregivers' NGO is mainly run by Ratna and Tanya. Apart from providing manpower support, Ratna is also generous with financial support. Aasha runs a residential rehab home for PwMI on no profit no loss basis. Aasha has opened daily need shops, run and managed by patients from the rehab centre. The patients who are nearing remission are employed by Ratna in her factory. Such recovered patients, during their sheltered employment at Ratna's factory, gain skills and confidence, which helps them find employment in the open market near their homes.

The mother and the daughter duo, committed to recovery, rehabilitation and employment of mentally ill, have started another NGO, Atmanirbhar exclusively dedicated to providing employment to PwMI, creating sustainable employment opportunities for them. Atmanirbhar runs retail stores that provide gainful employment to PwMI. Supervisory staff are engaged to provide support.

Sambandh Health Foundation, Gurugram: Sambandh Health Foundation was co-founded by Rita Seth, a caregiver of her elder brother Starting from promoting Family Self Help Groups, Sambandh has gone on to working with people living with severe mental disorders. It provides community-based mental health services and works towards the integration of mental health into primary care. In collaboration with the Haryana Government, Sambandh has started a pre-vocational resource centre, in Gurugram and has extended its services to villages around Gurugram. Sambandh organizes mental health literacy workshops and has developed partnerships with psychiatrists, PHCs, temples and dargahs, health and education departments of the state government, schools, other NGOs, frontline health workers, educational institutes and employers. Sambandh has ventured into a least restrictive community living option, for people in recovery, within a residential area in Gurugram. It has a live-in support staff, and no in-house, but only outreach support by professional staff.

Schizophrenia Awareness Association (SAA), Pune: SAA was founded by a Canada-based NRI, Late Dr. Jagannath Wani, a caregiver of his wife diagnosed with schizophrenia. SAA's focus is to create awareness about mental illness, minimize stigma and promote peer support groups. SAA has conducted sensitization programs for the press and has conducted sessions with health reporters on coverage of incidents involving persons with mental disorders. SAA runs a day rehab centre for PwMI. "Expressive Therapies"—music, painting, dance, singing and drama are used at the Centre. Arts Based Therapy (ABT) is used as a diagnostic tool for service users to come out with their unconscious concerns. Yoga is a daily activity. A diet expert volunteer reviews the food habits of the service users and their family caregivers and offers advice. Volunteers conduct skill learning activities. The items prepared by patients by way of learning are sold and they get paid monthly for the work done. The Centre conducts Group Animal Therapy and has conducted workshops on Forum Theatre (Theatre of the Oppressed). A residential facility mainly for service users from lower middle class and poor families at an affordable, subsidized cost and those discharged by mental hospitals but no home to go has started.

Peer Support Groups are promoted and run by SAA. Service users are taught the use of recovery tools developed by Dr. Abraham Low, founder of Recovery Inc., USA. SAA participates in consultations and advocacy related to PwMI and their families.

Manav Foundation, Mumbai: Meena Mutha is the caregiver of her daughter who, with a childhood learning disability, later developed severe mental illness. Meena is the founder of Manav Foundation, which provides treatment, support and care to PWMI and their caregivers. The Manav Foundation runs the Manav Rehabilitation Centre to provide rehabilitation services to those recovering from mental illnesses. The families are given psycho-education and the group talk therapy. The Manav Foundation provides financial aid to needy PwMI and has a "sliding" fee structure, which takes care of the family's economic condition. Therapeutic interventions include occupational activities, group therapies and rehabilitation guidance. Counselling services are provided to those with compromised coping conditions. Family caregivers are provided support at "Sahyog" a safe enabling space for the family caregivers to come together to share their experiences and learn from each other.

Parivaartan, Chandigarh: Parivaaratan was started by a group of family caregivers, under the guidance of late Dr. B. S. Chavan, Director Principal, GMCH located at Chandigarh for the welfare of PwMI and their families in UT Chandigarh. Parivartan creates awareness among PwMI and their families about welfare schemes and legal provisions relevant to them. It provides a platform to caregivers of PwMI for group activities and professional support. Programs are arranged for family caregivers of PwMI to equip them in handling of difficult situations at home and to take care of themselves. Parivartan runs Crisis Resolution and Home-Based Treatment (CRHT) Services to provide treatment to PwMI in case of emergency.

Prayatan, Chandigarh: Prayatan is an NGO run by a group of family caregivers of Chandigarh. Its founder president was Caregiver D. K. Sood and the current president is Caregiver R. P. S. Kapoor. Prayatan runs a Peer Support Group of families of PwMI and creates awareness among them about the need for treatment at an early stage of illness. It extends help to families in mental illness-related crisis and to families with limited social support and meagre income. Paryatan distributes free medicines to the PwMI from poor families. It runs kiosks to promote self-employment among PwMI. Many PwMI engaged in these kiosks have found private jobs. In collaboration with another NGO and the Govt. Hospital, Prayatan has been assisting in providing home-based treatment to the patients. Prayatan has created a residential facility for a few destitute patients, who have no place to go. Prayatan has also established a long stay residential home with modern facilities and medical care for patients and their caregivers on no profit no loss basis.

Pushpanjali Trust, Chandigarh: Pushpanjali Trust is founded by Rametras, a caregiving family. Creating awareness and dissemination of information on different aspects of mental health is Pushpanjali's key area of work. They do this through public meetings, webinars, articles in the newspapers and in social media.

Pushpanjali empowers individuals and families to advocate for themselves. Formation of peer support network is promoted by them as part of service users' recovery journey. Pushpanjali encourages PwMI to develop their own personal resources, friendships, and support to overcome barriers. Pushpanjali team also assists families to seek their right of community living for their family members with mental disability.

Citizens for Inclusive Living, Chandigarh—CIL is an association of caregivers and other stakeholders based in Chandigarh. It works for the dignity and welfare of the families having one or more family members with mental illness. The Association has campaigned successfully for a group home for PwMI within the community and succeeded in convincing the Chandigarh administration to build such a place. The group now intends to take up more such initiatives to convince neighbouring state governments to provide similar facilities in neighbouring towns.

Turning Point, Kolkata: Turning Point is an NGO engaged in rehabilitation of persons with mental illness through a Day-Care Centre. Ishita Sanyal, a caregiver of a family member with schizophrenia, is its founder secretary. For economic rehabilitation, the PwMI are trained with mock job interviews and encouraged to do computer certificate courses, so that they are restored back to the mainstream with self-supported earnings. PwMI with abilities in drawing, painting, writing, music or dance are helped to get jobs involving these skills. Handicrafts Training is given keeping in mind their ability, skill and aptitude. Those gifted with creative writing talents are encouraged and offered avenues for publication or jobs in news agencies or are encouraged to join mass communication courses. Each year Turning Point arranges a Cultural Program Nite with performances by the PwMI in music, dance, elocution, recitation, plays etc., and a grand Sports-Cum-Painting-Cum-Music Competition. The shows are featured in newspapers and TV channels, which creates awareness about mental health and reduces stigma. Turning point has also been instrumental in starting the first caregivers' peer support group in Kolkata.

The Altruist: The Altruist is an NGO founded by Milesh Hamlai, a family caregiver of his brother living with mental illness. The Altruist runs an intervention program "Dava & Dua" jointly with the Government of Gujarat to reach out those who come in search of cure for mental disorders at religious places. It is a combination of psychiatric medicine and faith healing implemented at Mira Data Dargah. Dava-Dua model provides an access to modern medicine without compromising patients' belief in religious and spiritual practices. The Altruist runs another program Aadhaar to rescue the wandering people with mental disorders in the cities of Ahmedabad and Vadodara. The Altruist Team rescues such wanderers, facilitates for them police protection, treatment at a government mental hospital and after treatment and recovery, reintegration with their families. Other initiatives by the Altruist include awareness programs on mental health for school teachers, family counselling, trainings and sensitization programs for police personnel, occupational training for recovered mentally ill persons, facilitation of disability benefits for mentally ill persons, free ambulatory service and admission in mental hospitals.

Atmaviswas Vidyalaya, Valsad (AVV): AVV was founded by Bipin Malia, a caregiver to his daughter, is a residential community home for persons with schizophrenia and other severe mental disorders. The AVV built at Valsad, Gujarat has infrastructure and facilities for 56 patients with open space for games and other activities. There is also a long stay home for the elderly patients runs an OPD for poor patients residing in nearby villages. Awareness programs are conducted for the neighbourhood community.

AMEND FACEMI, Bengaluru: Dr. Nirmala Srinivasan, a caregiver to her son, is the founder of the Association for Mentally Disabled (AMEND), which is a self-help group for the families of the PwMI. There are about 55 families in the membership of AMEND in Bangalore and around 20 more families located elsewhere. Meetings of family members are organized once a month to discuss issues of common interests. AMEND's focus is on emotional support and psychosocial education to the families and the community at large (Srinivasan, 2008).

Saathi FACEMI Vadodara: Saathi FACEMI is a caregivers' NGO established by Nand Kishore Shukla, who then was a caregiver of his late elder brother living with mental illness. With the help of like-minded caregivers, he formed an Association of the Relatives of the Chronically Mentally Ill Patients to help families who needed to visit the hospital with their dear ones. The caregiver members meet periodically in the space provided by the Govt. Mental Hospital Vadodara. Saathi, runs a shop in the premises of the mental hospital where daily essentials are sold by the PwMI admitted in the hospital. Till 2014, the caregiver office bearers of the NGO were going to the homes of the families to help them bring the uncooperative violent patients to the hospital. In 2015, due to the efforts of the NGO, "Aadhar" 24 × 7 helpline was launched by the Government which can be used by the families to seek ambulance help for picking up such patients. This arrangement is working well and is a big facility for the families.

Saathi organizes awareness programmes for the families and provides vocational training and help in their getting jobs when they are in remission. Saathi plans to open branches in districts of Gujarat to conduct voluntary services in the psychiatric wards of the civil hospitals with the help of local families.

Action for Mental Illness (ACMI), Bengaluru: ACMI is an advocacy initiative working for the rights and needs of persons with mental illness (PMI) and disorders was founded in 2003 with Dr. Nirmala Srinivasan, a caregiver as its co-founder. ACMI was a lobbying forum to bring about macro-level change in all aspects related to the rights and needs of persons with mental illness and their families. Advocacy followed by action was the hallmark of ACMI.

Currently, the NGO is not active.

Roshni, Delhi: Roshni founded by caregiver Rajeshwari Aiyer was formed as a peer support and advocacy group of family caregivers of PwMI. The objective of the NGO was to motivate family caregivers to share their experiences and support each other in a crisis.

Roshni worked as an advocacy forum to seek help from the government towards providing crisis intervention aids like ambulance services and other benefits and services as provided in the Mental Healthcare Act (2017). Roshni conducted peer support group meetings to provide a forum for sharing without restrain and stigma. Well-known mental health professionals were invited to address such meetings to provide guidance to the families. Roshni provided peer counselling, guidance on obtaining disability certificate, benefits available under various disability laws, formation of trusts for care receivers, information about services available in Delhi and elsewhere, facilitate support to set up day care centres, rehabilitation centres for PwMI as part of their recovery process and integration into the society. Due to old age and some other setbacks, Roshni's founder Rajeshwari Aiyer is now not able to do much running around and other members' involvement is minimal. As such Roshni is not able to function actively.

Research Advocacy, Support and Help for Mentally Ill (RASHMI), New Delhi: RASHMI a society, for families of PwMI was promoted by Paul Foundation, with R. K. Bhatia, a caregiver, as its chairman and chief functionary. RASHMI was active in advocacy work. It was a party in the writ petition filed in 2001 before the Supreme Court in connection with the death of 25 chained inmates in an asylum fire at Ervadi in Tamil Nadu. Rashmi submitted proposals to the Ministry of Social Justice and Empowerment seeking amendments in the Persons with Disabilities Act, 1995. It took up the issue of protection of the business units of PwMI, threatened under the Master Plan of Delhi. RASHMI took up the issue of developing special modules of vocational training programs for mentally ill with the Ministry of Labour and Employment. It also took up the issue of providing tax incentives to the employers of industrial establishments and organizations for giving employment to mentally ill and obtained necessary amendments in the family pension rules of Central Government employees for their wards living with mental illness. RASHMI was instrumental in the formation of National Federation for Mentally Ill (later registered as All India Federation for Mental Illness)—an all-India body for taking up the cause of families of PwMI. It provided helpline services and distributed reading material on mental health. For some time now, RASHMI is not in the news.

Saathi, Ahmedabad: With support from Dr. Ravindra Bakre, the then Superintendent of the Government Mental Hospital Ahmedabad, a family caregivers' NGO Saathi Ahmedabad was formed in 2005, by a group of caregivers led by two family caregivers, whose children lived with schizophrenia. The caregiver members met every Sunday morning in the OPD section of the Govt. Mental Hospital to discuss their problems and try to find out how best they could perform their duties as caregivers. Over the years, the attendance at the Sunday weekly meetings had started thinning and the group meetings had become irregular. During COVID period, the lockdown was imposed, due to which the group could not function. The NGO has remained inactive since then.

Torch Bearers, New Delhi: Rukmini Pillai, a caregiver of her daughter Nandita living with schizophrenia had formed an NGO, which was active in 1990s and the first decade of the current century. In those days Rukmani was known for her blogs, "A Mother in India" and "A Mother's Journey." In the last few years, the Torch Bearers and its founder are not in the news. She is reported to have settled down in Kerala.

Manorogi Kalyaan Sansthan, Lucknow: Manorogi Kalyaan Sansthan was founded by a group of caregivers in Lucknow and was registered as a society on 31 December 2009. Col. Satyaveer Singh Yadav, a caregiver of his son was its first president. The caregiver members were meeting periodically to discuss the issues concerning the caregiver families and their family members living with mental illness. Currently, they are not active.

Athma Shakti Vidyalaya, Chandigarh: Col. Ajay Mendiratta caregiver of his son with schizophrenia was much impressed with the concept of community living model, Fr. Hank Nunn had conceptualized for mentally ill at the Athma Shakti Vidyalaya, set up by him in Bangalore. Fr. Hank visited Chandigarh with his colleague and it was decided to start a half way home for mentally ill in Chandigarh on the same lines as Athma Shakti Vidyalaya in Bangalore. The project, however, did not take off due to ill health of Col. Mendiratta and also of Fr. Hank.

Survival of Family Caregivers' Initiatives?

As we can see from the aforesaid, some of the NGOs started by family caregivers did well till the founders were alive and in good health. After their departure or on their becoming non-functional, there were no anchors in the family or outside the family, to carry the work forward and such NGOs became dormant. It is important that founder family caregivers of such NGOs prepare succession plans and identify their successors in their lifetime to ensure smooth transitions. It is also observed that where an NGO's main activity is limited to promoting peer support groups and holding their periodic meetings, such NGOs mostly do not survive long.

Looking Ahead

Broad needs of the family caregivers include "medical" services (early identification, treatment, rehabilitation etc.), social support (financial, rehabilitation related, reservations in employment, tax relief, shelters for long-term stay, etc.) and focused support in their caregiving tasks (caregiving skills, self- care, handling emergencies).

Caregiving is a lifetime responsibility for the family caregivers and there can be multiple, unexpected situations requiring guidance in handling the same. What is needed is "Comprehensive, Continuous, Coordinated and Compassionate Care" (5 C intervention). It is possible to minimize the distress/burden/challenges through a number of measures from public education to minimizing stigma of mental disorders and discrimination, sharing caregiving skills with caregivers, respite support, financial supports for caregivers and ill persons, skill training facilities, reservations in jobs, support to voluntary organizations for community care facilities and self-care skills. It is important that such supports are accessible to caregivers by pro-active measures rather than the caregivers having to go hunting to find the services or avail of the benefits. It will be a positive development to see all of these aspects brought under a law similar to the RAISE Caregivers Act of 2018 of USA.

The following is an illustrative list of the actions that can be taken at different levels to provide support to family caregivers (Bakhshy, 2022; Srinivasa Murthy et al., 2022).

1. **Responsibilities of the Government (Central/State/UTs)**
   - Focus on population, mental health and self-care
   - Enactment of Family Caregivers' Act
   - Integration of mental health care in general health care
   - Amendments to MHCA 2017, to provide care for families
   - Wide range of community care facilities for PwMI
   - Uniformity in financial support to persons with mental disorders across states (currently it ranges from a low of Rs. 300/ to a high of Rs. 3000/)
   - Financial support to families caring for PwMI
   - Financial support to voluntary organizations of PwMI and their families
   - Public awareness about mental illness through mass media similar to other health conditions.
2. **Responsibilities of the Psychiatric Social Workers and the Mental Health Professionals**

   Focus on population's mental health

- Make self-care a part of all clinical contacts
- Focus on the needs of caregivers along with that of patients
- Documentation of the impact of caregiving
- Development and dissemination of caregiving skills to all caregivers
- Development and dissemination of self-care skills for emotional health
- Involvement of caregivers in planning services and research
- Advocacy with planners
- Helpline for caregivers at the local level.

3. **Responsibilities of the NGOs**
   - Focus on population mental health
   - Organize self-care programmes at local level
   - Understanding the local cultural and community strengths
   - Innovative services for local populations using community resources
   - Facilitating access of governmental benefits of respite support
   - Public mental health education and advocacy.
4. **Responsibilities of the Community**
   - Focus on population mental health
   - Organize self-care programmes at local level
   - Public education on local determinants of mental health
   - Engaging caregivers in planning of services
   - Inclusion of ill persons and families in all programmes
   - Setting up local-level support groups.
5. **Responsibilities of the Families**
   - Daily activities that support mental health

- Making caregiving a family activity
- Acquiring information about the illness of the family members
- Acquiring the caregiving skills to minimize burden of caregiving
- Planning for the future as a family goal
- Joining support groups.

6. **Individuals' Role**
   - Include daily activities that support personal mental health
   - Sharing the "live-in" experiences to decrease stigma and discrimination
   - Self-care to maximize the benefits if treatment and minimize the effects of treatment
   - Treatment adherence.

Conclusion

India has a rich tradition of caregiving as an important part of the society and as the preferred way of caring for the persons needing care in general and PwMI in particular. However, changes in the society, especially urbanization, migration, shifting from joint families to nuclear families, change in the employment status of women, are challenging the caregiving capacities of families. There is an urgent need to recognize the caregivers' contribution and to support the families in caregiving. These challenges have also been well documented. Since we are living in a dynamic situation, the responses too indeed have to be equally dynamic and appropriate. Fortunately, recent understanding of mental health, especially the advances in the self-care measures to promote mental health and minimize of mental disorders, allows for non-clinical interventions to address and mitigate emotional distress. The growing awareness of challenges of caregiving and the vital role of caregivers should result in developing user/family friendly services. There should be support to minimize the burden of care of the caregivers. The caregiver mental health should be an essential part of all mental health care. Such a multipronged approach covering services, support and strengthening of caregivers will realize the important role family caregivers play and extend greater recognition of the caregivers, minimize the negative impact and assure better quality of life for the PwMI and their caregivers.

We hope the lawmakers will realize the need for an Indian Family Caregivers Act, which should address all the needs of caregivers. This is both a challenge as well as an opportunity for the community, press, planners, politicians, professionals and voluntary organizations. Professional social workers indeed have a vital role to bring about these transformations in India.

References

Angothu H, Chatuervedi S.K. (2016). Civic and legal advances in the rights of caregivers for persons with severe mental illness related disability. *Indian Journal of Social Psychiatry, 32*, 28–34.

Ashadeep https://www.ashadeepindia.org/

Aasha Trust https://ashaf.org/

Atmaviswas Vidyalaya, Valsad (AV) https://atmaviswasrehab.org/new/

Bakhshy, A. (2021). *Mental illness and caregiving: Challenges, concerns and complications*. White Falcon Publishing.

Bakhshy A. (2022). The Indian family caregivers of persons with mental illness, Schizophrenia Awareness Association. Pune.

Chaddha, R. K. (2014). Caring for the family caregivers of persons with mental illness. *Indian Journal of Psychiatry, 56*(3), 221–227. https://doi.org/10.4103/0019-5545.140616

Janardhana, N., Raghunandan, S., Naidu, D. M., Saraswathi, L., Seshan, V. (2015). Care giving of people with severe mental illness: An Indian experience. *Indian Journal of Psychological Medicine, 37*,184–194.

Gangler, J. E., & Kane, R. L. (2015). *Family caregiving in the new normal*. Elsevier.

Gururaj, G., et al. (2016). *The national mental health survey of India*, 2015–16: Summary National Institute of Mental Health and Neuro Sciences, NIMHANS, Bangalore. Publication No.128.

Kapoor, R. L. (1994). Community involvement in mental health care. *The National Mental Health Journal of India, 7*(6), 292–294. PMID: 7841883

Kohmeyler, W. A., & Fernandes, X. (1963). Psychiatry in India: Family approach in the treatment of mental disorders. *American Journal of Psychiatry, 119*, 1033–1038.

Manas Foundation https://manas.org.in/

Mental Health Care Act. (2017). http://prsindia.org/uploads/media/Mental%20Health/Mental%20Healthcare%20Act,%202017.pdf

Mental Healthcare Act 2017. (2022). *Indian Journal of Psychological Medicine, 44*, 315–316.

Mental Health First Aid Australia. A guide for caregivers of people with mental illness. www.mhfa.com.au

Narayanan, H. S., & Reddy, G. N. N. (1968). Review of treatment in a family ward. *Indian Journal of Psychiatry, 14*, 123.

National Alliance for Caregiving. https://www.caregiving.org/

Prayatan, A. Mental Health Support Group, Chandigarh. https://parivartan.in.net/

Prabhu, G. (1995). Foreword-Innovations in psychiatric rehabilitation, Richmond Fellowship of India, pp. 5–8.

RAISE Family Caregivers Act of 2017. (2018, January 22). H.R. 3759, P.L. 115–119 Section 15.2. https://acl.gov/sites/default/files/about-acl/2018-10/PLAW115publ119%20-%20RAISE.pdf

Recognize, Assist, Include, Support, & Engage (RAISE). (2021). Family Caregivers Act Initial Report to Congress Prepared by: RAISE Family Caregiving Advisory Council, September 22, 2021. Washington. USA.

Rehabilitation Council of India (RCI) RCI Certificate Course in Care Giving: Syllabus and Guidelines. http://rehabcouncil.nic.in/writereaddata/caregsyll.pdf

Rochat, T. J., Redinger, S., Rozentals-Thresher, R., Yousafzia, A., & Stein, A. (2019). *Caring for the caregiver*. UNICEF.

Murthy, R. S. (2021). Self-care for mental health-the new frontier In G. Saha, (Ed.). Indian 'Different strokes' (2nd edn). Psychiatric Society.

Roshni Action For Mental Illness Delhi https://www.opencounseling.com/india/new-delhi/counseling-agency/roshni-action-for-mental-health-illness

Salamone et al. (2021). Pilot randomized controlled trial of the WHO caregiver skills training in public health services in Italy. *Journal of Autism and Developmental Disorders*. https://doi.org/10.1007/s10803-021-05297-x.

Sambandh Health Foundation, Gurugram. https://www.sambandhhealth.org/

Schizophrenia Awareness Association https://schizophrenia.org.in/

Sengupta, K., et al. (2021). World health organisation-caregiver skills training (WHO-CST) program: Feasibility of delivery by non-specialist providers in real world 20 urban settings in India. *Journal of Autism and Developmental Disorders*. https://doi.org/10.1007/s10803-021-05367-0

Seshadri, K., Sivakumar, T., & Jagannathan, A. (2019). The family support movement and schizophrenia in India. *Current Psychiatry Report, 21*, 95. https://doi.org/10.1007/s11920-019-1081-5

Shankar, R. (1994). Interventions with families of people with schizophrenia in India. In Family interventions in mental illness. In A. B. Hatfield (Ed.). New Directions for Mental Health Services (vol. 62, pp. 79–88).

Sood, M., Chaddha, R. K., Chawla, N., Sharma, M. R., et al. (2022). Understanding needs of stakeholders and outcomes desired from a home-based intervention program for "difficult to treat" schizophrenia and related disorders: A qualitative study. *Indian Journal of Psychiatry, 64*, 38–47.

Murthy, S. R. (2016). Caregiving and Caregivers: challenges and opportunities in India. *Indian Journal of Social Psychiatry, 32*, 10–18.

Murthy, S. R. (2020a). COVID-19 pandemic and emotional health-social psychiatry perspective. *Indian Journal of Social Psychiatry, 36*, S24-42.

Murthy, S. R. (2020b). Psychosocial and behavioural aspects of populations affected by humanitarian emergencies: Recent developments. *Current Opinion in Psychiatry, 29*(5), 280–285.

Murthy, S. R., Divya, B., Nischitha, S. (2022). Family Caregiving: Indian experiences and looking ahead. In Bakhshy A (Ed.) *The Indian Family caregivers of persons with mental illness.* Schizophrenia Awareness Association. Book rivers

Murthy, S. R., Divya, B., Nischitha, S. (2023). *Self-empowering for emotional health* (Caregivers' Manual). The Association for the Mentally Challenged, Bangalore.

Murthy, S. R., Divya, B., Nischitha, S., Srikanth (2023). *Loss, love and growth-stories of families caring for a person with special needs.* The Association for the Mentally Challenged.

Srinivasan, N. (2008). We are not alone-family care for persons with mental illness. Action for Mental Illness (ACMI).

Thara, R., Padmavati, R., Kumar, S., & Srinivasan, L. (1998). Instrument to assess burden on caregivers of chronic mentally ill. *Indian Journal of Psychiatry, 40*, 21–29.

The Hindu. (2021). The Annual Budget.

Torch Bearers Foundation. https://www.torchbearersfoundation.com

Turning Point, Kolkata. http://www.turningpoint.org.in/

World Federation of Mental Health. (2013). *Caring for the caregiver*. Woodbridge.

World Health Organisation (2001). *World Health report-2001: Mental Health-new understanding*: New hope. WHO

World Health Organization. (2019). Caregiver skills training (WHO-CST) program: Feasibility of delivery by non-specialist providers in real-world urban settings in India. WHO

World Health Organisation (2020). *Country profiles on mental health resources. Atlas 2020.* WHO

World Health Organization. (2022). World Mental Health Report 2022: Transforming mental health for all. WHO

Chapter 16
Three Decades of a Journey Towards Mental Health for All: The Story of IPH

Anuradha Sovani

Abstract The chapter outlines the journey of a social enterprise called Institute for Psychological Health, situated in the state of Maharashtra, India. The goal of the Institute is to work in the field of Mental Health, responding to the needs of the community and focusing on disability, distress and development through various ongoing activities that build awareness about mental health and psychological well-being, promote inclusion and reduce mental illness stigma. The story of IPH covers the beginning of IPH in March 1990, with no place to call its own, and a handful of like-minded mental health professionals spearheading a movement to promote well-being in the community of Thane, a township on the border of Mumbai city. The only association the city had with mental health or illness so far was the location of a Regional Hospital for long-stay psychiatric patients in its midst, ensuring nothing but stigma and fear associated with mental illness in residents' minds. IPH created a totally different vibe, one of easy footfalls, a welcoming atmosphere, and plenty of activities for young and old alike. It has since grown from one city to three, Thane, Pune and Nasik, from one venue in the city to four sites in the city of Thane and one each in the other two cities. This has been possible due to a vision beyond psychiatry seen as psychopharmacology, using a team approach towards positive mental health, and stigma reduction. A vision beyond surviving on donations or state funding, by adopting self-sustenance and backward integration to develop in-house services. The Institute serves at three levels today, helping to assist disability through a core spirit of inclusion, addressing client distress through professionally run services at all its sites, often at very low cost for those who cannot pay, and ensuring development for all those who are striving towards higher goals and self-improvement. Multiple support groups for patients as well as caregivers, all of them run free of charge for years, serve to meet the first goal; IPH projects focusing on activity centres for chronic ailments like schizophrenia will be described at length. Teamwork marks IPH efforts to manage client distress, with a strong team of over a hundred professionals: psychologists, psychiatrists, physiotherapists, occupational

A. Sovani (✉)
Department of Psychology, SNDT Women's University, Mumbai, India
e-mail: anuradhasovani@gmail.com

Institute for Psychological Health, Mumbai, India

M. Anand (ed.), *Mental Health Care Resource Book*,
https://doi.org/10.1007/978-981-97-1203-8_16

therapists, speech therapists, special educators, and career guidance professionals. Additionally, a strong workforce of *community volunteers* carries on all institutional activities ably and well. The chapter highlights various unique practices at IPH, tying them to their basis in psychological science. It dwells on important *lessons learned* in the 32-year journey; it marks off *challenge areas* where much work is still needed, and the *changes achieved* along the way. It also offers blueprints to other like-minded organizations, for developing inclusive attitudes, use of books and articles in the local language to promote awareness, and harnessing the wide reach of social media. The aim of the chapter is to add to the documentation of existing community mental health efforts in India, and also to point fledgling organizations in the right direction, cautioning them to learn through earlier mistakes made, and experiments that turned out to be successful. Possible negative aspects that hinder the process of institution building could also be a takeaway from the chapter. Or else it may motivate like-minded professionals to build something like IPH in their own vicinity.

Keywords Mental health · Well-being · IPH

What is IPH?

An NGO? A community mental health service centre? A Learning Centre? A social enterprise? A group of like-minded mental health professionals got together at the beginning of the year 1990, and decided that they would work towards a common goal, "Mental Health for All". The initial name thought of was Institute for Psychological Handicap, but then the error in this thinking became very apparent to the team, and they decided to go with Institute for Psychological Health.

As is well known, Thane city houses the Regional Psychiatric Long Stay Hospital of the Government of Maharashtra, and that was the association with the city for years together.

The "Thane Mental Hospital", as it is locally known, was established over 150 years ago, and no doubt responded to a need of the time, but residential care for the mentally ill can breed its own problems including institutionalization, and a revolving door presence of service users in and out of the institution. The huge number of patients in such an institution leads to anonymity and occasionally, neglect of personal needs; the high walls and strong security breed some amount of fear of the unknown in the community around.

Although Thane city was a strong cultural hub and a rapidly growing township bustling with activities of schools, colleges, social clubs and yoga centres, auditoriums, movie theatres, sports complexes, gymnasiums and in later years, malls and large housing complexes, the Thane Mental Hospital stigma never really detached itself from the city.

In this environment, the group of innovators decided that they would focus on wellness and well-being. They would focus on the Disorder of persons suffering from chronic conditions such as Obsessive Compulsive Disorder, Schizophrenia and Bipolar Disorder, releasing them from shackles of stigma through public awareness programmes, media-based pieces and support group activities.

The focus would be on the distress of persons suffering from more manageable conditions with a shorter duration, more treatable conditions such as anxiety and depression, common mental disorders in all their various forms, including exam anxiety. Help may also come in disguise, such as "personality contests" for youth as well as the ageing, which were really invitations to beat exam stress, set life goals and ensure happiness and confidence.

And finally, another important focus would be development. Helping sportspersons to achieve their best performances, students to become good public speakers, writers, and artists if they so wished; women in the community to achieve a healthy work-life balance and celebrate their personhood.

So, the overall aim of IPH, it was decided, would be to cater to the mental health needs of the community primarily by:

- Building awareness about mental health,
- Promoting inclusion, and
- Reducing mental illness stigma.

Initial Hurdles and Current Developments

Any new effort has to set certain basic requirements in place before launching into their intended activity. The three primary needs are space, money, and people. The IPH kitty was empty on all three fronts in 1990, and the only energy that could sustain the dream was a strong belief that this was a much-needed service, and somebody had to set it up at the earliest. Today, IPH can look back with satisfaction, having steadied the rocky boat and churning ahead, moving forward through constantly changing seascapes.

Space

One early decision that needs to be taken with regard to space and funding is whether to turn to government support, corporate funding, or charity. Since the IPH core team was sure that the first two were not options that would be taken, for either place or funding, they turned to large hearted local support systems, one of whom gave them one floor in their hospital building to use for one year, free of charge. The attraction was that there would be no monetary outlay. The challenge was to ensure that a viable self-sustenance option would get generated within the year, when this generous offer would end. To begin work without changing the existing structure or beautifying the place in any way was the default option and the team went with it.

In today's times, this seems like a naïve step. Most concerns do not venture to start work without making their workspace attractive, market it actively and ensure footfalls before launching out. 1990 was an era before social media, and advertising was expensive, hence not an option. The team was young and relatively inexperienced. They had had glowing student career paths and support from their former teachers and mentors but were yet to make a name in the medical-paramedical fraternity. On their side were their skill sets: professional mental health training and skills, writing, public speaking, creativity, and a strong conviction about their "Mental Health for All" mission statement.

This first year became memorable for flexi-use of the available space, interspersed with occasional comments from service users comparing the rather makeshift appearance of the rooms, replete with packing boxes and cheap furniture, with other more attractively presented mental health centres in the city and surround. The year flew past, seeing growing numbers in client base, and soon there was enough money to pay for rent in another location just across the road. Surprisingly, clients did not blink at the change of address, which was cleaned up personally by the team, and readied for occupancy. The rent was just barely affordable and the management not enormously friendly, but everything was taken in good spirit, and work began.

Of course, as will always be the case at that stage of life, each of the core team members had their personal life journeys which were ongoing, and each brought their share of joys as well as hurdles. But none of these stopped the IPH effort, which soldiered on. There is always a risk of building a Pollyanna-like, uniformly positive picture of bonhomie and friendship as any organization struggles through its fledgling years. By and large, the visions of all core team members matched, and were fuelled by the energy of youth and dreams. There were a few differences of opinion too, naturally, and some initial travellers left the caravan, either because they were not happy with decisions taken, or because life took them elsewhere across the globe.

Predictably, landlord-renter relationships are a rocky road, and these premises need to be vacated within a few years, and not in the happiest of circumstances. One also understands the innate fear and stigma in the mind of the owner of the premises, arising from the knowledge that the space is being used to treat people with some form of psychological illness. Stigma is a vitriolic and virulent entity, an enigma spreading its tentacles into society. Another place was readied at short notice, again in the close vicinity, and again through the goodwill of former clients, but this time not pro bono.

These premises were smaller, on the ground floor and could be partitioned with some creative planning, to generate the workspaces needed by the Institute. Some tiny cabins, a little library, and a relatively larger open space that could be alternatively used for support groups and public programmes. This venue taught the team that space need not be a barrier, and one can always work around what is available. Also, it gave pointers to the core team for exactly which spaces were non-negotiable and what were the true needs of the Institute, and this helped greatly while planning a permanent and self-owned home of IPH several years later.

During the years spent in this small location, the team often felt the space crunch and tended to grumble about it. Each professional wanted to do something new, something interesting, and there was never enough space. A visitor from abroad, a classmate and friend of one of the core team members and an erudite faculty member in a university setting abroad came one day to visit IPH. He sat in one of the tiny cabins, listening to apologies from his friend for the lack of space and amenities. Then he raised his head like a pointer hound, and sat quietly, allowing the vibe of the place to wash over him, so to speak. Then he smiled. "This place will do well", he prognosticated with a smile. "I have visited many organizations all over the world, and there is a certain buzz one hears around one when the place is busy and happy. I hear it here".

This last move also strengthened the resolve of the team to ensure that a space of one's own is a dire need. A place which one rightfully owned, from where one would not be thrown out on a whim. A steep demand, given property prices, and once again the innate reluctance to offer space for "an organization tending to the mentally ill"; but necessity steers resolve. Constant setting of funds towards this cause, and keeping eyes and ears open for any probable real estate becoming available, became a pattern. IPH was able to get a home of its own only seventeen years after it was established.

Today, three decades later, IPH owns premises in the centre of Thane city, spread over three floors and designed to suit the Institute's needs, with a large attractive mural thrown in for aesthetics, and beautiful nature photographs gifted by a close friend and well-wisher, in each room. The space, though not huge, accommodates windows bringing natural light into each cabin, a central foyer open to the top via a skylight which once again brings in natural light.

A book vendor dispensing publications from the IPH team nestles in one corner. There are conference rooms, personalized consulting rooms which are flexi-use, a common lunch room, reception and office spaces, a file room for the mandatory documentation backup, as well as rooms for specific activities such as Occupational and Play therapy, and Telephone Helpline, *Maitra*. Initially, space was also made for a Library and a Rehabilitation Centre, which were later accommodated into alternative premises for convenience. These are briefly described in the following paragraphs.

Once again, a tip to fledgling organizations is that one need not squeeze all activities into a single space, but rather allow them to sprawl out naturally and organically. Soon each space will develop its own life and purpose, and users grow into their own comfort level. The challenge then remains to keep communication alive between these spaces, and this will be addressed later in the chapter.

Of course, difficulties abound, and issues like lack of parking space, and complaints from other residents of the building where the current premises are located, can still disturb the flow of work. Some of these complaints may still stem from the core stigma associated with any mental health work, even after three decades of actively addressing the issue. Others are simply logistic difficulties like use of elevators and payment for common facilities such as generators, stairwells and basement. Most can be handled with the same calm, rational approach that one advocates to one's clients in therapy, combined with good relationships and bonhomie generated by continuously doing good work for the community.

Thane city now has three more venues used by IPH, some rented, others in collaboration with Government partnerships. One is a *Maitraghar*, once again flexi-use for accommodating guests on a short visit, a top-end recording studio for IPH productions, and space for seasonal activities such as Vocational testing and Career Guidance.

The second is a space shared with a State Government facility dedicated to rehabilitation and recovery: this houses *Saptasopaan*, which translates from Sanskrit as "seven steps to wellness" for the Elderly and also for Persons recovering from chronic mental illness, and has also made room for the IPH Library. This is a busy activity centre providing Psychological Nurturance and Cognitive Nutrition to a large number of senior citizens in Thane and surround, who visit regularly, avail the library resource and partake happily of the many new learnings regularly offered there, all designed to keep the brain nourished and active for over twenty hours per week. This was an outcome of a project on Satisfied Aging (SAGE), which explores factors contributing to healthy ageing (Wandrekar et al., 2016).

The adjoining space on the same premises also houses *Tridal*, a successful IPH experiment in cognitive and social rehabilitation of persons with chronic psychiatric conditions such as Schizophrenia. Tridal members are called *Shubharthis*, which means "people on the path to wellness" (Apte, 2018; Sovani, 2009).

Tridal stands on its own feet financially, sustaining its activity with popular products prepared by *Shubharthis* under the watchful eye of trained volunteers and supervised by mental health professionals. Tridal Center has received considerable help from generous grants from the Paul Hamlyn Foundation, India (PHFI).

The *Shubharthis* commute to Tridal by a minibus, donated by a well-wisher, register their daily presence biometrically and are fairly compensated for their work. Ups and downs in their mental health condition are a part of life, which become more tolerable with group support, and rich social activities including Film screenings, film festivals and discussions, yoga and cognitive stimulation games. The path is by no means as smooth as it sounds in this short paragraph. Every recurrence of their psychiatric condition brings pain and upheaval, but most have learned to recognize signs of disturbance early, and take help well in time.

There are several success stories from Tridal that come to mind. Some pertain to Shubharthis who were not even willing to sit in a circle for group exercises, and used to sit facing away from the rest, uncomfortable with social interaction, now participating in product sales at the Tridal counter. Others hail from the pandemic period, when *Shubharthis* adapted willingly to the online format, and stayed in touch with each other virtually, something which even people without any disability found hard to do. The nicest memory is of a Conference held jointly by IPH with a University Department where one of the core members was teaching.

Many psychologists and academicians attending the Conference, which was held on University premises, had not worked in clinical settings, and probably held an image in their mind, about "how people with psychosis look.....*different*". Tridal work was shared during the proceedings, and delegates were urged to go and buy products from the Tridal counter, one among many other displays of the Conference. Later the delegates came back and asked the core team member where the Shubharthis were, who prepared these products, since they wished to compliment them. They were utterly surprised to learn that the counters had in fact been manned by *Shubharthis!* It takes a lot of cognitive training to be able to decipher how much change to give back after a purchase is made, and we notched this experience up as a rehabilitation success.

Finally, a newly added rental space has launched the ambitious new experiment of a *Mental Health Hangout* (Sovani, 2019b). It is well documented by now that young people facing mental health issues require a safe space for healing and recovery, and social, emotional and vocational development (McGorry et al., 2013). Research has supported recovery-oriented services that promote safety and autonomy (Green et al., 2019). The Hangout awaits inauguration as this chapter is being written.

Activities around the central area of Schizophrenia research and rehabilitation have been a strong interest area for IPH, and the work at IPH has been presented regularly by the team at National conferences of Indian Psychiatric Association and Indian Association of Clinical Psychologists, and also on international platforms such as International Conference on Schizophrenia (IConS of SCARF) and conferences of the International Society for Psychological and Social Approaches to Psychosis (ISPS), and in collaborative work with International Universities under the Shastri Indo Canadian Grant.

Some Flagship Programmes and Satellite Centres

After resisting the concept of satellite centres for several years until its own model was established and free of glitches, IPH began two sub-centres in Pune and Nashik city, respectively. Both are doing well, and reaching out to the city and surround with similar programmes to the original set, but tweaked to suit local needs, e.g. Pune is a strong IT hub; Nashik is more a more agro-industrial belt, hence some niche content is being created for the users of each zone in Maharashtra. Currently, an IPH team is contributing actively to a 3-year effort of the Maharashtra State Faculty Development Academy (MSFDA) to reach out to campuses all over Maharashtra State and render them Emotion Friendly.

Some flagship programmes have come to define IPH, and they are held are various sites all over Maharashtra every year. One of them is ***Vedh,*** the annual career guidance event which is also mentioned elsewhere in the chapter. Each Vedh (an acronym for Vocational Education, Direction and Harmony, and also a Sanskrit word for taking aim) has a theme, and a theme song which is taught to the student audience on the first day and sung in unison.

People who have achieved excellence and a huge social stature by virtue of their career success are invited and interviewed on stage. The young audience is permitted written questions and also maintain diary through the event, which is evaluated and the best write-up and best questions rewarded by judges. The weekend event easily draws over four thousand people every year and is eagerly awaited every December in the city of Thane. Currently, this program is also conducted in over twelve major cities in Maharashtra. Avaahan, the media team and Aakalan, the learning centre, pitch in when such projects are under way, but more about that later.

Another unique programme conducted at IPH, perhaps the first ever in Asia, was the ***Dwij Puraskaar.*** This was an effort to reduce the stigma associated with mental illness, and actually convert it to a sense of pride at having achieved recovery. The accolades in this Award ceremony, held once a year at first, and then tapered off to once in two years and then even less frequently, as the need decreased, were given to the *Shubharthi* or person suffering from the condition, as well as to the caregivers, both from the family as well as professional caregivers.

There was a form to be completed by all, which was a unique feature since it required a person with mental illness to declare their history of struggle with the condition, with pride instead of shame, as is usually the case. The forms were carefully scrutinized and awards declared, which were first shared privately over the phone with the *Shubharthis,* to allow them the choice to finally decide that they were psychologically ready to accept the ***Dwij* award** on stage in the presence of a large audience.

The actual event was grand, and there was no question of shame as there was much pride in narration of the victory over mental illness in a stage interview that moved the audience and increased their respect towards those who had made it past the journey of recovery.

Perhaps a short description of one episode in a *Dwij* interview will help the reader understand the power of this model. On the well-lit, decorated stage were two people, the Director and Managing Trustee of IPH, an experienced, socially aware psychiatrist, writer and activist who conducts the live interview, and the little figure of a woman, about 30 years old, not very educated, simply dressed, and clearly shy of the arclights in this big-city auditorium focused on her.

She was the spouse of a person with schizophrenia, a man who had been ill since his age of 17 years, a fact that was never divulged to her or her family when they married, perhaps since nobody really understood what was happening to him. He grew steadily paranoid as his condition worsened, and there was violence, mistrust and chaos in their little home, while the children watched, terrified. He worked for a small district office as office staff, cleaning the place, fetching water for the officers, and making tea. Their extended family blamed her squarely, saying that she must be doing something wrong, or may have angered the gods in some way to bring such circumstances upon the family.

One watched her grow relaxed and confident as she told her story on stage. How she gently persuaded her husband to see the local doctor, then a psychiatrist, to treat his condition. How she spoke to people in his office and got them to allow her to work in his place while he underwent treatment. A couple of years passed, he grew steadily better under the watchful eye of a psychiatrist, a psychologist and his wife. She grew steadily more popular at office with her work ethic and her smiling and prompt service. The eight-hundred strong audience hung on to her words, and held their breath at the pause and turning point in her story.

> And then he was well", she said in the local language, "and I persuaded the office to take him back....my children and my house needed me. I took him with me to office everyday for a month, and let him slowly pick up the ropes while my children stayed with neighbours. Once I knew he could do everything well, I stopped going.

"What you did is what we call rehabilitation, "*punarvasan*" you know?" our Director asked her with a gentle smile, and a glance at the audience. "How did you know what to do, and how did you get all the steps so right?" The silence in the auditorium could be cut with a knife, and then she smiled. "What else was there to do?" she said with a modest shrug.

Other similar stigma reduction efforts include ***Manatarang*** **Film Festivals** and the **Manatarang Film Club** which is a monthly activity on the last Sunday of each month. The agenda of every club meeting is a short film screening of short films pertaining to resilience in the face of strife and psychological stress, and discussion thereafter. The audio-visual medium has great power and can convey a message that stays with you. The structure of each festival differs, e.g. some have used the popular Marathi film trilogy of "*Devrai*" which highlights schizophrenia, "*Kaasav*" which explains Depression, and "*Astu*" which unpacks Dementia. Others have used short films made in other states of India, or films from other regions of the world, with subtitles. If the festival is held on school or college premises, the student audience feasts on the content, and volunteer. Members of all the IPH support groups are always regular attendees.

Other "firsts" at IPH are the "***Maitra***" **telephone Helpline** manned by trained volunteers (Subramaniam, 2008), and the ***Manovikas*** **programmes** (Nadkarni, 2016), conducted by volunteers in the community, with a scripted stigma reduction and public awareness message. Maitra volunteers are selected and trained in a unique manner, and need to "report for duty" just for one slot a week, which makes the work doable. There are regular call-discussion sessions conducted by professionals, where difficult calls are discussed threadbare, a process made possible by detailed call notes maintained by each volunteer.

Workshops regularly conducted at IPH include "***Paalakshaalaa***", which is a parenting school, "***Bahar***", a search for a woman for her self-identity, and of course, the popular Stress Management and Anger Management workshops. **Paalakshaalaas** can focus on different age groups of children as per the felt need in the community at the time. Parents of toddlers have different issues in mind, and parents of teenagers have a different set of stressors. For instance, the pandemic saw the surfacing of major concerns about online primary school and issues with screen time.

The word "Bahar" literally means a season of abundance. Women in our society, and in a lot of communities around the world, devote their life to spouse, children and family care, and when they approach menopause, there is a sense of having lost years of their life to routine, a nagging empty nest, and doubts about their own creativity and purpose. **Bahar workshops** show them the magic of their life where they are now their own person, independent, and free to express and celebrate their existence in the way they see fit.

Long-term projects like ***Tridal, Saptasopaan*** and important verticals like ***Aavahan***, the Media team and ***Aakalan***, the Learning Center, are mentioned earlier in the chapter. IPH currently boasts more than 155 such activities in all. The material pertaining to all these can be easily traced on the IPH website, healthymind.org.

Funds

After settling in into its first rental space, IPH resolved to have a fundraiser. Going with the spirit of the times, and the young vibe around, it was decided that the event would be a first of its kind western music programme in the huge sports stadium that Thane city boasts. But when we make plans, it is said that some divinity up there laughs. The end of 1992 brought a huge upheaval to the political scenario of the country, and the peace of Mumbai city and neighbourhoods was rattled in the beginning of 1993. It took a catastrophe like a chain of bomb blasts across Mumbai to shelve this ambitious fundraiser, return all the money collected and lick the financial wounds left by payouts already made.

Playing to One's Strengths: Some Do's and Don'ts

If one has paid a price, it is wise to at least benefit from the lessons learned, and IPH learned the first big lesson: all future fundraisers must rely on in-house expertise, so that any event can be rescheduled depending on exigencies. Subsequently, over the last three decades, IPH has held and raised funds through Rights Conferences, Career Guidance Conclaves, Public lectures, Corporate trainings and Action research collaborations, and occasionally through programmes and mental health enhancement trainings for the general population, interweaving mental health with Music, Spirituality and Biographies of noteworthy Indian thought leaders.

The unique feature of any IPH fundraising programme is that it is always light on the audience pocket (Sovani, 2019a), draws resources from in-house expertise and caters to a previously identified local need. It also provides work and income from Tridal product sales and book sales of IPH publications, which are always available for visitors to the event. These interlinkages help showcase the activities going on at IPH and result in drawing more clients and volunteers to the organization.

The move to funded projects comes with a footnote of limited period funding aiming at self-sustenance for the activity when funding stops. No programme is sustained by charity in perpetuity, which often breeds complacence. This offers motivation to retain independence, and make each activity a profit centre.

Self-sustenance and Backward Integration

Another tip to fledgling organizations is to create in-house services and backward integration, so that those services also begin to earn from day one, and the institution is not dependent on outside expertise for its operational needs. The IPH *Sahachari* community kitchen is one such example; this initiative is a catering service run by spouses of persons with alcohol addiction, who attend an IPH support group of the same name for their emotional needs, and bolster themselves financially, also maintaining their dignity and self-respect, by catering for all public programmes of IPH and even accepting orders from other organizations.

Personnel

One of the biggest strengths of any mental health service provider is the professionals who offer these services. IPH began with literally a handful of like-minded professionals, most of them ready to work for next to no payment. Today, the Institute boasts over 110 professionals, with a promise that there would be a free choice of OPD timings, no unethical practices, no rent to be paid, secretarial support offered by IPH reception staff, and payments that cover the financial needs of these professionals. Every consultant has a choice in terms of how much time to devote to the organization, as well as to pick their own working hours.

The key to recruitment is that there are no official interviews, no head hunters. In an effort to blend professionalism with informality, observers who have worked with IPH "select" the Institute, and express a wish to work there. In turn, the current professional team is consulted to check if these applicants are a good fit to IPH philosophy; if there is a positive consensus, they are invited to join the team.

The backbone of IPH is the huge group of volunteers, ever energetic, ever smiling and always there for all major events to handle the work behind the scenes, and of course, for all celebrations to add to the joy. To quote late Professor N. N. Wig, a stalwart in the field of mental health "Mental Health is too important to be left to mental health professionals alone".

Activities and Feeder Centres

Many feeder centres have been created over the years: University departments from where former students approach IPH for internships and observerships, professionals who have availed of training under the *Aakalan* banner, professionals from client families and from the community at large who have previously participated in IPH community programmes and enjoyed the vibe.

As IPH credibility was established over a period of time, graduate and postgraduate students studying various aspects of mental health, viz. psychiatry, psychology, social work, occupational and speech therapy, physiotherapy, special education, etc., from across various universities from Maharashtra and the other states, some from overseas as well, come to visit IPH to understand its philosophy and working. Sometimes it is large community events that generate this interest and draw many volunteers and professionals.

The danger lurking behind large events such as those described above is the personal adulation that can follow. There is always a key person at the centre of such events, who draws the crowds, who carries with his or her name the glitter and glamour of fame. That is inevitable, and public events do need to be designed around a crowd-puller. But the lesson to be learned here by fledgling organizations is to always be mindful of creating a second line of talented people who can take over if the need arises, and still not result in monetary losses to the organization. Being at the centre of virtually every large ticket event in the year is not healthy for the central key figure either, and bodes ill in terms of health hazards and stress levels, which need to be managed carefully.

Team Approach and Personnel Selection

Those wishing to work at IPH are asked to join for a 2-month internship and work within the system without getting paid for that period. Those who lose interest automatically drop away, and those who stay and express interest in a long-term relationship are given a highly individualized welcome letter of commitment in lieu of an "appointment" letter. They are also included in many other activities besides their regular professional work, which gives them the opportunity to hone other skills and develop a taste for a variety of tasks: research, creative writing, designing logos, writing blogs and theme songs for events, creating poster content and editing newsletters, and many others. Training like this is hard to find elsewhere and acts as a magnet for young talent.

Team Building and Training

Community training and corporate training cross-subsidize one another, which is important for team building as all get to work in all settings and play to their strengths, and all team members get to hone newer skills. There is an open-handed sharing of all intellectual resources, and new joinees feel this trust and openness. There is no sense of competition or insecurity, and all new learnings and knowledge created are open source. Everybody gets to work under a common roof like a family, still maintaining their individuality. Once again, a warning to fledgling organizations is that all may not take to this format. Many young professionals prefer a formal and detached working environment to a setting resembling the warmth of an extended family. Finally, it is a matter of personal preferences, and team members will join or leave depending on their choice.

Administrative Model

IPH administration and accounts teams are once again an interesting mix of diverse people. They are, once again, not "recruited through HR". They are people qualified to do this work, who have volunteered from the community to do it for IPH since they have already served as volunteers before, or they have already enjoyed some programme that was offered by the Institute previously and have felt motivated to join up.

Or else they are people who have availed the mental health services at IPH through some stress points in their lives, and enjoy their wellness now; and of course, feel the urge to give back to society in some way by serving through the organization. Some of them may be hesitant to venture outside into a fiercely competitive world of work, but may find IPH a safe and relatively threat-free place where they can start working flexible hours and slowly build up confidence to shoulder more responsibilities.

There is also a unique and empathic, caring interface between professionals and administrative staff at the Institute. The professionals help admin to upgrade continuously by inviting them to attend some of the programmes designed to teach stress management, time management etc. or may devise special modules for them, Library science and English-speaking proficiency being some examples.

Learnings and Challenges

Some of the new learnings that came to the IPH team have been listed through the chapter, the major ones being, ensuring that fundraising is done with in-house talent, the importance of training the team in multi-tasking and the importance of developing strong in-house backup and support services.

The balance between professionalism and informality is another important learning, as is the importance of maintaining open sources. IPH still attempts to maintain the firm stand of not depending financially on any single source since that takes away from their autonomy.

Managing time well, keeping the connection and communication alive between all the teams and sub-centres, and keeping on updating and refining in house talent are some key mantras regularly reiterated by having regular online programmes for enrichment for all teams at the different sites, with creative nomenclature like Wonderstorm, and Launchpad GenNext.

Challenges include creating a second line of expertise. It is often easy to rest on one's laurels and begin to rely on the same well-honed "expert" resources within the organization because they make everything seem to smooth and easy. But one day, when for some reason they are abruptly unavailable, there must always be someone in readiness to step into their shoes, however hard they are to fill. As showbiz says famously, the show must go on.

Documentation of the host of ongoing activities is always a challenge and has remained one through the three decades plus of the IPH existence. There is never enough money to pay separately for researchers and documenters and scribes; yet, research and records are the only assurance that work is remembered till posterity, and efforts have to be taken to maintain accurate records. Media usage has simplified things a little, and also made for more transparency and accountability.

Planning activities in the 155 plus verticals that now exist in the IPH portfolio is no mean task, and delegation of work is a must. The answer will always lie in every member of the organization feeling as responsible for every task on hand, and a strong work ethic, a sense of accountability and constant search for excellence will ensure the long life of the institution.

Another challenge is to create a footprint that is National and International, while most activities of the institute are local and state level, largely in the local language Marathi. The pandemic helped ensure that interested people living abroad could participate in many of the online trainings. The innate resilience of the Institute caused it to flounder far less than most other similar organizations during the pandemic, although all activities did take a hit, and there were financial setbacks, which are now largely made up.

Philosophy

The philosophy of IPH is summarized in the motto, mental health for all. The unwritten bit is that it is "mental health by, with and for all". Mental health care need not be limited to only treating illness. Rather, it has to be about promoting wellness. Thus, awareness and prevention form a large part of the day to day activities of IPH. The trajectory starts from awareness, leads to involvement and then participation until empowerment is achieved.

Every activity under the rubric of mental health activity has to be embodied as a social enterprise, a thriving, self-sustaining activity which is not just about profit making, but which looks after the welfare of service users as well as service providers, so that both remain motivated to carry on this activity which will ultimately contribute to community and society building. Funds generated from industry and community programmes can sustain subsidies to support groups and other free community events, as well as low-cost services.

Publications, creative writing, newspaper columns, film making, viewing and discussion, public lectures and live discussions, plays and music programmes can crossbreed and create a synergy, an energy source to motivate young professionals and keep community interest in mental health alive.

Activities that apparently have different thrust foci, such as psychiatric illness, addiction and its management (Nadkarni, 2015), management of physical health, lifestyle and nutrition, child and parent well-being, educational and research enterprise, and many others can all find common ground in order to achieve a pre-decided goal: That of mental health for all.

To quote from a 3-year-old issue of *Manas*, the IPH newsletter which reinvented itself from hard copy to a virtual format:

"By believing passionately in something that still does not exist, we create it. The non-existent is whatever we have not sufficiently desired" (Nikos Kazantzakis, nineteenth century Greek writer).

Acknowledgements The author acknowledges inputs and suggestions by Dr. Anand Nadkarni and Dr. Shubha Thatte, Founder Trustees of Institute for Psychological Health.

References

Apte, S. (2018). *Roj Navi Suruvaat* (Marathi: A new beginning every day) Manovikas Prakashan.

Green, R., Mitchell, P. F., Lee, K., Svensson, E., Toh, J-W., Barentsen, C., Copeland, M., Newton, J. R., Hawke, K. C., & Brophy, L. (2019). Key SPIES ET AL. 451 features of an innovative sub-acute residential service for young people experiencing mental ill health. *BMC Psychiatry*, 19, 311. https://doi.org/10.1186/s12888-019-2303-4

McGorry, P., Bates, T., & Birchwood, M. (2013). Designing youth mental health services for the 21st century: Examples from Australia, Ireland and the UK. *British Journal of Psychiatry Supplement, 54*, s30–s35. https://doi.org/10.1192/bjp.bp.112.119214

Nadkarni, A. (2015). *Muktipatre (Marathi: Letters of deliverance)*. Akshar Prakashan.

Nadkarni, A. (2016). *Manovikas* (Marathi). Akshar Prakashan.

Paul Hamlyn Foundation India IPH projects. https://www.phf.org.uk/grants/?select-region_country%5B0%5D=india&current-page=13

Sovani, A. (2009). *Shubharthis* in India: Destigmatizing schizophrenia, a move towards Inclusion. In C. Marshall (Ed.) *Disabilities, insights from across fields and around the world*. Praeger Press

Sovani, A. (2019a). Mental health management in low resource settings. *In Ms. How and Me.* Chapter 30. Notion Press

Sovani, A. (2019b). Triggering conversations about mental health. In *Nation-building, education and culture in India and Canada*. Springer.

Subramaniam, S. (2008). *Of human bonds: The Maitra story*. IPH Publication.

Wandrekar, J., Nigudkar, A., Thatte, S., & Sovani, A. (2016). Successful aging and self perceptions, *Bombay Psychologist, 31*(1 and 2), 1–4.

Chapter 17
Destitution, Mental Illness and Law: Issues, Challenges and Possibilities

Mohd. Tarique

Abstract A sizable number of destitute live on the streets and many suffer from mental health issues. Some end up on the streets after either being abandoned by the family or as a result of wandering around in the state of illness, while others developed illness due to the extreme abuses faced on the hostile street. The State mechanism, i.e., legal framework to address homeless persons with mental illness is about first turning them invisible and then punishing under Beggary laws. If homeless are vulnerable, more vulnerable are the homeless people with mental illness. Even more vulnerable are those mentally ill homeless who are caught under beggary laws. At present, anti-beggary laws exist in more than 20 states and two Union Territories. The features of these anti-beggary laws in different states are almost similar. Almost all states criminalize mental illness as the term 'beggar' has been defined in such a manner that 'homeless mentally ill' person wandering about is legally considered a 'beggar' and therefore punished. Person arrested under the Beggary Law can be kept in custody for a period ranging from 1 to 10 years and for an indefinite period under special circumstances. Most civil interventions too exclude people by its design. Koshish has been working to end this criminalization of mental illness. Following 'Systems Approach', organization collaborates with the state in offering rehabilitation services while opposing them on law. Over the years, thousands have been supported but more importantly, the intervention has demonstrated an alternative and is impacting policy-level reforms. Koshish is not an expert on mental health but it has managed to make these institutions visible. Basing its interventions on fundamental needs of empathy and compassion, Koshish has established that institutions of mental health are not the only ones that need reforms.

Keywords Koshish · Mental illness · Law and destitution

Mohd. Tarique (✉)
Koshish, Tata Institute of Social Sciences, Mumbai, India
e-mail: tarique.tiss@gmail.com

M. Anand (ed.), *Mental Health Care Resource Book*,
https://doi.org/10.1007/978-981-97-1203-8_17

Understanding Homelessness

There are a large number of people who are forced to live on the streets. They are the most visible yet the most invisible residents of our cities. We see them on an everyday basis but rarely acknowledge their existence and that is how they remain invisible to us. They remain as invisible from our vision as from the policies and programmes. The terms 'we' and 'us' here are used both for the state as well as the citizens. There are a range of reasons how and why people end up being on the streets and live a life of destitution. Some of the key reasons remain distress migration, breaking down of families, failed relationships, employment requirements, caste-based violence, natural disasters, development projects, failed agriculture, historical practices and traditions like with several denotified tribes, health factors including mental illnesses or disabilities. These are just a few reasons to mention here.

For the homeless, life, on the streets is extremely tough and vulnerable, full of exploitation and abuse. What remains common to most of these people is the enhanced vulnerability and absence of structural support to overcome those vulnerabilities. Worst, most of these people face a legal response that further pushes them down and deeper into the cycles of helplessness and destitution.

Most Indian states, at least 24 of them have laws on beggary that penalize the state of destitution. The features of these anti-beggary laws in different states are almost similar. Broadly, all are criminalizing in nature, where people, irrespective of their physical, economic, and psychological condition are arrested and punished for begging.

The way beggary has been defined in most of these laws, anyone wandering about aimlessly (read person with mental illness) or appears to be living off alms (read most elderly or persons with disability), pretending to be selling articles or performing arts (read certain de-notified tribes giving street performances, acrobatics etc.) is technically considered a 'beggar' and therefore be liable for penal action under the law. The people who need state's assistance, who need to be protected, taken care of and who need treatment are made to serve the sentence under these anti-beggary laws.

Mental Health, Homelessness and Law

For the homeless, life on the streets is extremely tough and abusive; full of exploitation and hostility. The worst affected within the homeless population are probably those suffering with mental health issues; their vulnerability is much higher. Despite having severe mental health-related issues, they have extremely limited or no access to treatment.

Many people end up on the streets after either being abandoned by the family or as a result of wandering around in the state of illness, while others may have developed mental illness due to the extreme forms of abuse and violence encountered while living on the streets.

The worst affected are those mentally ill homeless people who are caught under the beggary law. Section 17.2 i (d) of the Act, while defining what 'Begging' means, says, 'having no visible means of subsistence and wandering about or remaining in any public place in such condition or manner, as makes it likely that the person doing so exist by soliciting or receiving alms'. This one clause is enough to get any person with mental illness or even otherwise, arrested.

The law provides for detention ranging from 1 year to a 10-year period as punishment for begging with 1–3 years detention for first-time offence and 3–10 years for repeat offence. Also, under special circumstances, if Superintendent of the Certified Home concludes that the person is incurably helpless and would not be able to come out of begging, this detention could be extended for indefinite period after a Special Appeal process. Speaking specifically in the context of mental illness, most people would run the risk of an indefinite detention. With no control on their illness, it is certain that they would be punished as 'repeat-offenders'. So, a person with mental illness who is detained for 1 year for wandering around aimlessly, can be sentenced for any period of detention upto 10 years for 'having not recovered' from illness and further be detained for a life time.

Sadly, this life time detention is done as a favour to the person. The assumption here is that the person does not have a way to sustain himself/herself and therefore state grants sanction for his/her stays in a custodial institution for an indefinite period. What remains ambiguous here is legal identity that is created/maintained while granting this; person lives in a custodial institution as an offender. Most homeless persons with mental illnesses are at risk of being processed under this clause. If the aim is to provide relief and care, why does state need to detain such persons in institutions that are custodial in nature? Why can the state not provide for voluntary centres where care and treatment with efforts made at rehabilitation?

The legal status of a person sent to Beggars Homes is that of an offender who is sent to the institution to serve the detention period. Therefore, often the person is not put on the required treatment. Once the detention period is over, the person is released out of the institution gates. With nowhere to go mostly and no control on one's life as a result of increased illness or helplessness, person is back on the street, with higher vulnerability and greater possibilities of abuse and exploitation.

Koshish—Civil Society Experiment

Koshish was initiated by Tata Institute of Social Sciences, Mumbai as its field action project as a response to this criminalization of destitution happening in the form of Beggary Prevention Legislations. Different situations of vulnerabilities are processed under these laws as offences. Persons with Mental Illness, Elderly and abandoned, disabled, persons from de-notified communities, transgender, persons affected with leprosy etc. are all included and the way beggary has been defined, all these categories of people technically become Beggars who can be arrested. It was to oppose and end this 'criminalization of poverty' that Koshish came into being for.

Approach: Following 'Systems Approach' and collaborative practice, Koshish has intervened to demonstrate the strong community-based rehab model that can be followed upon once law is repealed. It is important to create support system for the community and for that, Koshish has attempted to build alliances and networked with a large number of agencies working on issues of urban poverty or allied areas.

Started in Mumbai in 2006, programme expanded to Delhi in 2009 and in 2012, it was extended to Bihar. With the firm belief in 'Systems Approach', project has worked in collaboration with the states through the custodial institutions and civil society organizations through community-based intervention, with efforts to facilitate rehabilitation of persons processed under the Beggary Law, bringing overall change in custodial conditions and facilitating people's exit from state of destitution.

Koshish offers whole range of programmes and services right from the street outreach to legal aid to people processed under Beggary law to sensitization of different government agencies to capacity building to advocacy for policy changes and reforms. Amidst several other programmes, Koshish works extensively with persons with mental health issues. There are two crucial intervention models that Koshish has developed based on its experience with this population over the years. Both the models are based on fundamental need and capacity of every human being; need to be loved and accepted and compassion and empathy to understand other person's suffering and pain.

Based on the belief that every person deserves a life of dignity, these models have challenged the convention structures and shown extremely satisfying changes. One model is implemented at the institutional level where people with mental illness are brought to beggar homes and spend their detention period. The other model is carried out with homeless clusters in the communities where we work with. In the following paragraphs, we will unpack both the interventions and attempt to understand how both these models can easily be replicated for different locations and profile of people simply because of the principles of engagement that these interventions follow as design.

(a) My Space—Institutional Care Model: This is Koshish's intervention in the custodial institutions. The concept of 'My Space' revolves around the inner strength and capabilities of the person. The intervention draws its strength from fundamental nature and need of human beings. People display tremendous grit to fight the odds and survival instincts. While working in these institutions, we saw a completely different side of human existence.

The extremes of lives people on streets live with are very disturbing. 'My Space' programme has its roots in the disturbing life story of one such female client that we worked with several years ago. Waheeda (name changed) had been in the Beggars Home for more than 8 years when Koshish social worker first met her. She was about 35 years old then. She informed that she has lived her entire life in the institutions. She was a child with polio below her waist and was abandoned at some point of time that she did not remember very clearly. All she remembered was about staying at a child care institution for about 10 years till she grew into an adult and was shifted to another shelter home for women. She was in that institution for about 6–7 years and then lived on streets for couple of years before being brought to Beggars Home under the Beggary Prevention Law.

Those who are aware of custodial institutions and their functioning would know and understand the control and discipline that govern the lives of people there. The control is exercised to such an extent that every aspect of one's life is decided by the set rules and control of the authorities; so much so that things like sleep or eating are also decided by the authorities. The realization that someone had been living her entire life in this manner where minutest choices are also not made by her was very unsettling. While sharing her experience of staying in different institutions she spoke about how she wouldn't be allowed to sleep outside the hours allocated for sleeping. Even for sitting in the barracks, people had to follow caregivers' instructions. One wondered how could someone live entire life under such fear and control; the loss of agency of self and individuality with prolonger stay in institutions could literally make a person lifeless. Something had to be done to alter this.

This disturbance is what caused the birth of 'My Space'. This was conceived as a place that would allow some degree of freedom and space for self-determination within the custodial setup.

Thanks to a sensitive official, when this concept was shared with the authorities, it was not only agreed upon, directions were also issued for the required administrative changes. Within the larger custodial environment, this one barrack was dedicated to this initiative that was started as an experiment but grew into one of the core interventions and catalyst in the rehabilitation process.

'My Space' is a specially created space within the Certified Institution where people experience the joy of being themselves, being free. We have this special barrack where residents come for a fixed period every day and engage themselves in the activities of their choice. Though we have a structured training and educational programme running but largely it depends on the wish of the residents. They do whatever they wish for: sing, dance, run, play, sleep or simply not do anything. No one tells them what they should be doing. For these few hours when these residents are at 'My Space', they are not governed by the rules of the institution but their likings and choices. Whole idea of this place is to ensure freedom and space of choice not just in physical sense but also emotionally and psychologically. In their otherwise controlled lives, 'My Space' became a part that was theirs, that did not require any permissions, that did not bring any control or directions. One could leave everything behind and just do what heart desired.

People usually say that persons with mental illness are dangerous…they get wild…have no sense of what they do and so on. The fact is that they understand life far better, they understand relations in a most unpretentious way, they value another person, a smile is enough to make them trust you. They love you more than you would love them.

The response to the 'My Space' has been phenomenon, way beyond what we expected. We started this experiment simply to break the control that was exercised on the lives of people but it turned out to have much deeper impact. We experienced that women would simply want to sleep, especially on their first few days of coming to 'My Space'. We realized it was the absence of fear of being beaten up or reprimanded for sleeping at odd hours. It was also a painful reminder of how custody deprives people of things as basic as 'sleep'. Women would start with sleeping but gradually start engaging with different activities. It is here that many women had their first interactions with fellow residents of the institutions.

'My Space' ensured an environment where there was no fear and that triggered recovery for large number of women. Many women who had not spoken or shared anything for several years began to speak. They started recalling their past; they started hoping for a different future. Simply by removing fear Koshish was able to make people regain control on their lives. Once they started revisiting their past, many women were able to recall their families, the addresses and so on. Those who needed psychiatric intervention, showed willingness to get treated and once on medication, results were surprisingly quicker; the healing was much faster and organic.

So far 'My Space' has facilitated reintegration of several hundred men and women into their families; many of them after more than a decade. An extremely simple concept, based on love and compassion, coupled with necessary treatment, My Space has resulted in recovery and rehabilitation of such cases that were thought to be untreatable. Simply by accepting people the way they are, showing that they matter and offering them human warmth, 'My Space' has been able to counter the ill effects of years of illness, abuse and neglect.

While it is unfortunate truth that many families dump these people, especially women for treatment at hospitals and then, never return, we also met families who left the ill person after going through deep turmoil and crisis for survival. They reached a point where looking after mentally ill person became unaffordable in several ways, not just financially. 'My Space' enabled us to support such families in supporting their family members. It has been an extremely fulfilling learning where we understood how absence of comprehensive mental health care system is resulting in families abandoning patients in the family. Unfortunately, this vital reality gets shadowed in the hype of stigma and awareness aspects. While stigma and awareness around mental illness remain key factors, it is time to accept that availability, access, and affordability of mental health care facilities is much bigger reality.

What keeps this programme relevant even after a decade and half, is the inner strength that all of us possess as humans. Despite mental illness, people can build new relations, they are able to reciprocate warmth and affection extended to them. They might be incoherent or fail to remember their past life and families, they have the capacity to build new ones.

With little support, they can start anew. We are witness to their capacities in doing that. The patience and faith that they have in relations is tremendous, their belief in human goodness is unbelievable.

(b) Ehsaas—Community-Based Care Model: It is scary to see the high prevalence of mental health issues within the communities living on the streets. Though it is not at all surprising given the excessive level of abuse, exploitation, and stress that people on the streets are forced to live with. Given the complexity of the people facing the double jeopardy of homelessness and mental illness, comprehensive intervention was required.

Ehsaas is the extension of the work, Koshish has already been doing with institutional setups in different states. Ehsaas was initiated with specific focus and goal of addressing widespread prejudices around mental illness and develop a mechanism that addresses the mental health issues with a prevention approach. While the broader goal is to address the issues homeless communities face regarding mental health, idea is to facilitate their daily struggles vis a vis citizenship including their engagement with the state and thereby reduce the factors that cause or trigger mental health issues.

With this intervention, we implement the community-based programmes to address different vulnerabilities of the homeless population. The idea is to address mental health issues through range of other services that impact the vulnerabilities and therefore the mental health.

Stigma and discrimination toward individuals experiencing mental disorders is a pattern all over. However, with homeless population, this gets worse because of the Beggary law where illness itself is treated as an offence. Further, state action like evictions or exclusion from scope of government schemes adds to their plight. Life becomes an everyday struggle where survival itself becomes a challenge. The resultant stress and pressure often break down people but unfortunately, there is very little or no support available for people to cope or address this pressure. Denial of services comes largely from the denial of identity amounting to denial of existence. This intervention aims to break this feeling of 'being unwanted' or 'being a burden' a message that is constantly communicated to homeless citizens. The community project aims to change this experience of 'being unwanted' that homeless communities live all through and build a narrative that they are not only 'not unwanted' but play a constructive role in running or functioning of our cities.

Often the early signs of illness either go unnoticed or the families have no resources or access to seek treatment. Also, the access to treatment is affected by the stigma attached with mental illness. This is where Koshish wanted to build a strong community-level prevention programme. We not only wanted to break this stigma but also build community-level volunteers who understand key aspects of mental health and work towards ensuring healthy mental health for the members of the cluster through the mental health responders.

We run community support programmes with the homeless clusters with focus on youth. While the end goal is to address mental illness, the design focuses on mitigating the factors that often cause distress and may trigger mental health issues. Ehsaas is a set of comprehensive services offered in the community, with various groups, trying to check and reduce the vulnerabilities they are faced with. It includes education programme for children, vocational training and support with livelihood, mentorship for youth, sessions on gender equality, developing peer-support group, legal assistance in interface with police/municipal actions, facilitation for citizenship entitlements like banking services, voter cards, health services, pensions etc. The ultimate purpose for this community intervention is to spread mental health well-being within the homeless population.

Some of the key aspects of community intervention are:

a. **Counselling**: Primary support that the intervention offers the communities is professional counselling that enables people to deal better with the issues and complications. This is not restricted to medical situations but acts as a broader support available to community where it feels supported and cared for. Counsellor also works towards deconstructing the mental health and how it is understood within the communities.
b. **Peer Support Group**: We began with forming a collective of persons, especially women who were trained in identifying early signs of illness. These people now anchor as 'Peer Support group' that not only spreads awareness about the issue but also facilitates other community members' access to care services whenever there is a need. Most importantly, this group of community volunteers prevents any sort of violence facing persons with mental health issues in the community.
c. **Education**: Children are the worst victim where not only the present but future is also ruined. With parents facing crisis, children are forced to beg or live as destitute or unguided lives, getting thrown into lives of uncertainty and anxiety. The trauma caused due to the life they live is bound to cause severe mental health issues. Also, children are exposed to violent situations at a very early age while living on streets. Fear, uncertainty, violence, deprivation; everything contributes and adds to their difficult and often disrupted upbringing.

   Children's education is a crucial aspect of this framework. Education is used as a tool to address this situation. It has worked to a large extent and provides these children with a real opportunity and acts as a barrier for mental illness. Due to the historical factors as well as the socio-economic situation of the present, children from these communities are deprived from receiving education. Education is one certain way that has changed the lives of children who were mostly forced into destitution.

   There are many children from the communities that have traditionally been into vocations of selling small articles or rag picking. Once children are prepared to cope up and adjust with the mainstream education, they are admitted into government schools for formal education. We continue to offer support classes so that children adjust well in the regular schooling. Working closely with teachers and school administration is another crucial aspect of this intervention. This is done in order to ensure that children are treated respectfully and with care.
d. **Livelihood**: Absence of stable and socially acceptable livelihood has been identified as one key factor causing stress and anxiety in homeless communities. The uncertainty about employment often pushes people into alcohol and other kind of substance abuse. Ehsaas focuses on creating the opportunities for livelihood for the community people, especially the youth. This includes vocational training, special inputs whenever required and career guidance and facilitation. We also work towards facilitating independent working or self-initiatives.
e. **Capacity Building Through Relevant Training and Life Skills**: For persons affected with mental health issues, vocational training and life skills serve as factors that reduce families 'resistance towards the person's acceptance in family.

The purpose therefore is to provide certain life skills that build person's capacity to handle threats and pressures of staying within the family setup.

We have developed a process that involves a cycle where first a person is prepared mentally to get ready to work and earn livelihood. This is also the phase where one's emotional stability is assessed and social skills are developed. This is then supplemented by trainings with life skills, which enable the person to deal effectively with the challenges of everyday life.

f. **Facilitating Access to Government Schemes**: There are several existing schemes that should have been extended to homeless communities. However, people's inability to fight the resistance from systems created for delivery of those services results in constant exclusion and marginalization. Community programme focuses towards increasing the access to government services and schemes, (especially health, education, and elderly care).
g. **Sanitation and Living Environment**: As part of the community intervention, one of the goals has been to motivate the community to improve their living surroundings. While there is a clear neglect that the community faces from the authorities, leading to the unhygienic conditions, there has also been a need for the community to take more responsibility. Improved sanitation and living environment have resulted in better health in the community.
h. **Health Referrals**: Health is one of the first compromise that a homeless person makes. In many cases, situation is such that any long-term intervention can be initiated only after immediate health situation has been addressed. Therefore, health referrals are one of the primary components. This is done by leveraging government facilities shouldering the responsibility with better access to health services.
i. **Emergency Support to Families**: Often we have seen that family's own condition is extremely weak and vulnerable and they are unable to take care of ill person despite the willingness to do that. Family might be all caring and concerned about its person but may have very limited or no capacity to support the treatment. Also, there are incidents that create serious survival issues for the family. In such situation, we reach out to family and offer support to take care of emergency. This includes emotional support, connecting with relevant agencies or financial support (towards medicines, food, travel etc.). First effort, however, is to get them support through government systems.
j. **Recreational Programme**: Recreational Programme assumes far greater significance in the context of the depressing environment of the community sites and the abusive background that most people face. The recreational activities are intended to facilitate client's social skills and repair the emotional strains that he or she may have suffered. Through these programmes, we convey understanding, acceptance, and support for the homeless persons.
k. **Institutional Placement**: All possible attempts are made to reintegrate the abandoned/destitute clients with their families wherever possible. However, there are situations when family no more remains an option for the client to return to. This is due to various reasons. In some cases, families are unwilling to accept them while in other clients do not want to return to their families. Few clients do

not have any family at all, while still others are there who do not remember the details of the family to be traced back.

In such situations, institutional placement comes up as an effective alternative, especially for women, unless the person is capable enough of independent living. So, we develop individual plan according to specific needs (training, employment, temporary shelter, medical care etc.) and shift them in shelter homes or institutions catering to those needs.

Relevance for 'Systems Approach'

Despite being a small organization, Koshish has been able to create successful impact both at the field intervention as well as policy changes. This has been possible due to the 'Systems Approach' practised by the organization. We needed a strategy through which we would reach to the maximum people possible. Government structures are certainly the best resource in this regard. Civil Society Organizations and passionate individuals can and have been making significant impact but the problem that we are faced with is huge. Response, too, needed to be in accordance.

We may evolve best practices but it is extremely difficult for any single organization to reach out to every person requiring support. Most thought-out and successful approach might fail to address the need as the scale and numbers go up. The issue of mental health is complex and must not be addressed as tokenism and therefore even to think of the alternatives, continued and sustained efforts are essential and this sort of continuity is possible with the committed and serious government involvement.

The issue with the government, despite having the required resources, is the lack of personal investment and compassion in their execution of programmes. This investing of self is as critical as any other resources, rather it is more crucial. Government systems, unfortunately, lack personal and humane approach, at least mostly, if not always.

Answer lies in the union of the two. Civil society groups evolve the strategy/approach and then government collaborating and ensuring that it is adopted as part of its programme and covers the entire population needing support. This is exactly what Koshish followed. We work closely with state government as well as central government in order to create enabling programmes for the homeless and destitute citizens. In fact, all our programmes are being implemented in partnership with state governments.

Many of us have our reservations when it comes to working with the government setup. It may not be without reasons also. Experience has been that though government talks of partnership, in actual, relationship is rarely of equality. For an effective and healthy partnership to evolve, equality is central requirement. Unfortunately, this is where government tends to go wrong.

Secondly, and more obvious one, is the difference of approach, positions, and philosophies. People involved in NGOs are largely driven by their passion and sense of affection towards the people suffering and this is where they find it difficult to relate with the government institutions as partners.

Now, this is what we must work towards to break. Civil society needs to trust the government and vice versa. We must realize that there are certain cores which should remain non-negotiable but broader flexibility must be there to accept each other as partners working for a common cause.

Compassion and skills of the Civil Society Organizations coupled with the resources and machinery that the government has can produce wonders. We must work together provided both government as well as NGO partners share equal authority and responsibilities. Government must realize that it is not only the resources that matter when it comes to the rehabilitation. To address the needs for mental health care, one needs very high degree of skills and motivation. The expertise and the skills that social workers bring in must be acknowledged and valued by the government.

Through our experience at Koshish, we can say it is possible. We have been supported and encouraged by some extremely beautiful officers in the different institutions governed by the state. Be it civil hospital, beggars' home, or regional mental hospital, everywhere we have found officers who invested themselves thoroughly, gave their best and ensured that the required support was made available.

We are not the experts in mental health but we are linking up various institutions of government and ensuring that unavailability of support groups should not mean unavailability of treatment for these people. We are opposing the beggary law but at the same time, engaging with the government helping them understand the futility of continuing the draconian legislation on beggary. We need to work towards creating an environment where the resistance for each other is replaced with acceptance, common understanding and shared compassion for our people.

Investing in Youth

One of the core strengths of the organization has been its 'Youth Engagement' programme. If organization has succeeded in reaching out to significantly high numbers, it was, to great extent, because of our young 'Friends of Koshish', as they are called. In our engagement with youth, we attempt to build them into strong support for the cause but more importantly, develop them into citizens with compassion and acceptance for the poor.

We have consciously invested in youth as we involve them as ambassadors for our work. We want them to change the narrative around homelessness where apathy and neglect rule the description. We reach out to the youth in multiple ways including through orientation sessions/talks in colleges and universities, special night walks, internships and volunteer opportunities. While their immediate form of engagement is through activities related to our direct work, there is constant dialogue on values that matter. Youth, equipped with values of compassion and empathy are the best bet for bringing any kind of change towards inclusive world. Koshish considers it a responsibility to engage and invest in young people where the fears are removed, ground realities exposed, doubts cleared and decision left on them.

An extension of youth engagement is team building process. It is important to understand that given the extremes homeless people go through in life, dealing with their situation is not easy for the staff/personnel dealing with them and it is essential that strong system is built for their support as well. Koshish invests significantly in supporting its teams and ensures the best mechanisms of support for them legally, financially, and emotionally.

Call for Solidarity

Lives of the homeless citizens with mental illness are often cornered due to the widely prevalent biases, apprehensions and stigma attached with the mental illness. Largely seen as unproductive and difficult to work with, this is the population that needs extended period of support as compared to any other settled group since their capacity to adjust is lesser, learning is slower and abuse is far more devastating and traumatizing. However, with serious and constant efforts, with adequate individual planning, assessing person's strength and personality, chances for stable rehabilitation grow manifold.

Empathy and Compassion is all that we need to trigger the change. Rest everything follows. There is a lot of credibility that the organization has built through its continuous work and display of results. It has shown to the government that it is possible to rehabilitate without punishing and criminalizing them. While we fight the states criminalizing people's vulnerabilities, we also do not want them to be in that situation of vulnerability. With the social capital that the organization has successfully built over the years, there is a real possibility of leveraging that to build strong support for the cause. Idea is to connect with as many stakeholders as possible and educate them on the realities of the life that homeless people are forced to live.

Mental health is not our forte but what we have managed to do is that we have made these institutions visible. We have brought out the fact that institutions of mental health are not the only ones that we need to look at while addressing or providing for mental health care needs. People who had been removed and taken out of sight, we have brought them back and hope that more effective intervention is carried out by the people who know it best. We seek support and collaboration from every possible agency that can help restore dignity into the lives of homeless persons.

We all must continue with our efforts, in whatever form, whatever manner. Whatever strategy or approach we might follow; we must walk together to ensure the availability of our collective strength.

Fight must be kept on!

Chapter 18
Embrace All.... No Labels Attached: Reflections by OYA Foundation

Raheen Jummani

Abstract The present chapter provides experiential insights from 'Open Your Arms Foundation' (OYA), an organization dedicated to Mental Health that focuses on a holistic approach by providing psychological counselling/therapy, remedial education, workshops and training. It traces the initial journey of OYA when the main challenge was to mitigate the taboo against mental health and familiarize everyone with the concept of mental well-being. Through case vignettes, the chapter endeavours to illustrate few success stories about OYA's creative approaches that had an enormous impact on the lives of the clients. It also covers the unique and budding project *Pankh* and another new initiative *OYA's Changmakers* comprising of the alumni with the ideology of paying it forward; giving to the society what they received in their testing times.

Keywords Mental health · Therapy · OYA foundation

> Started the expedition towards the unknown as a lone traveller, but along the way, kept meeting people and the ensemble kept growing: Akela hi chala tha jaanib e manzil magar, log saath aate gaye aur karvan banta gaya – Majrooh Sultanpuri.

The journey of learning and experimenting started way back with a thought of repaying to the society the warmth it has bestowed in abundance. The notion of making mental health services available to all no matter what age, class, religious background and no matter what social status emerged as the need of the hour.

After learning psychology and understanding the concept of human behaviour, the perception that mental health services are required by each and every individual at some point in their lifetime became more evident. Working with several NGOs for more than 7 years (2002–2009) who cater to different population, from different strata of the society; we realized the need for mental health services to be easily available. With this mindset, we came up with the idea of developing a mental health service centre. Through loads of brainstorming, discussions, analysis and understanding, we came to a conclusion that if we develop a centre, our services will be confined between

---

R. Jummani (✉)
OYA Foundation, Mumbai, India
e-mail: raheenjummani@gmail.com

M. Anand (ed.), *Mental Health Care Resource Book*,
https://doi.org/10.1007/978-981-97-1203-8_18

four walls and our vision to maximize our reach will be faded. It will be difficult for the marginalized population to come down to one centre from their nooks. This led to the conceptualization of an NGO, having a team of mental health professionals and other support staffs who cater to the mental well-being of the people; especially focusing on the marginalized population and other weaker sections of the society who are often left unheard.

We knew and we understood that for certain sections of the society mental health services were readily available but for some population it was far from reach. Firstly, these services were not easily available to the marginalized group and secondly, it is not affordable to them. That's how the idea of an NGO model came into picture to provide subsidized or free services to the weaker population. If they need counselling it is available here, if they need therapy, it is available here. We had the intent; we had the idea but what should we name our setup? Took us weeks of discussions with our mentors and core group of people—we believed in the power of the hug which acts as a symbol of acceptance—the power of accepting people without hesitation towards their backgrounds and standard of living. The name 'Open Your Arms Foundation' was then coined with a simple ideology of accepting people unconditionally and embracing them truly. The expedition began in 2010.

The focus population of Open Your Arms Foundation are children, youths and teenagers so we thought that it can also be a fundoo name which the focus group would really like. When we introduced this name to our beneficiaries, they gave it a very cool and happening acronym 'OYA' foundation.

Open Your Arms Foundation is an organization dedicated to Mental Health, which focuses on working with different population and people belonging to different strata. Catering to the society by providing psychological counselling/therapy, remedial education, workshops and training. It works with an integrated approach, having a unique model—a combination of psycho-therapies and creative therapies.

'Mens sana in corpore sano'—'A healthy mind in a healthy body', having staunch credence in this phrase we laid the foundation of our organization's vision and mission statements.

Vision—Psychologically empowering every individual with learning and coping capabilities to lead a mentally healthy life.

Mission—Create a child-friendly environment in the society by using simple and creative methods to bring out the best in children, adolescents, youths, adults; and help them deal with various issues they face in contemporary society and family life.

The vision and mission are to create and help sustain a child-friendly and mentally healthy environment. To achieve this, along with children, the organization works in conjunction with their support system consisting of family members, caregivers, teaching and other staffs where children reside in child-care homes. When we work with the children or teenagers, it is pivotal to work with their support system as we cannot help the children in isolation. Hence, Open Your Arms Foundation works with the entire support system of a child. If a child is in school, we work with the teachers, staff, the principal, the management and the parents. If a child lives in a child-care institution we also work with the care-takers, guardians, social workers and the staff members of the child-care institution.

In the initial years, the main challenge was to mitigate the taboo against mental health and familiarize everyone with the concept of mental well-being. The emphasis was to bring the receptors to a stage where they can easily speak. This was done by shaking the shackles of denial. Our area of services also comprises of handling traumatic repercussions resulting from child-sexual abuse and rape. It is a strenuous task to make the survivors regain their confidence, understand their self-worth and build their self-esteem.

Our perspective is to initiate counselling therapies through group sessions, which in-turn leads to individual sessions. A group session helps to create a non-threatening environment releasing an aura that all the children are in the same boat and boosting them to be a part of individual sessions where the detailed case history can be ascertained.

We call our team as the 'Band of Believers' because we strongly trust in the quote 'Believe it achieve it!'. A usual day at OYA starts with positive affirmations to ourselves as our healing is also one of the priorities. This is followed by understanding the focus group, and when we want to understand the audience, we cannot go with set thought process and own titles; it involves planning the sessions, choosing the best creative therapy or psychotherapy with flexibility in our mind towards change as we work in a dynamic environment. Our tasks continue with conducting sessions, documentation, discussions and sharing with other team members or mentors, feedback sessions and moving forward with the lessons learnt. We never leave without paying gratitude to our team members and ourselves. Each one in our organization competes with their own self at individual level for self-growth and at the same time motivates their companions in the squad. Mental wellness starts with you first, we have regular counselling therapy and training sessions for our team members as well. Self-introspection and self-talk are highly encouraged at OYA as it helps us to understand ourselves better which in turn aids in healing others. The spirit of 'Believe it achieve it' not only runs in our team but is also imbibed by our beneficiaries; one such life story of our alumna is expressed in her words:

> Believe it ... achieve it', is the way I think about my life and work daily.
>
> I am Annie (name changed to maintain confidentiality), 28 years old OYA's 'Belie-Chiever'. Today I am glad, that I got this opportunity to write about my life, thanks to the OYA Foundation. This is a 'wow moment' for me, not just because I would like my story to be told and heard, but because I would like to inspire every girl with my story and to have the spirit to achieve their dreams.
>
> I belong to a lower middle-class family. My mother worked as a household maid and currently my father is an auto-rickshaw driver. I have two siblings. I completed my schooling from a BMC school. I used to get scholarship for my education from an NGO. I have been able to complete my education through scholarships alone as we faced financial difficulties. In the past, my mother was the only earning member of my family for a long time and my father stayed in the village for farming. My mother carried out all the financial responsibilities towards me and my siblings single-handedly. My mother came from a small village and could not complete her education. She could only study till the 3rd grade and got married at a very young age, after which her life has just been a series of constant struggles - struggles

for fulfilling the responsibilities of her family, for taking care of her children, for attaining her rights, for almost everything. What got her through all her struggles was a strong desire to help her children complete their education and make them capable individuals who could achieve anything they dream of in life.

Very often, you find the young generation looking up to an actor or a sportsperson as their idol in life. However, my idols have been the heroes in my real life rather than the 'reel life'. The first one to play that role in my life has been my mother. She always teaches me to think big and motivate myself to win. I remember, accompanying my mother to her work along with my siblings when I was about 9–10 years old. She would clean utensils, wash clothes and cook food for other people and at the same time have us around at work and look after us; as it was out of question for her to leave us alone at home where we lived. I never felt ashamed of the work my mother did. She always taught us that no work was inferior or superior and that one must have love and respect towards their work.

I was a bright student throughout my school and college. I worked hard and did well at school despite all obstacles. Complaining was never an option. As hard work always pays off, I always found help through scholarships to continue my studies. Throughout my schooling years, I took part in many cultural activities and social activities. I was always excited about my hobbies of dancing, singing, acting, and anchoring.

The turning point of my life was when I changed my school in the 7th grade. I attended after-school classes, where I met with **my second Idol and my role model: my Counsellor Didi, my teacher and my mentor**. She came into my life like an Angel who helped me achieve every dream I ever dreamt of in my life. Some people come into your life as blessings and she has definitely been a blessing for me.

It was Counsellor Didi who recognized the potential in me and gave me several opportunities to showcase my talent to the society. She gave my hobbies a purpose and helped me bloom with her guidance, love and care. When I was in the 9th grade, she had faith in my abilities and gave me the opportunity to anchor an important event on the occasion of Navratri for the very first time in my life, and that too in the presence of the Minister of Child and Women Health Care, who appreciated my abilities and felicitated me. That was a very proud moment for me and Counsellor Didi. It was only because of her support that this was possible for me. She always encouraged me to do something extraordinary and creative that would help me explore myself. She was with me for about five years; but those five years meant the world to me and I enjoyed every bit of that time with her. She plays a major role in my life to help me achieve all my dreams and goals. She is not my biological mother, but our relationship is as special as that of a mother and daughter. She gave birth to the new phase of my life. Under her constant love and care, I grew from a sapling and became a beautiful plant. When I was studying in the 10th grade, Counsellor Didi gave me an opportunity to be the voice of a female fetus in a mother's womb in a short film made for spreading the social message of 'Save the Girl Child'. I received such a wonderful opportunity because of her. She has been a constant support in my life. She has always given me the courage to get out of my shell and try the things I never thought of doing. She has always been instrumental in building confidence in me with her powerful words—**'Yes, you can do it'. It's only because of her, that today I believe in Miracles- I believe in the power of Intent**.

After I completed my schooling, I opted for the Science Stream in college. Once, I completed my 12th grade, Counsellor Didi suggested that I opt for Nursing, based on my potentials and interests. I completed my Nursing Degree from a renowned government college - G T Hospital. Today, I am a successful Registered Nurse. Since the past seven years, I have been performing my duties as a nurse very sincerely and ethically and I enjoy helping each and every one of my patients by providing the care they need. My mom feels extremely proud of me that I completed my Nursing Degree and even own a house today all because she made me so capable with her constant love and hard work.

I have faced many ups and downs in my life due to financial problems and due to the discouraging ways of the society, but I never felt discouraged or disappointed. I always reminded myself that if you want success in your life, then focus on the goals and not the obstacles, push yourself and rise up again day after day because no one else is going to do it for you but 'You'! Grab every opportunity you get to make your future brighter and to change your destiny.

I just want to tell everyone that '**Today might feel bad, Tomorrow may seem worse, but the day after tomorrow will be the best. So never let your failures get to you and give up**'. God has given equal opportunities to everyone. You just need to be aware of your abilities and potentials, accept the challenges that life throws at you and fight fiercely to achieve your dreams. You are the only artist of your own life. You can't waste your precious life by waiting for somebody to come into your life and make your life more graceful and colourful, mould yourself, your behaviours, and your personality in such a manner that someday someone would be inspired by you and consider you their Role Model.

Lastly, I would like to thank the entire team of OYA Foundation for the lovely opportunities they provided me with. It was a one-of-a-kind experience for me. Thank you OYA for all your support."

Our sessions are distinct and unique as these are not necessarily like the typical sessions carried out in a closed room. Our experiences have made us change our ways of conducting the sessions because change is inevitable. This includes—a talk with a walk in the nature, a talk while painting, a session while gardening, dance movement therapy sessions etc. We have also designed sessions for girls at NGOs or shelter homes where we encourage participation in different activities eventually motivating them and making them believe in their talent, their capabilities and their self. Each activity like drama, dance and art makes them have faith in their power; the healing begins from here. This reminds us of one of our sessions' success story of a girl Sally (name changed to maintain confidentiality). She was a survivor of child sexual abuse by her family member. She was in extreme level of trauma, distress, low self-esteem, physical and mental pain. She was under our counselling sessions on regular basis. She got in touch with her real self and understood her worth after she actively participated in the drama therapy sessions. The theme of the session was Self-Acceptance. Through each session, she could slowly and gradually accept herself and ascertain her dignity. After 17 counselling sessions and the final drama presentation where she was the lead; **for the first time she fell in love with herself and post that there was no looking back**. At present, she is a successful chef and a super mom, inspiring her clan and setting an example of developmental outcome.

Our programs in schools focus on students, parents/family members, teachers and even the non-teaching staff. Initially, when we started, we had a difficult time in breaking the barriers and myths about mental health concerns and learning difficulties. It was a popping hurdle to make the parents cognizant of the issue called learning disability. We started with regular awareness sessions, involving the parents and family members actively. It was a huge challenge to get adults out of their repulsive stage and accept the reality. Many of us were touched with the storyline of the Bollywood movie 'Taare Zameen Par'; but practically the attitude of everyone is that it is always okay if it's about other's child, it's not okay if it's with our own child.

The school dynamics and the mental health concerns of school students are very different. A student's life involves many phases, experiences and moments of achievements and failures. When we first commenced services in our partner schools and approached the students as a counsellor, they were reluctant to talk to us. The major factor to cease them from coming us was trust, 'How can I trust someone I don't know and open up with them?'—was their pondering question. Also, some of the children had their episodes with counsellors who had just come to them, heard their trials, wrote some reports, did some techniques and left them in mid-way. Some of the students had no knowledge about counselling. Slowly and gradually when we started interacting, we realized there is a lot of hesitance, reluctance and disbelief towards us. We re-grouped with our Band of Believers and mentors to diagnose the obstacles and empathize with the students by eliminating the roadblock. To initiate the process of counselling and eventually leading it to healing, the **prime aspect is trust** and if there is no trust then holistic healing cannot be accomplished. We designed a framework wherein we initiated our interactions with very non-threatening activities. We started with playing games with them, having fun programs and conducting fun-cum-learning sessions to build the rapport, break the ice and create the connection; that worked miraculously. We customized the activities and programmes by including life skills which were carried on by adding the enjoyment factor. Over the time, the students started trusting us and showing their belief in us. The process became easy for us to seep into their problems and they subsequently learnt many things; the best part was that we develop their faith in us.

While doing majors in psychology, there was always a feeling that there were so many concerns as a school student, and things would be so different if there was a counsellor back then or an adult friend whom we could confide in, who will not judge, add labels or be biased. When we started working on the School Projects, we decided we will not call ourselves counsellors but an '**Adult Buddy/Friend**' who is not interested in their grades or performances but concerned only about them as individuals with their own unique identity. After a few years, we were successful in overcoming the hindrances and becoming a friend to the school parents as well. Parents came up to share their heart out, attend sessions and heal simultaneously; gearing up to re-live and make the parenting journey beautiful.

One of the ex-students from our partner school had penned down her experience as below:

> I'm Kate (name changed to maintain confidentiality), an ex-student of ***High School. I'm not sure if you remember me but I remember you well as our counsellor cum friend who used to come to our school on alternate days to help anyone in need of counselling. I even remember the workshops conducted by you and your team for both parents and students. I just came across a certificate which is extremely close to my heart, which is the one which I won along with my team on national girl child's day. I was in 8th standard that time. Today I'm in my third year of LLB at Government Law College. I love public speaking and yours was the very first event where I won my first ever debating certificate. I remember your team's efforts towards educating us regarding how important it is to embrace every essence of being a girl, how to grow up to be a strong woman and how to stand up for what is right. Your focus on mental health too inspired and helped many. I couldn't thank you properly back then. Today as I glance through my certificate and write this message to you, I want

to thank you for inspiring me back then. **You indeed opened your arms for all of us and stretched it wide enough to inspire and empower. I shall always remember you.**

None of us get wherever we are alone. There's always someone who inspires and motivates us in every action of theirs. I'm sure whoever knows you or has ever met you, might have felt the same. It's so important to teach our children about mental health and well-being.

Open Your Arms Foundation owes majority of its learnings from all their experiences, involvements and interactions over the years with commercial sex workers, their daughters, street children, slum children, child sexual abuse survivors, rape survivors, child labourers, parents, elders, elders living with Alzheimer's and Dementia and their families, HIV affected and infected adults and children, artisan women and their children and domestic violence survivors. All of them have taught us the most important aspect—**The Attitude of Gratitude**. Whatever situation a person or a child has been in or is going through, the power of love and care spreads unconditionally. To have such consciousness to embrace the sense of gratitude is enough to plant the seed of positivity. **Harmony is crucial—at heart and at mind**. Our bodies are beautiful entities which can surprise us by achieving and performing endeavours which are unimaginable when the heart and the mind are in harmony; whereas, when one fails, the other follows.

Our alumna essayed her story of harmony of mind and heart:

My name is Nancy (name changed to maintain confidentiality) and I am 27 years old. I want to express my heartfelt thanks to OYA and Counsellor Didi because of their support and motivation, I am able to write my story today and be a reason to motivate everyone. Lots of love to OYA from me and my family.

I was seven when my mother passed away. We were three sisters who no one was ready to take care for but my maternal grandmother lovingly took the responsibility of handling all three of us. She wanted to educate us, but she did not have enough means to send us to school. Due to which she had put us in a child-care organization from where I completed my education till 10th Grade. However, difficulties didn't seem to leave our side; while I was studying for the 10th Grade, my grandmother was detected with Cancer. We could sail through these testing times due to the timely help of this organization for our education and treatment for our granny. I will always be grateful to them. After passing my 10th Grade, I was helped by another similar institution for my further studies and became my home during that period. It was then, that I gained plenty of opportunities to grow and learnt various life-skills like cooking, tailoring, communication and various other skills. Counsellor Didi of OYA was our counsellor there and was a great emotional support. She noticed my ability to express through art and always kept providing me with great platforms to do so. Once, during an Art-Based Therapeutic activity, we were asked to draw out how we felt about our journey of emotional well-being with the OYA organization. And my expression of love for OYA on that humble piece of paper became OYA's Logo. Counsellor Didi's faith in my artistic skills has helped me believe in my abilities and pursue them further.

Although, I had support from the institution where I lived and they helped me to grow, being physically distant from my sisters and my grandmother made me feel a sense of emptiness that I could only fill on being united with them again. Hence, I made the decision to step out during my 14th grade, rented a place where we sisters and our grandmother could live together under one roof, and look after each other. Being together with my family filled my heart with happiness again. But the financial challenges we faced to see this dream come true required me to take up jobs in Cafes while I was still trying to complete my education. It became very challenging to manage a job, education, and household responsibilities altogether at that tender age, fortunately, I completed my graduation.

> Even, while I had moved out of the institution where I had come in touch with OYA, Counsellor Didi stayed in touch with me and continued to be my emotional support and source of encouragement. She saw that my art had never left me as I loved taking the responsibility of designing menus and boards for the cafes I worked at. She helped me do so in the field I cherished so much. She was instrumental in helping me to get admission at a college for a course in Interior Designing and in finding donors to help me pay my fees.
>
> Today, I am happily married and my husband is in the field of Event Organising. I am about to complete my course in Interior Designing and looking forward to a long and happy married life where my husband is not only my partner for life but also a partner in work as I help him with decorations for events and parties. After juggling through all the struggles, today I could finally see all my dreams come true and it could have never been possible without the support I received from the child-care institutions and OYA; I am very grateful to all of them. I wish OYA Heartiest Congratulations for completing 10 beautiful years of service to mankind and I wish for OYA to complete 100 years of bringing hope in the lives of many.

Our budding project started in 2021 is 'PANKH'—a group home maintained for the 18+ girls who have exited child-care institutions. The perspective of this project is to provide a platform to the young girls to prepare themselves before being left on their own in the competitive world. The goal is to support the girls to complete their higher education and help them in acquiring their talent and career-based jobs. Our outlook is concentrated in guiding them to tactfully manage their studies, work and home chores concurrently. By managing all the tasks, they learn budgeting, responsibility planning, rationing, self-dependence and at the same time being available as a family to other mates when the other is in need of any assistance. The group home is set up next to our residence and the girls are a part of our family. All the family gatherings, festival celebrations and parties are not complete without having our girls making merry with us. The idea was to give a homely environment to the girls who do not have anyone in their families or have to stay away from them due to certain problems. So, our parents are their parents now, our uncles and aunts are theirs as well; all the children and youngsters are their friends and play together in free time.

In 2022, we introduced an initiative called 'OYA's Changmakers' consisting of our alumni with the concept of paying it forward; giving to the society what they received in their testing times. Changemakers is a group consisting of 15–20 girls who have been a part of our counselling sessions when they were in our partner schools or resided in NGOs/child-care institutions. The girls have exited these respective organizations and are either living individually, are married or living in group homes. The changemakers conduct different fun-based learning activities and life skill sessions in other NGOs and institutions. Other activities like cooking for senior citizens in elder care homes and conducting activities for them are also taken up by the girls. Their motto is to impart their learnings and experiences and pay it forward to the souls who crave for such affection. They also focus on giving a direction to the children and young population in their moulding years. At present, the group has organized 12 sessions and events and are looking forward to actively reach out to more and more people. We at OYA see the changemakers as the fruits flourished through the years of counselling and relationship building.

By narrating OYA's origination, work done by the team, experiences gained, surpassing hurdles and feedback from the beneficiaries; we come to a conclusion on the doctrine that **'It's easy to judge, difficult to understand'**. Understanding requires compassion, patience and a willingness to believe that good hearts sometimes choose poor methods. **Through judging we separate; through understanding we grow**. The fear of being judged pushes back people from openly speaking about their mental health. Giving a hand to someone drowning in their plight is what counselling and therapy is all about. One should definitely talk about their mental health and treat it with counselling and psychotherapy where required leaving behind the dismay and assumptions; it helps to accept yourself and your environment which in turn reduces stress, anxiety and depression. **Positivity and self-love is bloomed when your confidence is raised**.

Concluding Excerpts from OYA's Experience

- Every child is a unique flower, let their fragrance spread.
- Pay attention to the non-verbals, they have the loudest screams.
- Upgrade your perception with power of intent.
- Have an outlook of boundless acceptance for others as well as for yourself.
- Nurture your thoughts with positivity.
- It's okay to do less when you are coping with more.
- Self-admiration is a symbol of self-respect.
- Clearing mental clutter, clears the soul.
- Talking about your trauma allows you to move out of it.
- Uplift each other with grace.

Chapter 19
Conclusion

Meenu Anand

Abstract The concluding chapter of *Mental Health Care Resource Book: Concepts and Praxis for Social Workers and Mental Health Professionals* accentuates the need for escalating the canvas for mental health care to include social-ecological niche of Psy professionals. It strives to advance an architype, based on the person-centred, human rights-based approach towards caring for persons with mental health challenges. It offers the *Key Take Aways* from this tremendously eclectic and valuable resource book that revolves around normalization of the discourse on mental health while promoting the local and contextual grassroots narratives and stigma reduction. In the most exclusive manner, the chapter also envisions the futuristic roadmap ahead for transforming mental health care and envisages the professional contribution by social workers in diversifying mental health care.

Keywords Mental health care · Social work · Roadmap

Mental Health Care Resource Book: Concepts and Praxis for Social Workers and Mental Health Professionals has highlighted the ubiquity and importance of socio-cultural narratives on mental health. Accentuating the need for escalating the canvas for mental health care to include social-ecological niche of Psy professionals, it has emphasized the professional contribution by social workers and other mental health professionals in order to diversify mental health care beyond the hegemonic realm of medical professionals.

The book is a clarion call to adopt a transformational, inclusive and practical approach to mental health care, with rights and sustainability at its centre. Based on theoretical foundations, covering gamut of professional skills in the field, it has acknowledged multifaceted contests in the milieu of mental health. Backed by evidence from the grassroots, it has endeavoured to present the socio-cultural and holistic narrative covering multifaceted stakeholders including clients, caregivers and diverse set of mental health professionals. The book has strived to advance an

M. Anand (✉)
Department of Social Work, University of Delhi, Delhi, India
e-mail: meenuanand75@rediffmail.com

M. Anand (ed.), *Mental Health Care Resource Book*,
https://doi.org/10.1007/978-981-97-1203-8_19

architype, based on the person-centred, human rights-based approach towards caring for persons with mental health challenges. The book would be advantageous to social workers, psychologists, academics, research scholars/students from a wide range of disciplines, nurses, policymakers as well as practitioners. It also resolves to influence decision-makers to meet the mental health care-related challenges and fill the prevailing voids in the field.

Key Take Aways

Socio-cultural factors as prerequisites in mental health: The book has been a powerful reminder of how societal factors, such as gender disparities, discrimination, negligence, lack of cognizance and stigma, pose challenges and barriers with regard to mental health care. Social support is a prerequisite to enable an individual to lead full, equal, inclusive and independent life. As a consequence, need of the hour is to address the root causes of mental disorders related to socio-cultural contexts viz. gender, caste, social status, race/ethnicity. The ideas related to gender roles, race, sexuality and class strongly inform and perpetuate how people understand mental health from an intersectional perspective.

Thrust on De-medicalization: The biomedical approach to subjective suffering necessitates the person's experience to be decontextualized and abridged to the 'clinical picture' while amputating the probable causes for the person's diverse manifestations, e.g., adverse childhood experiences, traumas, experience of multiple oppressions, etc. There are sundry indicators of psychic and emotional pain as natural to the human experience and thus alternate ways of 'healing' are a must. Accepting the pathologization of human agony without a critical view in place is outright perilous for individual well-being, struggles for social justice and human rights in the society. Since mental health issues have significant detrimental personal, familial, regional and global consequences, de-medicalization with a diversified contribution across Psy Professionals is an urgent necessity (Cantón, 2022).

Normalizing the discourse on mental health: There is an ongoing global mental health crisis, with a growing number of people facing mental health issues such as short- and long-term stress. Since mental health exists on a complex continuum, with experiences ranging from an optimal state of well-being to enervating states of great suffering and emotional pain; it is intricate to expound the notion of mental health. The book has tried to reiterate that promotion and prevention are indeed required across the life course to strengthen the discourse on mental well-being and endurance, to 'normalize' conversations concerning wellness, prevent the early development and manifestations of mental health conditions, and, as a result, diminish the need for mental health care. Raising mental health literacy at the family, school, and community levels, early childhood development and group activities for children's well-being, destigmatizing mental disorders, and fostering discourses on well-being and happiness are all indispensable.

Promoting grassroots narrative: Investing in mental health for all promotes public health and, from a human rights standpoint, can facilitate social and economic progress. Promoting community mental health at the 'local' level, with a focus on improving community structure and connections, as well as capacity building, can help deinstitutionalize and promote a culture of care, understanding and sharing are indeed need of the hour.

Transforming Mental Health Care: The Roadmap Ahead

- **Soliciting peer support**

Peer support groups represent a very tangible tool that can make an enormous difference in a person's life. As 'safe spaces', peer-led support groups can allow the acknowledgement of suffering and provide a platform for sharing the pain as well as knowledge, provide emotional support, create opportunities for social interaction, offer practical help or engage in advocacy and awareness raising (WHO, 2022). The benefits of peer support include personal (such as poise, self-esteem, enablement, camaraderie), practical (information, flagging), social (social inclusion, challenging dishonour and discernment, challenging blockades specific to relegated groups) (Faulkner & Kalathil, 2012). Furthermore, these can lead to collective learning, flourishing as well as constructive action.

- **Integrating 'lived experience' in knowledge production**

The lived experience "*one of healing and transformation through psychic pain and extreme distress*" is extremely critical to be amalgamated in the course of knowledge production (Cantón, 2022, p. 209). Persons with mental disorders are often excluded from knowledge production in the field of mental health owing to their challenged state of faculties of 'reason' (Taggort, 2022). Valuing 'experiential knowledge' also called as 'lived experience' is indeed the way forward in order to enact instrumental changes. There is distinction in valuing and giving importance to survivors' lived narratives and incorporating the 'first-person' pragmatic understanding in creation as well as production of knowledge on the subject.

- **Person-centred practice**

The person-centred practice as advocated by Beresford and Slasberg (2023) implies the ideas of person-centred planning, and independent living and focuses on the individualized support that people need to live their lives on equal terms. This requires taking into account the individual variables such as the nature of the person's impairment and its severity, duration, familial support and resources. Key elements for such practice as expounded by Beresford and Slasberg (2023) include:

> Putting the person at the centre, rather than fitting them into services, treating service users as individuals, ensuring choice and control for service users, setting goals with them for support, emphasizing the importance of relationship between service users and practitioners, listening

> to service users and acting on what they say, providing up-to-date/ accessible information about appropriate services, flexibility (p. 101).

The person-centred practice is also essential from the rights-based approach and is non-negotiable for psychosocial rehabilitation of persons with mental disorders.

- **Solidification of community structures**

Access to eminent mental health care and cognizance cannot be separated from research and system development, learning and teaching, and community engagement with critical players (Uwakwe, 2019). There is a need to promote community-based mental health care encompassing a network of unified services, e.g., integration of mental health services in general health care; participation of key stakeholders in awareness on mental health, training services that deliver mental health care in non-health settings, engagement and training of local grassroots functionaries like ANMs, Anganwadi and ASHA workers, etc. Community-based network of accessible, affordable and quality services and support can also enable in stigma reduction in addition to creating an enabling environment for promotion of mental health and well-being.

- **Decolonizing knowledge**

The anti-psychiatry movement stresses on the need for eclectic and novel approaches in understanding mental health care rather than getting wedged in the fetters of psychiatry. The decolonial thinking and practice must focus on the person and his/her context, engage in local and locally-determined action; understand mental distress and the specific symbiotic social and personal issues. It is imperative to develop a stock of non-medicalized approaches and models that may help in moving beyond the terrain of symptomatic treatment and focus more on providing meaning to subjective experience, enabling and promoting holistic recovery. Beresford and Slasberg (2023) propound a model based on rights, social and holistic approach rather than individualized understandings and approaches. There is a need to build on collectivist methods to understand, organize and make changes while striving to develop wider coalitions beyond 'mental health'.

- **Putting the spotlight on mental health activism**

There is an increasing demand for a rights-based, sustainable and just system in the form of promoting mental health activism, which should be largely centred on the idea that people should have the agency to make informed decisions about their mental health (Uwakwe, 2019). Beresford and Slasberg (2023) expound:

> What stands revealed is a Cinderella service in the shadow of health care, often associated with the perpetuation of dependency in its clientele, and marginalization in its workforce. Its patronizing and disempowering logic, preoccupation with funding constraints over rights and the meeting of need, are a salutary reminder of its limitations in the face of the growing numbers of older and disabled people globally. This sets the scene for an internationally inadequate policy which can only have increased significance in a context of rapidly changing and polarized demographics globally (Beresford & Slasberg, 2023, p. 22).

Activism in mental health care can provide an outstanding pulpit to build meaning and find inspiration to share one's suffering by actively sharing personal stories, engaging with communities and finding a purpose that transcends one's individual experiences (Cantón, 2022).

- **Engagement of caregivers**

I strongly feel that the mental health movement must engage with the equivalent experience of caregivers in addition to those facing mental health difficulties. The unique evidence-based learnings and experiential insights of caregivers with regard to care giving, nurturing, availing services, encountering diverse challenges and dealing with systemic barriers must find voice and be amalgamated in mental health care. The carers can play a vital role in supporting as well as strengthening the interventions for mental health services, aid in policy making and vice versa (Pearsall & Yates, 2004).

- **Social workers as key players**

Social work emerges as one of the front runners in mental health care owing to its strength in the uniqueness and eclecticism as a helping profession. A distinguishing feature of social work profession is the knowledge of understanding the intricate affiliations people have with their environments (Heller & Gitterman, 2011) in addition to multifaceted skills of working with people at micro, mezzo and macro levels. Applying professional values that nurture well-being, healing, growth and constructive changes in individuals, families, social groups, communities, social workers enrich the ecological perspective with the broader focus on assessment, intervention and appraisal. The International Federation of Social Workers' asserts that '*social work intervenes at the points where people interact with their environments*' thereby denoting their role in '*the empowerment and liberation of people to enhance well-being*' (International Federation of Social Workers, 2000). With multipronged interventions at individual and structural levels, they enable enhancement of social functioning while endorsing purposeful behavioural patterns as well as more efficient policies (Kerson et al., 2005).

As *pioneers of new thinking, anti-discrimination and social approaches*, social workers are the professionals 'most closely associated with social care' (Beresford & Slasberg, 2023). The clientele of social workers is eclectic and encompasses from individuals from the general population to those who are under difficult circumstances with distinct socio-emotional needs.

Social work as a profession is committed to issues of social justice and multiplicity. As strong advocates for social justice and equivalence, social workers are particularly competent to work with persons with mental health challenges and the socio-cultural conditions that surround and impact them. The social work role has always encompassed advocating rights of the client (Porter, 1996) as against the authority of the State. Grounded in the psychosocial as well as alternate models of providing mental health care, strong practice-based professional skills, social workers can indeed be the front runners in provision of multidisciplinary mental health care to persons with mental health challenges across the life course in addition to providing support to their families. Enabling the client's access and negotiate their social and physical milieus is a distinguishing feature of social work practice (Heller & Gitterman, 2011). Therefore, their contribution is vital especially in early interventions, assertive outreach, challenging inequity, respecting diversity, identification of persons in need and promoting well-being and building positivity around mental health (Gould, 2010).

The strength of social work entails bringing together the understanding of biopsychosocial factors, their knowledge about the biological rudiments of mental conditions and their expertise in knowledge of psychological and environmental influences, the impact of social factors on an individual, his/her family as well as the community (Heller & Gitterman, 2011). I sturdily feel that strength-based practice will be the key to future interventions that will entail building on collaborations, empathic understanding of unique strengths/values of individuals that indeed forms the very basis for person-centric interventions. In addition, it will also necessitate promotion of autonomy, agency and dignity of people with thrust to the socio-cultural context while building community-based resources (Pulla & Francis, 2015).

Social workers can play effective and numerous roles as advisors, navigators, brokers, service providers and designers of holistic social care systems (Gould, 2010) that promote advocacy on mental health from a rights-based perspective.

- **Engagement of multidisciplinary professionals**

Psy professionals, with skills outside of psychiatric medicine, can make a significant contribution in mental health care. Services can only be given by working as a team, by means of supporting one another and playing complimentary roles to each other's knowledge base and areas of professional practice. Mental health care can benefit and progress beyond the constricting scope of the biomedical approach by honouring the skills and perspectives of diverse experts involved in care planning and ensuring the key participation of individuals with lived experience of mental distress.

Concluding Remarks

Mental health care is at a unique juncture with heightened need for speckled professionals with diverse specialties, skills and novel methods. This resource book has dwelled into the theoretical perspectives, unveiled practice skills adopted by mental health experts and amalgamated voices from the Indian grassroots. In a progressively rapidly changing world comprising of new demands and pressures, there is indeed a need for a more flexible and well-trained workforce. It is therefore imperative that mental health care embraces the cultural shift towards adopting a psychosocial narrative and the opportunity is seized to widen the scope and create fresh opportunities towards contribution by social workers to enhance research and mental health activism. Stigma obliteration through objective and evidence-based information on mental health and illness through the adoption of community-based preventive approach from a rights-based perspective will go a long away in this direction. Exploring new and emerging arenas for provision of mental health care including music, creative arts (Keen, 2005) can be novel opportunities in the future. What is required is to develop an understanding of 'local' context and develop culturally relevant solutions and demonstrate their effectiveness through reinvigorated community networks.

While providing mental health care services to people with mental health issues, social workers bring skills, expertise, competence and values to the forefront. Through their work in a multidisciplinary environment, understanding of psychosocial needs of people across the life-cycle, and a value base that illustrates anti-discrimination and anti-oppression; social workers can develop an effective leadership that aims to create an embracing, proactive familial as well as community environment in addition to creating a cadre of local leaders at the grassroots as well as advanced practitioners at the national and international levels.

References

Beresford, P., & Slasberg, C. (2023). *The future of social care: From Problem to Rights-Based Sustainable Solution.* Edward Elgar Publishing Limited.

Cantón, M. I. (2022). Why we must talk about de-medicalisation. In P. Beresford & J. Russo (Eds.), *Routledge International Handbook of Mad Studies* (pp. 205–216). Rutledge.

Faulkner, A., & Kalathil, J. (2012). *The Freedom to be, the Chance to Dream: Preserving User-led Peer Support in Mental Health.*UK: Together.

Gould, N. (2010). *Mental Health Social Work in Context.* London and New York: Rutledge.

Heller, N. R., & Gitterman, A. (2011). *Health and Social Problems: A social work perspective.* Rutledge.

International Federation of Social Workers. (2000). *Definition of Social Work.* http://www.ifsw.org/en/f38000138.html

Keen, A. (2005). Using music to facilitate social work intervention. In T. Heinonen & A. Meeri (Eds.), *Social work in health and mental health: Issues, developments, and actions* (pp. 85–106). Canadian Scholars' Press Inc.

Kerson, T. B., McCoyd, J. L. M., & Chimchirian, J. M. (2005). Spanning boundaries: An enriched ecological perspective for social workers practising in health and mental health care. In T. Heinonen & A. Meeri (Eds.), *Social work in health and mental health: Issues, developments, and actions* (pp. 8–25). Canadian Scholars' Press Inc.

Pearsall, A., & Yates, L. (2004). *Good practice in adult mental health.* In T. Ryan, & J. Pritchard (Eds.). London and Philadelphia: Jessica Kingsley Publishers.

Porter, R. (1996). *The social history of madness: Stories of the insane.* London: Phoenix.

Pulla, V., & Francis, A. (2015). A strengths approach to mental health. In A. Francis, V. Pulla, M. Clark, E. Susana Mariscal, I. Ponnuswami (Eds.) *Advancing social work in mental health through Strengths based practice.* The Primrose Hall.

Taggort, D. (2022). "Are you experienced?" The use of experiential knowledge in mental health and its contribution to Mad Studies. In P. Beresford & J. Russo (Eds.), *Routledge international handbook of mad studies* (pp. 154–165). Rutledge.

Uwakwe, R. (2019). Foreward. In S. Bährer-Kohler, & B. Bolea-Alamanac (Eds.) *Diversity in global mental health*. Springer Briefs in Psychology (pp. ix–xii). Switzerland: Springer. https://doi.org/10.1007/978-3-030-29112-9_2

World Health Organization. (2022). *World mental health report: Transforming mental health for all*. https://www.who.int/publications/i/item/9789240049338